Recent Developments in AIDS

Volume I

Recent Developments in AIDS
Volume I

Edited by **Abby Calvin**

FOSTER ACADEMICS

New Jersey

Published by Foster Academics,
61 Van Reypen Street,
Jersey City, NJ 07306, USA
www.fosteracademics.com

Recent Developments in AIDS: Volume I
Edited by Abby Calvin

International Standard Book Number: 978-1-63242-344-3 (Hardback)

Printed in China.

Contents

Preface

In a world where diseases and disorders aplenty and medicine to treat them are also available; there are still a few diseases and syndromes that defy man's attempt to subdue it, instead they are becoming more dangerous. HIV-AIDS or Human Immunodeficiency Virus / Acquired Immunodeficiency Syndrome is one such syndrome that threatens a large part of the world's population. Scientists generally agree that the two strains of HIV-AIDS, have probably been transmitted to humans through chimpanzees. Not really taken seriously as first, it has grown into a global phenomenon. Not much attention was given when it first started appearing on the medical radar and that was the drawback. Much more could have been done if awareness about AIDS had been clear from the beginning. Even now, when there is always a danger of AIDS popping up somewhere in our lives, awareness and knowledge about it is not as widespread as it should be. Factors such as unprotected sexual practices and using used syringes for vaccination are few of the most common reasons of AIDS infection. There is also a certain trauma associated with this syndrome that is unfair and most often misplaced. Sufferers of HIV need help, support and better healthcare policies instead of being derided for something that cannot be changed now.

The research and data collated in this book are drawn from leading researches around the world on HIV-AIDS. I would like to thank those who work tirelessly towards raising awareness about AIDS and applaud those who suffer from it for their bravery in the face of such adversity.

Editor

The Syndromic versus Laboratory Diagnosis of Sexually Transmitted Infections in Resource-Limited Settings

Musie Ghebremichael

Harvard Medical School and Ragon Institute of MGH, MIT and Harvard, 400 Technology Square, Room 857, Cambridge, MA 02129, USA

Correspondence should be addressed to Musie Ghebremichael; musie_ghebremichael@dfci.harvard.edu

Academic Editors: K. Arasteh, G. D'ettorre, and A. Guihot-Thevenin

Sexually transmitted infections (STIs) are highly prevalent in sub-Saharan Africa, where there is a severe HIV epidemic. Thus, accurate recognition and diagnosis of STIs are essential for successful HIV prevention programs in the region. Due to lack of trained personnel and adequate laboratory infrastructure in the region, information regarding the profile of STIs relies essentially on self-reported or physician-diagnosed symptoms. The main objective of the study was to assess the effectiveness of the syndromic diagnosis of STIs, which is often used as a proxy for laboratory diagnosis of STIs in sub-Saharan Africa and other resource-limited settings. The study builds on previously collected data from a community-based survey in Northern Tanzania. We found no significant agreements between patient-reported STIs symptoms and laboratory-confirmed STIs tests. The reported STIs symptoms had high specificity (range = 85–99%) and poor sensitivity (range = 2–17%). Knowledge gained from our study will have significant public health implications, and can help improve the syndromic diagnosis of STIs.

1. Introduction

AIDS is a major public health challenge in sub-Saharan Africa, and the prevalence of other STIs in the region is high [1, 2]. An estimated 22.9 million people infected with HIV live in sub-Saharan Africa, and approximately 1.2 million deaths from AIDS occurred in sub-Saharan Africa [3]. There is compelling evidence that STIs affect the transmission of HIV. STIs facilitate the sexual acquisition and transmission of HIV infection and HIV infection increases the risk of other STIs [4, 5]. Hence, the recognition, treatment, and prevention of STIs to reduce the risk of HIV transmission should be a public health priority, especially in sub-Saharan Africa where antiretroviral therapy may not be readily available. More than two-thirds of patients living with HIV in sub-Saharan Africa have no access to antiretroviral therapy [6].

STIs can be diagnosed in a number of different ways, including laboratory and syndromic diagnosis. Laboratory diagnosis is the most accurate method of making a diagnosis. However, it is expensive and is not feasible in many settings as it requires sophisticated laboratory facilities and qualified personnel who can perform technically demanding procedures. Moreover, laboratory diagnosis of STIs is time-consuming and results often cannot be made available at the same visit, thereby causing a delay in treatment initiation. For these reasons, the syndromic diagnosis of STIs remains the only feasible option in some resource-limited settings. Syndromic diagnosis of STIs is based on the identification of a group of symptoms and signs that characterize a clinical condition [7, 8]. It is simple, cost effective, and capable of yielding rapid diagnosis for immediate treatment. Moreover, this technique can be implemented at all levels of the health care system. Despite these advantages, it has several limitations: syndromic diagnosis relies on subjective judgment, cannot detect asymptomatic infections, and may result in overdiagnosis/overtreatment and potential drug resistance [9–11].

Due to a lack of trained personnel and adequate laboratory infrastructure in sub-Saharan Africa, information regarding the profile of STIs relies essentially on self-reported or physician-diagnosed STIs. However, there is still no consensus on its performance and several studies from the region have reported inconsistent results. The mixed reports might be due to the fact that the studies were carried out in particular groups that are not representative of the overall population, such as STD or antenatal clinic attendees [12–14]. Therefore, there is a public health need to evaluate the validity of the syndromic diagnosis of STIs using population-based studies from the region, that is, the urgent need for a comparative study of syndromic and laboratory diagnosis of STIs in sub-Saharan Africa. The main objective of the study was to evaluate the performance of syndromic diagnosis of STIs in comparison with laboratory-confirmed STIs.

2. Materials and Methods

2.1. Study Design and Study Sample. The study participants consisted of 2,019 women who were enrolled in a community-based survey, which was conducted from November 2002 to March 2003 in the Moshi Urban District of the Kilimanjaro Region. The Kilimanjaro Region, located in Northern Tanzania adjacent to the Kenyan border, is one of Mainland Tanzania's 20 regions and is experiencing a mature generalized stage of the HIV epidemic. Tanzania, with a population of 34.5 million, has about 7% of its adults infected with HIV [15]. In the Moshi District of Northern Tanzania, the prevalence of HIV infection is about twice that of the national average.

Study participants were selected to participate in the survey based on a two-stage sampling design. During the first stage of sampling, a total of 150 clusters were selected from the Moshi Urban District. In the second stage of sampling, a number of households were randomly selected from each of the 150 clusters and 2,019 women who were residents of the households were enrolled. A detailed description of the study protocol, data gathering instruments, and procedures and laboratory methods has been previously published [16, 17].

2.2. Study Variables. Demographic and socioeconomic characteristics including age, education, ethnicity, religion, and occupation were obtained. High-risk behaviors including alcohol abuse, age at first sex, number of sexual partners, and frequency of condom use were obtained. Symptoms of STIs including abdominal pain, abnormal genital discharge, foul smell in the genital area, excessive genital secretions, swelling of lymphnodes in the genital area, itching in the genital area, burning pain on micturation, pain during intercourse, and genital ulcers were obtained. Blood and urine samples were obtained from 1,418 and 1,440 women, respectively, who agreed to further testing for STIs. The blood samples were tested for HIV-1, HSV-2, and active and past syphilis. The urine samples were tested for chlamydia, gonorrhea, *Trichomonas*, and *Mycoplasma genitalium*.

2.3. Statistical Analysis. Descriptive measures (such as mean, median, standard deviation, interquartile range, frequencies, and percentages) were used to summarize the data. Sensitivity and specificity together with their corresponding 95% confidence intervals were calculated to assess the predictive accuracy of each STIs symptom. Exact binomial confidence intervals were used to estimate confidence intervals for rates

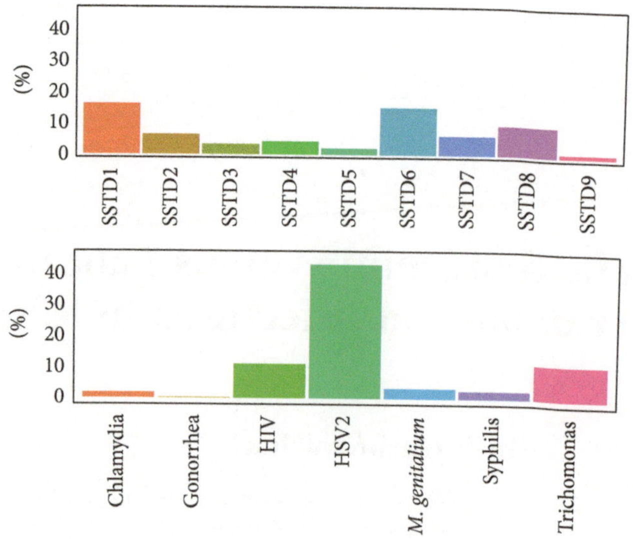

Figure 1: Prevalence of self-reported STIs symptoms and laboratory confirmed STIs (SSTD1: abdominal pain, SSTD2: abnormal genital discharge, SSTD3: foul smell in the genital area, SSTD4: excessive genital secretions, SSTD5: swelling of lymphnodes in the genital area, SSTD6: itching in the genital area, SSTD7: burning pain on micturation, SSTD8: pain during intercourse, and SSTD9: genital ulcers).

of STIs, sensitivities, and specificities. Kendall's tau-b was used to measure agreements between patient-reported STIs symptoms and laboratory confirmed STIs. The reported numbers of STIs symptoms were summed to obtain the total number of STIs symptoms for each participant. Receiver operating characteristic (ROC) curve was then constructed using sensitivity and specificity obtained from every possible symptom threshold. The area under the ROC curve (AUROC) was used to evaluate the overall diagnostic accuracy of the syndromic diagnosis of STIs. Bootstrap-based confidence intervals were calculated for the AUROC.

3. Results

We restricted our analysis to women who were tested for STIs; a total of 1,520 women were tested for STIs. The median age was 28 years (IQR = 23–35), and median age at first sex was 19 years (IQR = 17–21). The majority of study participants had pre-secondary education (77%), had not used a condom in the prior 12 months (77%), had one sex partner in the last three years (84%), and had a husband/partner (61%). Fifty percent of the women tested positive for at least one STI.

Figure 1 displays the rates of STIs symptoms and tests among the women included in the analysis. The prevalence rates of HSV-2, HIV-1, and *Trichomonas* were 43%, 11%, and 11%, respectively. The prevalence rates of the other STIs were below 5.0%. Among the tested women, 30% reported at least one STIs symptom. The most prevalent STIs symptom was lower abdominal pain (16%), followed by itching in the genital area (15%), pain during intercourse (9.4%), abnormal genital discharge (6.3%), burning or pain on micturation (6%), excessive genital secretions (4.1%), foul smell in genital

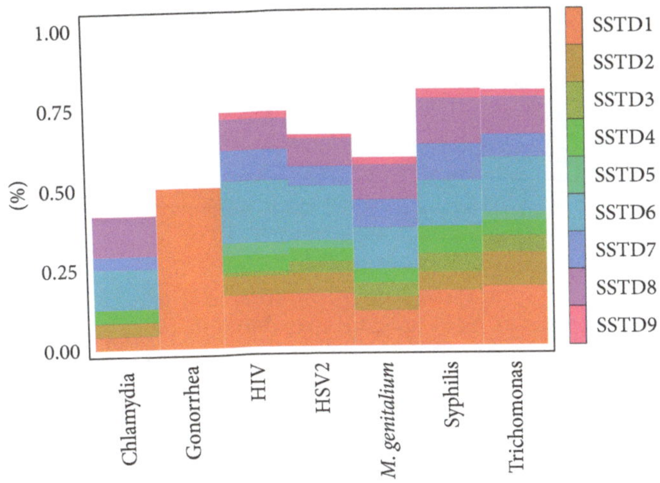

FIGURE 2: Prevalence of self-reported STIs symptoms among women tested positive for STIs (SSTD1: abdominal pain, SSTD2: abnormal genital discharge, SSTD3: foul smell in the genital area, SSTD4: excessive genital secretions, SSTD5: swelling of lymphnodes in the genital area, SSTD6: itching in the genital area, SSTD7: burning pain on micturation, SSTD8: pain during intercourse, and SSTD9: genital ulcers).

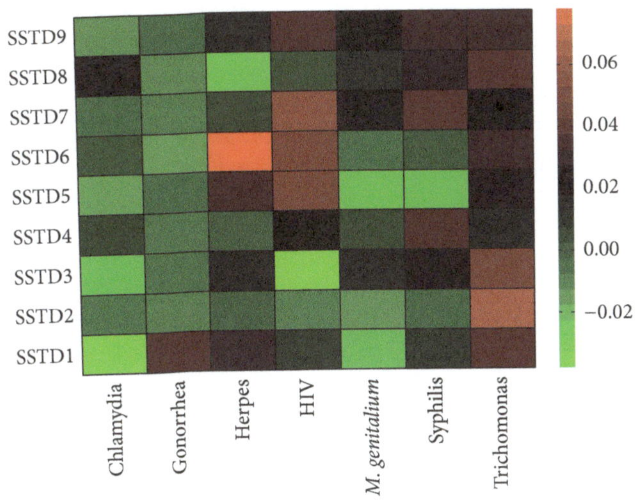

FIGURE 3: Heat map of Kendall's tau-*b* correlation coefficients between STIs symptoms and laboratory confirmed STIs (SSTD1: abdominal pain, SSTD2: abnormal genital discharge, SSTD3: foul smell in the genital area, SSTD4: excessive genital secretions, SSTD5: swelling of lymphnodes in the genital area, SSTD6: itching in the genital area, SSTD7: burning pain on micturation, SSTD8: pain during intercourse, and SSTD9: genital ulcers).

area (3.2%), swelling of lymphnodes in genital area (1.9%), and genital ulcers (1.1%). The prevalence of STIs symptoms among women tested positive for each STI is presented in Figure 2. Multiple STIs symptoms were reported with almost all the laboratory-confirmed STIs. Lower abdominal pain was a common symptom of several infections.

Figure 3 displays a heat map of Kendall's tau-*b* correlation coefficients used to measure agreements between patient-reported STIs symptoms and laboratory-confirmed results. Kendall's tau-*b* value of 1 implies perfect agreement and values less than 1 imply less than perfect agreement. The Kendall's tau-*b* coefficients were low (range = −0.04–0.08), showing no significant associations between each STI symptom and the laboratory-confirmed STI results. When the symptoms were combined together and summed, the level of agreement between STIs symptoms and tests remained low (Kendall's tau-*b* = 0.07, 95% CI: 0.02–0.12).

Figure 4 displays the sensitivity (true positive rate) and specificity (true negative rate) of each STI symptom, where sensitivity is the ability of an STI symptom to correctly identify women who have laboratory-confirmed STIs and specificity is the ability of an STI symptom to correctly identify women without laboratory-confirmed STIs. The individual STI symptoms had very low sensitivity (range = 2%–17%) and high specificity (range = 85%–99%). The less sensitive STI symptoms identified individuals as being disease-free when in fact they were not. Moreover, the more specific STIs symptoms identified individuals as being disease-free when they were disease-free. Figure 4 also displays the sensitivity and specificity of the combined STIs symptoms, which was defined as a positive response to at least one of the reported symptoms. The sensitivity and specificity of the combined STIs symptoms were 0.33 [95% CI: 0.30–0.37] and 0.73 [95% CI: 0.70–0.77]. The combined STIs symptoms correctly identified 33 out of 100 women with laboratory-confirmed STIs and resulted in a 67% false negative rate. Similarly, the combined STIs symptoms correctly identified 73 out of 100 healthy women and resulted in 27% false positive rate. Figure 5 displays the area under the receiver-operating curve (AUROC). The AUROCmeasures the overall diagnostic accuracy of the STI symptoms. The closer the AUROC value is to 1, the better the syndromic diagnosis of STIs is. The AUROC was 0.53 (95% CI: 046–0.62); that is, the syndromic approach had a 53% probability of correctly distinguishing a healthy from an infected woman. The 95% CI included 50%, indicating that there is no gain in predictive accuracy by using STIs symptoms. The syndromic approach showed no advantage over random guess (a random classifier has an AUROC of 0.5).

4. Discussion

Our study aimed to evaluate the accuracy (performance) of syndromic management of sexually transmitted infections (STIs) among women in sub-Saharan Africa. It included 1,520 women who were enrolled in a community-based survey from the Moshi Urban District of Northern Tanzania. Half of the women tested positive for at least one STI, while 30% reported at least one STIs symptom. The most prevalent STI among the study participants was HSV-2 (reaching 43%), followed by HIV and *Trichomonas* infection rates of 11%. The prevalence rates of other STIs were *Mycoplasma Genitalium* (3.2%), syphilis (2.5%), chlamydia (1.8%), and gonorrhea (0.2%). The most prevalent STI symptom was lower abdominal pain (16%), followed by itching in the genital area (15%), pain during intercourse (9%), abnormal genital discharge (6%), and burning or pain on micturation

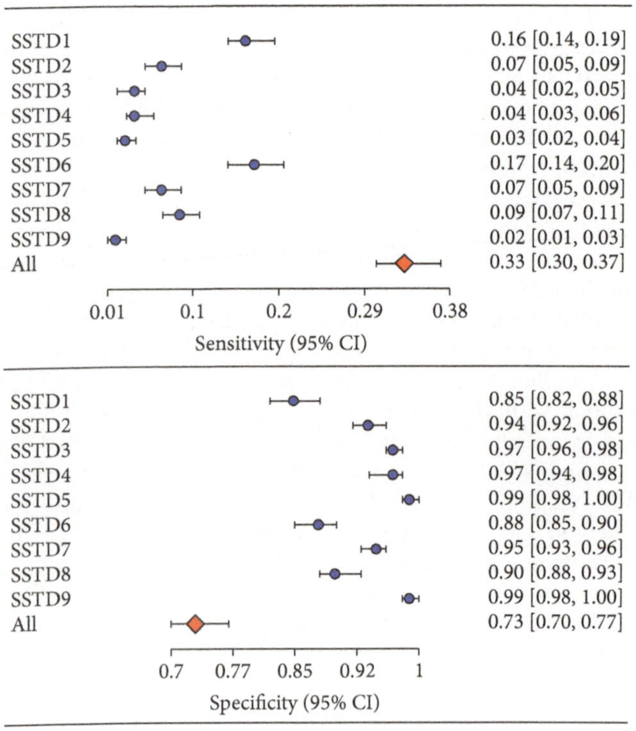

FIGURE 4: Sensitivities and specificities of STIs symptoms together with their 95% exact confidence intervals (SSTD1: abdominal pain, SSTD2: abnormal genital discharge, SSTD3: foul smell in the genital area, SSTD4: excessive genital secretions, SSTD5: swelling of lymphnodes in the genital area, SSTD6: itching in the genital area, SSTD7: burning pain on micturation, SSTD8: pain during intercourse, and SSTD9: genital ulcers).

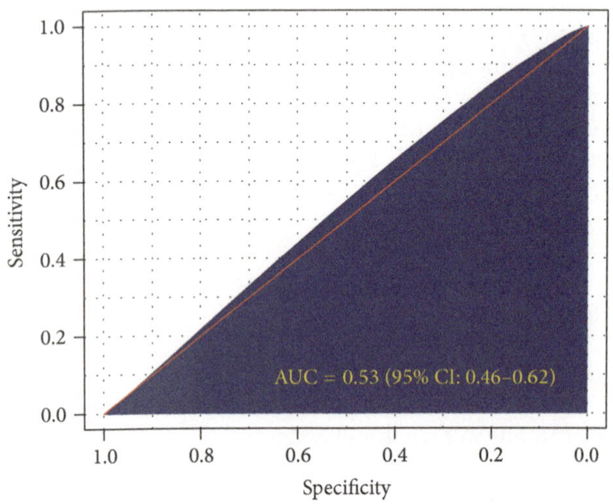

FIGURE 5: The receiver operating characteristics (ROC) curve. The shaded region represents the area under the ROC curve.

(6%). The prevalence rates of the remaining STIs symptoms were below 5.0%. We found no significant associations between patient-reported STIs symptoms and laboratory-confirmed STIs tests. Furthermore, we found that the individual STIs symptoms had high specificity and poor sensitivity. The sensitivity (specificity) of each symptom independently ranged from 2 to 17% (85–99%). The less sensitive STIs symptoms identified women as being infection-free when in fact they were not (high false-negative results). The more specific STIs symptoms identified women as infection-free when they were infection-free (low false-positive results). When the individual STIs were used together, the combined STIs symptoms showed poor sensitivity of 33% and moderate specificity of 73%. Nearly 67% of the infected women were missed and almost 27% of the women who report STIs symptoms were infection-free. The choice of less sensitive versus more specific tests depends on whether one wants to exclude a dangerous disease or avoid a dangerous therapy. A test's sensitivity (specificity) becomes particularly important when one is seeking to exclude a dangerous disease (to confirm a diagnosis that requires dangerous therapy).

Several previous studies from sub-Saharan African countries and other parts of the world have reported inconsistent results on the performance of STIs symptoms. Clark et al. [18] evaluated the diagnostic performance of self-reported STIs symptoms among high-risk men and women in Peru. The authors reported that the STIs symptoms had low sensitivity and high specificity consistent with our findings. Low sensitivity and high specificity of self-reported STIs symptoms were also reported in a Chinese study by Yin et al. [19]. A study by Mukenge-Tshibaka et al. [13] among female sex workers in Benin reported poor sensitivity of the STIs symptoms. Studies in Egypt and India [20, 21] among women attending antenatal, family planning, and peripheral government clinics reported high sensitivity and low specificity of STIs symptoms. In a study conducted in South Africa among women attending STD clinic, the sensitivity of STIs symptoms varied greatly, ranging from 0% to 88%, in detecting different infections [14].

Our study has several strengths compared to previous studies. It is a large population-based study, enhancing its generalizability. Most studies on the association between STIs symptoms and tests have been carried out in particular groups that are not representative of the overall population, such as STD or antenatal clinic attendees, or sex workers [13, 14, 20–22]. However, this study also had some limitations that may have influenced our findings. First, only women who agreed to be tested for STIs were included in the analysis, thereby ignoring the possible systematic differences between women who consented to be tested for STIs and those who did not. Analysis of the complete cases can be biased if there was a systematic difference between cases with observed data and those with unobserved data. For example, if women without or with fewer STIs symptoms consented to be tested, this might have led to an underestimation of the true association between STIs symptoms and tests. Second, some of the reported symptoms could have been caused by infections not measured in the study. This might have also led to an underestimation of the true association between STIs symptoms and tests. Third, the accuracy of the information given may be affected by the sensitive nature of information regarding symptoms of STIs. Thus, the self-reported STIs symptoms might have introduced social desirability and recall biases and were likely to be underreported.

The syndromic diagnosis of STIs is often used in resource-poor settings where laboratory diagnosis is limited. It is simple, cost effective, and capable of yielding rapid diagnosis for immediate treatment. However, it should be validated using population-based data and periodically evaluated.

Conflict of Interests

The author declares that there is no conflict of interests regarding the publication of this paper.

Acknowledgments

The author thanks the women of Moshi Urban District of Tanzania for their participation and staff at the National Bureau of Statistics in Tanzania for conducting the survey. The study was supported by Grants from Harvard University Center for AIDS Research (HU CFAR NIH/NAIDS P30-AI 060354).

References

[1] J. Z. Killewo, A. Sandstrom, U. B. Raden, F. S. Mhalu, G. Biberfield, and S. Wall, "Prevalence and incidence of syphilis and its association-with-HIV-1 infection in a population-based study in the Kagera region of Tanzania," *International Journal of STD and AIDS*, vol. 5, no. 6, pp. 424–431, 1994.

[2] A. Kamali, A. J. Nunn, D. W. Mulder, E. van Dyck, J. G. Dobbins, and J. A. G. Whitworth, "Seroprevalence and incidence of genital ulcer infections in a rural Ugandan population," *Sexually Transmitted Infections*, vol. 75, no. 2, pp. 98–102, 1999.

[3] UNAIDS, UNAIDS World AIDS day report, 2011.

[4] S. R. Galvin and M. S. Cohen, "The role of sexually transmitted diseases in HIV transmission," *Nature Reviews Microbiology*, vol. 2, no. 1, pp. 33–42, 2004.

[5] J. N. Wasserheit, "Epidemiological synergy: interrelationships between human immunodeficiency virus infection and other sexually transmitted diseases," *Sexually Transmitted Diseases*, vol. 19, no. 2, pp. 61–77, 1992.

[6] UNAIDS, Report on the global AIDS epidemic. Joint United Nations Programme on HIV/AIDS (UNAIDS), 2010.

[7] World Health Organization, *Sexually Transmitted and Other Reproductive Tract Infections: A Guide to essential practice*, WHO, Geneva, Switzerland, 2005.

[8] World Health Organization, *Guidelines for the Management of Sexually Transmitted Infections*, WHO, Geneva, Switzerland, 2001.

[9] W. K. Bosu, "Syndromic management of sexually transmitted diseases: is it rational or scientific?" *Tropical Medicine and International Health*, vol. 4, no. 2, pp. 114–119, 1999.

[10] L. Lush, G. Walt, and J. Ogden, "Transferring policies for treating sexually transmitted infections: what's wrong with global guidelines?" *Health Policy and Planning*, vol. 18, no. 1, pp. 18–30, 2003.

[11] Family Health International. HIV/AIDS prevention care in resource-constrained settings, 2001.

[12] A. Pettifor, J. Walsh, V. Wilkins, and P. Raghunathan, "How effective is syndromic management of STDs? A review of current studies," *Sexually Transmitted Diseases*, vol. 27, no. 7, pp. 371–385, 2000.

[13] L. Mukenge-Tshibaka, M. Alary, C. M. Lowndes et al., "Syndromic versus laboratory-based diagnosis of cervical infections among female sex workers in Benin: implications of nonattendance for return visits," *Sexually Transmitted Diseases*, vol. 29, no. 6, pp. 324–330, 2002.

[14] C. Mathews, A. van Rensburg, and N. Coetzee, "The sensitivity of a syndromic management approach in detecting sexually transmitted diseases in patients at a public health clinic in Cape Town," *South African Medical Journal*, vol. 88, no. 10, pp. 1337–1340, 1998.

[15] Tanzania Commission for AIDS (TACAIDS), 2005.

[16] U. Larsen, J. Mlay, S. Aboud et al., "Design of a community-based study of sexually transmitted infections/HIV and infertility in an urban area of Northern Tanzania," *Sexually Transmitted Diseases*, vol. 34, no. 1, pp. 20–24, 2007.

[17] M. Ghebremichael, E. Paintsil, and U. Larsen, "Alcohol abuse, sexual risk behaviors, and sexually transmitted infections in women in moshi Urban district, Northern Tanzania," *Sexually Transmitted Diseases*, vol. 36, no. 2, pp. 102–107, 2009.

[18] J. L. Clark, A. G. Lescano, K. A. Konda et al., "Syndromic management and STI control in urban Peru," *PLoS ONE*, vol. 4, no. 9, Article ID e7201, 2009.

[19] Y. P. Yin, Z. Wu, C. Lin et al., "Syndromic and laboratory diagnosis of sexually transmitted infection: a comparative study in China," *International Journal of STD and AIDS*, vol. 19, no. 6, pp. 381–384, 2008.

[20] F. Elkhwsky, A. Fawzi, A. Hany et al., "Validation of the syndromic management of sexually transmitted diseases in antenatal and family clinics in Alexandria.," *Journal of the Medical Research Institute*, vol. 28, no. 1, pp. 86–91, 2007.

[21] K. Ray, S. Muralidhar, M. Bala et al., "Comparative study of syndromic and etiological diagnosis of reproductive tract infections/sexually transmitted infections in women in Delhi," *International Journal of Infectious Diseases*, vol. 13, no. 6, pp. e352–e359, 2009.

[22] S. Gilani, "Syndromic management of pelvic inflammatory disease," *Journal of Medical Sciences*, vol. 18, no. 1, pp. 8–10, 2010.

2

Understanding the Profile of Tuberculosis and Human Immunodeficiency Virus Coinfection: Insights from Expanded HIV Surveillance at a Tuberculosis Facility in Durban, South Africa

Rubeshan Perumal,[1] Nesri Padayatchi,[1] Kogieleum Naidoo,[1] and Stephen Knight[2]

[1] *Centre for the AIDS Programme of Research in South Africa (CAPRISA), University of KwaZulu-Natal, Durban 4000, South Africa*
[2] *Department of Public Health Medicine, University of KwaZulu-Natal, Durban 4000, South Africa*

Correspondence should be addressed to Rubeshan Perumal; rubeshanperumal@gmail.com

Academic Editors: E. M. Fenyo, G. Hardy, and R. E. Jeeninga

Background. Expanded HIV surveillance in TB patients forms part of the World Health Organization framework for strategic collaborative activity. Surveillance helps understand the epidemiology of the local dual epidemic and enables design of a tailored response to these challenges. *Methods.* We conducted an observational, cross-sectional study of anonymous unlinked HIV testing for 741 consecutive TB suspects attending an urban TB facility during a seven-week period in 2008. *Results.* A total of 512 patients were found to have TB. The mean age was 35.7 years, and 63% were male. The prevalence of HIV was 72.2% (95% CI: 68.2–75.9) in all TB cases, 69.8% (95% CI: 65.3–74.2) in pulmonary tuberculosis (PTB), 81.6% (95% CI: 72.9–90.3) in extrapulmonary disease, and 66.8% (95% CI: 60.7–72.9) in those without TB disease. HIV prevalence in TB patients was higher in females than males and in younger age groups (18–29 years). The sex ratio of PTB patients correlated with the sex ratio of the prevalence of HIV in the respective age groups ($P < 0.05$). *Conclusion.* The use of a rapid HIV test performed on sputum anonymously provides an opportunity for HIV surveillance in this high-burdened setting, which has the potential to lend valuable insight into the coepidemics.

1. Background

In South Africa, the global epicenter of both tuberculosis (TB) and human immunodeficiency virus (HIV), the menacing convergence of these diseases: one viral and one bacterial, one emergent, and one ancient, presents a near insurmountable challenge to health, social, economic, and developmental welfare [1]. These dual epidemics threaten to undo the health care gains of the past decades in an already ailing health care system. Women now account for nearly a half of all global infections and 77% of all women living with HIV are in sub-Saharan African [2]. Acquired immune deficiency syndrome (AIDS) accounts for more deaths in women than all causes of maternal mortality combined [2]. While the global incidence of HIV is decreasing, new infections among young women aged 15 to 24 years have steadily increased in South Africa, which is due to multifactorial and complex biological, social, economic and behavioural factors.

The World Health Organization (WHO), in an effort to address the challenges of HIV associated TB, has proposed a framework of strategic collaborative activities for TB and HIV services which foster a more comprehensive approach to the synergistic dual epidemics [3]. In settings of generalized HIV and AIDS epidemics, like South Africa, WHO recommends expanding HIV surveillance to include TB patients.

Anonymous unlinked testing for HIV by means of a noninvasive sputum antibody test has been proposed as a means of HIV surveillance within South African TB facilities. This approach is cost-effective, sustainable, and feasible for rapid expansion of HIV surveillance in South Africa.

Comprehensive HIV surveillance is central to understanding the epidemic, the unique challenges in each country, the trajectory of the epidemic, resultant morbidity and mortality, and the impact of interventions. The WHO initiated unlinked, anonymous testing (UAT) through sentinel seroprevalence surveys amongst antenatal attendees as the global standard for HIV surveillance where heterosexual transmission is dominant. In UAT, blood drawn for routine purposes in the health care setting are stripped of patients-identifiers, unlinked from patient records, and tested for HIV [4]. This method has the primary advantage of eliminating nonresponse bias typically associated with other HIV surveys where consent is required. Since then this method has been the universally adopted standard throughout the world and serves as the methodological basis for comparing the prevalence of HIV across the globe, especially in generalized epidemics.

As an additional surveillance activity to antenatal surveys, HIV surveillance among TB patients is strongly recommended, especially in countries like South Africa where TB and HIV are deleteriously intertwined coepidemics. Expanding HIV surveillance to include TB patients will serve as an indicator of the level and maturity of the epidemic, as well as an indicator of the effect of HIV on health services [5].

The WHO guidelines for second generation HIV surveillance reiterate the need for additional data on HIV trends, not obtained from antenatal clinic surveys [6]. These guidelines promote a comprehensive HIV surveillance system, to better understand HIV trends and the factors that drive the epidemic in a country, by focusing on flexible surveillance in specific high risk populations to improve prevention and care activities [6].

The specific objectives of HIV surveillance among TB patients in generalized HIV epidemics are (a) to inform the targeting of resources and planning of activities for people with HIV associated TB and for monitoring the effectiveness of these activities; (b) to increase political, professional, and civil society awareness of coepidemics; (c) to assess the need for collaboration between HIV and TB programmes on formulation and implementation of a joint TB-HIV strategy; (d) to provide information on the HIV and AIDS epidemic and its impact on TB patients; and (e) to quantify the need for providing antiretroviral (ART) to TB patients [7].

One of the main challenges in conducting HIV surveillance among TB patients is the ethical concerns primarily surrounding the use of anonymous, unlinked testing. In settings with increasing availability of ART, there is considerable controversy about the ethical validity of anonymously testing for HIV where emphasis should be placed on counseling and testing for HIV and the provision of ART to patients who require it [8]. However, in general, testing without informed consent, for the purpose of surveillance, has been considered ethical if anonymous, unlinked testing is employed [7]. Moreover, in generalized epidemics with a high burden of TB-HIV coinfection, such as South Africa, the benefits of surveillance justify its inclusion as an additional method of surveillance. HIV surveillance among TB patients in the South African context using unlinked, anonymous testing will increase the epidemiological utility of the data by eliminating participation bias and will occur as part of a response to the public health emergency characterised by TB-HIV coinfection.

An existing challenge to anonymous, unlinked testing for HIV among TB patients is the lack of routine blood testing in TB on which HIV testing can piggyback. This has fuelled concerns as to whether the inclusion of routine bloods in TB will be driven by the covert intention to introduce anonymous, unlinked HIV testing, rather than out of a real need in the patient's interest. The use of novel methods for HIV testing on sputum specimens is rapidly gaining momentum in response to such concerns. Sputum, in contrast to blood, is routinely collected from TB patients, discarded after its use, and is being shown by an expanding evidence base to be useful in the diagnosis of HIV [7, 9–12]. The main ethical proviso regarding HIV surveillance among TB patients is that consent may only be omitted if samples are taken from routine specimens and testing is anonymous and is not linked to patient identifiers. Additionally, all TB patients included in HIV surveillance activities should have access to Voluntary Counseling and Testing (VCT) for HIV infection.

This paper explores anonymous unlinked HIV testing of TB suspects as a means to understand the local coinfection epidemic and the need to integrate services.

2. Method

2.1. Study Design. An observational, analytic, cross-sectional study design was used.

2.2. Study Site. The survey was conducted at an out-patient tuberculosis facility in Durban, South Africa. The clinic, situated in the central business district adjacent to a transportation nodal point, provides diagnosis and treatment of TB for those who reside or work in Durban. Sputum microscopy and HIV testing are conducted in the on-site laboratory.

2.3. Study Sample. The study sample included all adult patients presenting for TB diagnostic services who provided a sputum specimen during the study period.

2.4. Laboratory Method. OraQuick HIV 1/2 antibody testing was performed by a trained technician as per manufacturer guidelines on all sputum specimens prior to discard, irrespective of its suitability for TB microscopy [13].

2.5. Statistical Analysis. All data was processed and analysed using SAS Software (SAS 9.1.3, SAS Institute, Inc., Cary NC). For all statistical comparisons, the 5% significance level was used; correspondingly, 95% confidence intervals were used to describe effect size. All data was assessed for normality, and nonparametric tests were used where necessary. HIV prevalence for TB cases and suspects was calculated and selected demographic risk factors associated with the patients HIV status were measured using chi-squared tests for categorical

TABLE 1: Age and sex characteristics of study survey cohort.

Age group Years	Female n (%)	Male n (%)	Total n (%)	P value
<20	21 (7.7)	15 (3.2)	36 (4.9)	<0.05
20–29	89 (32.5)	100 (21.4)	189 (25.5)	<0.05
30–39	94 (34)	183 (39.2)	277 (37.4)	0.21
40–49	48 (17.5)	108 (23.1)	156 (21.0)	0.09
≥50	22 (8.0)	61 (13.1)	83 (11.2)	<0.05
Total	**274 (37.0)**	**467 (63.0)**	**741 (100)**	

Overall age (n = 741) mean: 35.7 years (95% CI: 34.9–36.5).
Males age (n = 467) mean: 36.9 years (95% CI: 35.9–37.9).
Females age (n = 274) mean: 33.6 years (95% CI: 32.2–35).

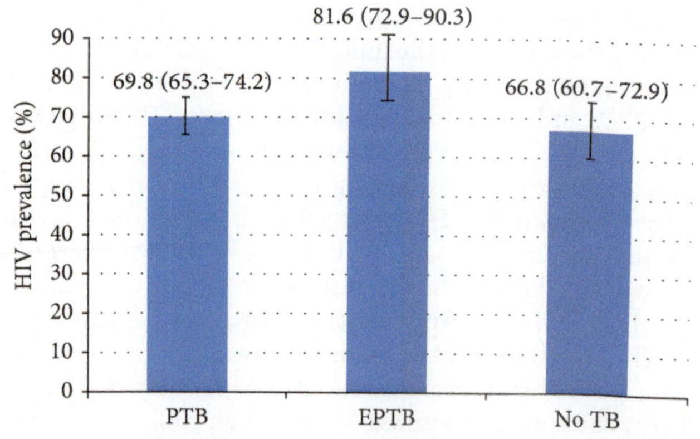

FIGURE 1: HIV prevalence (95% confidence intervals) in those with pulmonary tuberculosis (n = 407), extrapulmonary tuberculosis (n = 105), and without tuberculosis disease (n = 229) at the clinic, 2008.

data (participants age categories, gender, and visit type) and analysis of variance techniques for continuous variables (age).

2.6. Permissions. Ethical approval was obtained from the Biomedical Research Ethics Committee of the Africa University of KwaZulu-Natal (Reference number BFC031/08). Permission to conduct the study at a municipal health facility was obtained from the eThekwini Municipality Health Unit.

3. Results

3.1. Age and Sex Characteristics of the Study Sample. The mean age of the survey population was 35.7 years (SD ± 11.3 years). The mean ages of males and females were similar (36.9 versus 33.6 years, P = 0.234). Two-thirds (467/741) of the study sample were male. Of the total, 622 (84%) were between 20 and 50 years old, an identical proportion in both males (84%) and females (84%) (Table 1). Only 15 (3%) of the males were younger than 20 years old, compared to 21(8%) of the females (P < 0.05). There was a significantly higher proportion of males than females over 50 years of age (13% versus 8%, P < 0.05).

3.2. HIV Prevalence. A total of 229 (31%) TB suspects did not have a diagnosis of TB confirmed, of which 153(66.8%, 95% CI: 60.7–72.9) tested sputum HIV antibody positive. The balance of the study population of TB suspects, 512 (69%), was diagnosed with TB, of which 369 (72.1%, 95% CI: 68.2–76.0) were HIV positive. There was no statistical difference in HIV prevalence between these two groups (P = 0.15). The prevalence of HIV was 69.8% (95% CI: 65.3–74.2) and 81.6% (95% CI: 72.9–90.3) in those with pulmonary and extrapulmonary TB, respectively (Figure 1).

The HIV prevalence in TB suspects accessing the clinic varies by age, sex, and by the presence or absence of TB disease. In those without TB disease, the age- and sex-specific HIV prevalence reflects a similar pattern to the general population. Females have a higher age- specific HIV prevalence in all age groups except those 50 years and older, have an earlier peak prevalence than males (20–29 years versus 30–39 years), and have a higher peak prevalence (83.3% versus 75.6%) than males (Figure 2).

TABLE 2: Correlation between the change in the male-to-female sex ratio in all PTB and HIV associated PTB and ratio of sex-specific HIV prevalence across age groups.

Age group	Total M : F (all PTB)	HIV + M : F (HIV + PTB)	ΔM : F (change in ratio)	Male : female HIV prevalence
<20	0.8	0.4	−0.4	0.5
20–29	1.0	0.9	−0.1	0.9
30–39	2.5	2.6	0.1	1.0
40–49	2.7	2.4	−0.3	0.9
≥50	5.3	7.5	2.2	1.4

Pearson's correlation, one-tailed, r = 0.87, df = 3, and P < 0.05.

In those diagnosed with TB, the age-specific HIV prevalence in females was higher than in males in age groups under 20, 20–29, and 40–49. However, the peak prevalence (86%) of HIV in females occurred in the 40–49 years age group as compared to a peak male HIV prevalence of 87% in the 30–39 years age group. Females with and without TB (overall) have higher age- specific prevalence than males with and without TB in the younger age groups, while the males have higher age-specific prevalence than females in those 50 years and older.

The male-to-female sex ratio in all patients with pulmonary TB ranges from 0.79 in the under 20 years age group, to 5.3 in the greater than or equal to 50 years age group (Table 2). The representation of males increases across the increasing age groups. In HIV associated pulmonary TB, the male-to-female ratio ranges from 0.38 in the under 20 years age group to 7.5 in those 50 years and older. The proportion of females increases in the age groups less than 20 years, 20 to 29 years, and 40 to 49 years. In these age groups, the prevalence of HIV among females is higher than the HIV prevalence among males. There exists a significant positive correlation (r = 0.87, P < 0.05) between the change in the sex ratio between all those with PTB and PTB associated HIV and the sex ratio of HIV prevalence across the age groups.

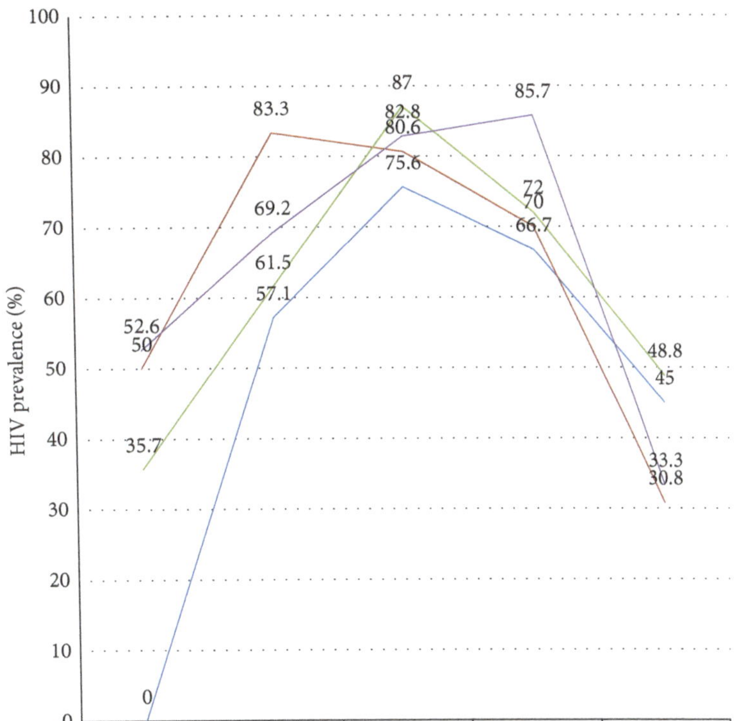

	<20	20–29	30–39	40–49	>50
No TB male	0	57.1	75.6	66.7	45
No TB female	50	83.3	80.6	70	30.8
All TB male	35.7	61.5	87	72	48.8
All TB female	52.6	69.2	82.8	85.7	33.3

FIGURE 2: HIV prevalence by age group, sex, and TB status in the study cohort.

4. Discussion

The primary objective of this study was to provide an estimate for the prevalence of HIV among attendees at an urban TB facility in Durban, South Africa, using a novel sputum-based HIV antibody test. The paucity of such information in the past has limited the ability of health services to exploit the opportunities presented by the changing epidemiology of TB and HIV in this setting. Analysis of the age and sex distribution of HIV associated TB in this study reflects the impact of a maturing HIV epidemic on TB in South Africa. Only 37% of TB patients were female, and the male-to-female ratio of 1.7 is lower than global and historic trends [14, 15]. Globally, in 2007, there was a 2 : 1 male-to-female ratio of cases notified to public health authorities [16]. Nonetheless, in low income countries, TB kills more women than all causes of maternal mortality combined. There was more pulmonary TB in females than in males under 30 years in this study. This increased burden of TB in young women has been attributed to biological, social, and methodological factors. Young women have up to 34% higher risk of progression to TB disease than men up to the age of 30 years initially attributed to reduced immunity associated with the stresses of pregnancy [16]. However, this hypothesis was not supported by a case-control study which demonstrated that pregnancy was not an exposure associated with TB disease [17]. In addition, young women have lower cumulative TB infections in adolescence, inferring that new postadolescence infection might be significantly greater amongst women. New infection with TB carries a greater likelihood to progress to TB disease, and to do so more rapidly. Females are more likely to encounter health services during their reproductive years, increasing their likelihood of having TB diagnosed. Similarly, the lower prevalence of TB disease in older women compared to men may reflect their differential access to healthcare due to a combination of complex social, economic, cultural, and logistical factors. This may be particularly true in settings such as South Africa where active case finding is too poorly implemented to rectify possible undernotification of women and their possible underrepresentation at health facilities. This age-sex trend of TB is similar to WHO estimates for other African countries with a high HIV prevalence where there are more female than male cases notified up to 25 years. The estimate was confirmed in this high HIV-burdened setting, with a male-to-female ratio of 0.9 in cases of pulmonary TB under 30 years of age.

The disproportionate burden of HIV on young women has largely been attributed to intergenerational sex of young women with older men, who are likely to have multiple concurrent sexual partners [2, 18, 19]. Young women have a 7-fold increased risk of acquiring HIV when in relationships with men between 5 and 7 years older [20–23]. The exact reasons for the increased risk of acquiring HIV in young women are not yet understood but include increased transmissibility from males to females, anatomy, condom use, sexual networking, poverty, education, economic autonomy, power imbalances between men and women, gender based violence, access to sexual and reproductive health services, and political and sociocultural issues [2]. The pattern of a higher HIV prevalence among young women in comparison to men in the same age group is now being reflected in the age-specific trends of TB. The impact of HIV on TB is reflected in the age-specific HIV prevalence figures generated by this study and confirms that HIV is shaping the evolving epidemiology of TB in this setting.

With nearly 70% of all TB patients being coinfected with HIV, it is not surprising that the age and sex distribution of TB is increasingly resembling the distribution of HIV in this region of hyperendemicity. The male-to-female ratio among HIV negative individuals was 1.98 while the male-to-female ratio among those living with HIV drops to 1.58. The increased representation of females in comparison to males in HIV associated pulmonary TB is significantly correlated with the sex-specific HIV prevalence figures in those age groups. There is a clear indication that HIV is driving the increased representation of females among TB patients with age groups in which females have the higher HIV prevalence containing a greater number of females with TB. A previous study in this setting demonstrated a significantly higher burden of TB disease among women in the 20 to 29 years age group, in keeping with predictions by mathematical models on the impact of HIV on TB in areas of dual hyperendemicity [24]. Whether this is due to biological or structural reasons is uncertain, but the greater representation of females at TB facilities in high HIV settings has multiple programmatic implications. A growing recognition of the gradually changing face of TB in this setting will allow for the exploitation of the opportunities presented by this evolving epidemiology. The unique opportunity to seek out synergies between TB-HIV and women's health services must be seized. The broadening of services may serve to appropriately orientate the existing TB services with regards to the changing demographic profile of patients to augment women's health services, to respond to the need for comprehensive primary health care services, and, most importantly, to acknowledge the presence of multiple pathologies in an individual patient that cannot adequately be addressed by a vertical programme design.

5. Conclusions

The demographic profile of TB patients mirrors the patterns observed in those living with HIV and suggests that HIV infection does fuel the TB epidemic in this setting. The increased number of young women, in particular, at TB services presents the opportunity to design more demographically sensitive TB services which include a more comprehensive health service package. The benefit of including women friendly reproductive health services at TB facilities requires further evaluation. Overall, this survey demonstrates the possibility of using a novel HIV antibody assay on sputum and an anonymous survey design for achieving additional HIV surveillance in a generalized HIV epidemic with TB endemicity. A better understanding of both of these epidemics and how they interact is crucial to optimise a consolidated comprehensive public health response. The richness of data that is generated is a clear indication of the potential benefits that may accrue from better understanding the confluence of these dual epidemics. The idea of an expanded surveillance programme for HIV in TB facilities is a direct response to a call from WHO to optimize the position of health systems to understand, appreciate, and react to the emerging destructive synergy between TB and HIV epidemics.

This study has highlighted that the problem of TB-HIV coinfection is not a homogenous entity but rather a composite of many complex subepidemics. This is largely due to the various drivers of HIV and TB which have differential effects on various strata of the population, most notably subpopulations by age and sex. A striking feature of the TB-HIV coepidemic is the direct influence that the epidemiology of HIV has had on the evolving TB epidemic, with young women representing a significant proportion of TB facility attendees. The majority of TB patients are now also in the economically active age group. The hyperendemicity of TB and HIV in South Africa coupled with the existing demographic distribution of the coepidemics has serious implications for the social, health, and economic status of the nation and threatens to be a significant limitation to national growth and development. Vertical programme designs have failed to demonstrate that they are capable of responding to the synergism of multiple morbidities in individuals. A more integrated approach is more attractive as it promises the possibility of increasing clinical and operational efficiency. This is the central theme of the WHO call for closer collaboration between TB and HIV services. However, the guiding tenet of all health care initiatives is to ensure that programmes are responsive to the needs of patients and that any intervention is tailored to respond to those needs while being informed by the unique epidemiology of the local epidemic. The local epidemic, as demonstrated in this study, is characterised by a broad cross-section of patients, with the majority of coinfected individuals in the economically active age group, and with the majority of women in their reproductive years. There are therefore several opportunities to maximize the impact of any healthcare contact with these individuals when they present to a TB facility. Sexual health services, in particular, would be well positioned in TB facilities and could aim to provide sexual health education, positive prevention, condom promotion, screening for sexually transmitted diseases, and the treatment thereof.

This study has confirmed that the burden young women face in terms of their heightened vulnerability for HIV infection has been translated to an increased vulnerability for TB. Existing TB programmes do not adequately reflect the needs of young women in their design. Women's health and basic reproductive health services would have a significant target audience at TB facilities. This might include access to family planning, Pap smear evaluations, and targeted interventions for young women such as microbicide gels in future. A more comprehensive service may lead to greater public access, more equitable access for all patients, a more convenient and satisfying service, and better health overall. New TB service design must begin to reflect the presence of young women as a significant group burdened by the disease.

Conflict of Interests

The authors declare that there is no conflict of interests.

Authors' Contribution

The study was conceptualised by Nesri Padayatchi, Rubeshan Perumal, and Kogieleum Naidoo. The implementation of the study was overseen by Kogieleum Naidoo and Rubeshan Perumal. Data collection and analysis were performed by Rubeshan Perumal. The paper was prepared by Rubeshan Perumal and Stephen Knight. All authors contributed to the editing and finalization of the paper.

Acknowledgments

The authors extend their appreciation to Natasha Samsunder for coordinating the laboratory activities and Lise Werner for assistance with the statistical analysis.

References

[1] K. H. Mayer and C. D. Hamilton, "Synergistic pandemics: confronting the global HIV and tuberculosis epidemics," *Clinical Infectious Diseases*, vol. 50, supplement 3, pp. S67–S70, 2010.

[2] Q. A. Karim, S. Sibeko, and C. Baxter, "Preventing HIV infection in women: a global health imperative," *Clinical Infectious Diseases*, vol. 50, supplement 3, pp. S122–S129, 2010.

[3] World Health Organisation, *Interim Policy on Collaborative TB/HIV Activities*, World Health Organisation, Geneva, Switzerland, 2004.

[4] O. Bolu, A. Anand, A. Swartzendruber et al., "Utility of antenatal HIV surveillance data to evaluate prevention of mother-to-child HIV transmission programs in resource-limited settings," *American Journal of Obstetrics and Gynecology*, vol. 197, supplement 3, pp. S17–S25, 2007.

[5] World Health Organisation, *Guidelines for Conducting HIV Sentinel Serosurveys among Pregnant Women and Other Groups*, World Health Organisation, Geneva, Switzerland, 2003.

[6] World Health Organisation, *UNAIDS. Guidelines for Second Generation HIV Surveillance*, World Health Organisation, Geneva, Switzerland, 2000.

[7] World Health Organisation, *Guidelines for HIV Surveillance Among Tuberculosis Patients*, World Health Organisation, Geneva, Switzerland, 2004.

[8] S. Rennie, A. N. Turner, B. Mupenda, and F. Behets, "Conducting unlinked anonymous HIV surveillance in developing countries: ethical, epidemiological, and public health concerns," *PLoS Medicine*, vol. 6, no. 1, Article ID e1000004, pp. 30–34, 2009.

[9] E. F. Bowen, P. S. Rice, N. T. Cooke, R. J. Whitfield, and C. F. J. Rayner, "HIV seroprevalence by anonymous testing in patients with Mycobacterium tuberculosis and in tuberculosis contacts," *The Lancet*, vol. 356, no. 9240, pp. 1488–1489, 2000.

[10] R. J. O'Connell, T. M. Merritt, J. A. Malia et al., "Performance of the OraQuick rapid antibody test for diagnosis of human immunodeficiency virus type 1 infection in patients with various levels of exposure to highly active antiretroviral therapy," *Journal of Clinical Microbiology*, vol. 41, no. 5, pp. 2153–2155, 2003.

[11] R. L. Hamers, I. H. De Beer, H. Kaura, M. Van Vugt, L. Caparos, and T. F. Rinke De Wit, "Diagnostic accuracy of 2 oral fluid-based tests for HIV surveillance in Namibia," *Journal of Acquired Immune Deficiency Syndromes*, vol. 48, no. 1, pp. 116–118, 2008.

[12] R. L. Hamers, I. D. Beer, H. Kaura, M. Van Vugt, and T. F. Rinke De Wit, "Oral fluid HIV rapid testing in Southern Africa is suitable for population-level surveillance but may not be so for individual diagnosis (invited response to scott et al: can oral fluid testing be used to replace blood-based HIV rapid testing to improve access to diagnosis in South Africa?)," *Journal of Acquired Immune Deficiency Syndromes*, vol. 51, no. 5, pp. 648–649, 2009.

[13] E. A. Talbot, N. M. Hone, H. J. Moffat et al., "The validity of HIV testing using sputum from suspected tuberculosis patients, Botswana, 2001," *International Journal of Tuberculosis and Lung Disease*, vol. 7, no. 8, pp. 710–713, 2003.

[14] C. Dye, "Global epidemiology of tuberculosis," *The Lancet*, vol. 367, no. 9514, pp. 938–940, 2006.

[15] World Health Organisation, *Global Tuberculosis Control: Epidemiology, Strategy, Financing*, World Health Organisation, Geneva, Switzerland, 2009.

[16] C. B. Holmes, H. Hausler, and P. Nunn, "A review of sex differences in the epidemiology of tuberculosis," *International Journal of Tuberculosis and Lung Disease*, vol. 2, no. 2, pp. 96–104, 1998.

[17] M. A. Espinal, A. L. Reingold, and M. Lavandera, "Effect of pregnancy on the risk of developing active tuberculosis," *The Journal of Infectious Diseases*, vol. 173, no. 2, pp. 488–491, 1996.

[18] S. H. Vermund and L. Van Damme, "HIV prevention in women: next steps," *Science*, vol. 331, no. 6015, p. 284, 2011.

[19] Human Sciences Research Council, *the South African National HIV Prevalence, Incidence, Behaviour and Communication Survey, 2008-The Health of Our Children*, Human Sciences Research Council, Cape Town, South Africa, 2010.

[20] S. Gregson, C. A. Nyamukapa, G. P. Garnett et al., "Sexual mixing patterns and sex-differentials in teenage exposure to HIV infection in rural Zimbabwe," *The Lancet*, vol. 359, no. 9321, pp. 1896–1903, 2002.

[21] A. Pettifor, C. Macphail, H. Rees, and M. Cohen, "HIV and sexual behavior among young people: the South African paradox," *Sexually Transmitted Diseases*, vol. 35, no. 10, pp. 843–844, 2008.

[22] A. Pettifor, K. O'Brien, C. MacPhail, W. C. Miller, and H. Rees, "Early coital debut and associated HIV risk factors among young women and men in South Africa," *International Family Planning Perspectives*, vol. 35, no. 2, pp. 82–90, 2009.

[23] A. E. Pettifor, H. V. Rees, I. Kleinschmidt et al., "Young people's sexual health in South Africa: HIV prevalence and sexual behaviors from a nationally representative household survey," *AIDS*, vol. 19, no. 14, pp. 1525–1534, 2005.

[24] A. B. Kharsany, C. Connolly, A. Olowolagba, S. S. Abdool Karim, and Q. Abdool Karim, "Increasing burden of pulmonary tuberculosis in young women," *South African Medical Journal*, vol. 96, no. 6, pp. 524–525, 2006.

3

Rapid Tests versus ELISA for Screening of HIV Infection: Our Experience from a Voluntary Counselling and Testing Facility of a Tertiary Care Centre in North India

Bhanu Mehra, Sonali Bhattar, Preena Bhalla, and Deepti Rawat

Department of Microbiology, Maulana Azad Medical College, New Delhi 110002, India

Correspondence should be addressed to Preena Bhalla; preenabhalla@gmail.com

Academic Editors: S. Dube, W. Fu, L. Gray, M. Monsour, and M. Patel

Early and accurate diagnosis of human immunodeficiency virus (HIV) infection is essential for timely identification of patients needing antiretroviral therapy and for instituting HIV prevention strategies. The primary methodology for HIV testing has shifted from enzyme linked immunosorbent assay (ELISA) to rapid diagnostic tests (RDTs) in recent years, especially in resource limited settings. However, the diagnostic performance of RDTs is a matter of concern. In the present study the performance of an RDT being used as the initial test in serial testing based algorithm for HIV diagnosis was compared with ELISA. Seven hundred and eighty-seven sera, tested at the voluntary counselling and testing facility employing a serial testing algorithm (based on SD Bioline HIV-1/2 3.0 as the first test), were subsequently tested with Microlisa-HIV for anti-HIV antibodies. The first test missed 9 HIV reactive samples and also registered 5 false positives. The sensitivity, specificity, and negative and positive predictive values of the first test were 77.5%, 99.3%, and 98.8% and 86.1%, respectively, taking ELISA as the standard test. Our study highlights that RDTs fare poorly compared to ELISA as screening assays and that reactive results by RDTs need to be confirmed by western blot for a positive serodiagnosis of HIV infection.

1. Introduction

Approximately 35.3 million people across the world are infected with human immunodeficiency virus (HIV) [1]. Early and accurate knowledge of HIV serostatus of an individual is the cornerstone of HIV prevention and therapeutic intervention. In addition to allowing timely initiation of antiretroviral therapy of the HIV infection, early diagnosis also provides an opportunity to limit the spread of HIV from the infected individuals to the naive population.

Detection of anti-HIV antibodies as a marker of HIV exposure is the most widely used approach for serodiagnosis of this infection. Enzyme linked immunosorbent assay (ELISA) has been a preferred screening procedure in this regard [2]. However the labour intensive and time consuming format of the assay as well as the requirement of instrumentation and technical expertise has resulted in a shift from an ELISA based approach to rapid diagnostic tests (RDTs), particularly in resource constrained settings. While some studies have reported the performance of RDTs and ELISA to be comparable [3], results from others have raised concerns regarding sensitivity and specificity of the rapid assays [4–6].

With regard to HIV testing, two testing algorithms are commonly described: parallel and serial. While in parallel testing samples are tested simultaneously by two different tests, in serial testing they are tested by a first test, the results of which determine requirement of any further testing [7]. Thus for HIV testing strategies employing a serial testing algorithm, the selection of testing technologies as well as the order in which they are employed is crucial for obtaining accurate results. Since the first test is the screening test, it should be highly sensitive and the subsequent tests need to be highly specific so that all true negative test results are identified as negative and false positives do not occur. In India, the voluntary counselling and testing (VCT) facilities are employing strategy/algorithm III for diagnosis of HIV infection as per the guidelines laid by the National AIDS

TABLE 1: Characteristics of human immunodeficiency virus (HIV) tests as per kit literatures.

Test	Principle	Specimen volume required	Antigen employed	Time to test result	Specimen type	Sensitivity	Specificity
SD Bioline HIV-1/2 3.0	Lateral flow immunochromatography	10 μL	gp 41 and p24 for HIV-1 and gp 36 for HIV-2	5–20 minutes	Serum, plasma	Not specified	Not specified
Pareekshak HIV-1/2 Triline card test	Lateral flow immunochromatography	10 μL	gp 41 and C terminus of gp 120 for HIV-1 and gp 36 for HIV-2	20 minutes	Serum, plasma	100%	99.49%
Pareekshak HIV 1/2 rapid test kit (Trispot)	Immunoconcentration	2 drops	HIV 1 and HIV-2 r (recombinant)-proteins	Immediate	Serum, plasma	100%	100%
Microlisa-HIV	Indirect ELISA	10–20 μL	gp 41 and C terminus of gp 120 for HIV-1 and gp 36 for HIV-2	>1.5 hours	Serum, plasma	100%	99.5%

HIV: human immunodeficiency virus; ELISA: enzyme linked immunosorbent assay.

(acquired immunodeficiency syndrome) Control Organization (NACO) [8].

In the present study the authors have evaluated the performance of the RDT being used as the first/screening test in serial testing based algorithm for HIV diagnosis being followed at the VCT centre of a tertiary care health facility and compared it with the standard ELISA based approach for screening of HIV infection. In addition, all the positive results by the 3 RDTs and by ELISA were confirmed by a confirmatory test (western blot) to identify any false positives that may have occurred.

2. Materials and Methods

2.1. Study Population. This study is from the VCT facility of a tertiary care teaching hospital in North India. Sera from 787 consecutive patients tested at the VCT centre in September-October 2012 were included in the analysis.

Patients enrolled at the VCT facility first underwent a pretest counselling, following which a written informed consent was obtained for HIV testing and blood sample collected by trained technical personnel.

2.2. Evaluation Protocol. Sera were separated and tested by serial testing algorithm whereby samples reactive by the first test were subsequently tested by the second and third tests to confirm the positive result. The first test employed was SD Bioline HIV-1/2 3.0 (SD Biostandard Diagnostics Private Limited, Gurgaon, Haryana, India), a lateral flow immunochromatographic assay. Sera nonreactive by the first test were considered negative for anti-HIV antibodies whereas those that were reactive were subsequently tested with both Pareekshak HIV-1/2 Triline card test (Bhat Bio-Tech India Private Limited, Bangalore, Karnataka, India), lateral flow immunochromatographic assay, and Pareekshak HIV 1/2 rapid test kit (Trispot) (Bhat Bio-Tech India Private Limited, Bangalore, Karnataka, India), immunoconcentration based assay. All the specimens were processed as per instructions in the kit insert. In the second phase of this evaluation, all the sera (both HIV reactive and nonreactive) were retested by Microlisa-HIV (J. Mitra and Company Private Limited, New Delhi, India), an enzyme immunoassay based on the principle of indirect ELISA. The evaluation was conducted in a blinded fashion with the RDTs and ELISA performed by different technical personnel and the status of the sera as per the RDT based algorithm not revealed to the personnel performing the ELISA. All the samples reactive by Microlisa-HIV were retested by the same ELISA kit to confirm the result. All samples that were ELISA positive were confirmed by western blot (J. Mitra and Company Private Limited, New Delhi, India), as were the ones that were positive by RDTs alone. The serostatus as determined by western blot was considered as the final result. The characteristics of the RDTs and ELISA employed in this analysis are summarized in Table 1.

2.3. Statistical Analysis. The sensitivity and specificity calculations and estimation of negative and positive predictive values of the first/screening RDT were done by comparing its performance with Microlisa-HIV (reference technique). Sensitivity of a test is defined as the ability to correctly identify the infected individuals; specificity as the ability to correctly identify the uninfected individuals; negative predictive value as the proportion of those with a negative test result who are uninfected and positive predictive value as the proportion of those with a positive test result who are actually infected. Sensitivity was calculated as true positives/(true positives + false negatives) × 100; specificity as true negatives/(true negatives + false positives) × 100; negative predictive value as true negatives/(true negatives + false negatives) × 100 and positive predictive value as true positives/(true positives + false positives) × 100.

Table 2: Diagnostic performance of SD Bioline HIV-1/2 3.0 in comparison to Microlisa-HIV (reference standard).

Test 1 (SD Bioline HIV-1/2 3.0)	Microlisa-HIV	
	Reactive	Nonreactive
Reactive	31	5
Nonreactive	9	742

HIV: human immunodeficiency virus.

Table 3: Sensitivity, specificity, and predictive values of SD Bioline HIV-1/2 3.0 (taking Microlisa-HIV as the reference).

Test	Sensitivity	Specificity	Negative predictive value	Positive predictive value
SD Bioline HIV-1/2 3.0	77.5%	99.3%	98.8%	86.1%

HIV: human immunodeficiency virus; ELISA: enzyme linked immunosorbent assay.

3. Results

All the 787 sera were tested for anti-HIV antibodies by at least one rapid test (SD Bioline HIV-1/2 3.0). Thirty-six serum samples were reactive by the first test. On subsequent evaluation of all the 787 samples by Microlisa-HIV, 40 HIV reactive samples were identified (all confirmed as positive by western blot), 9 of which had been reported as nonreactive by SD Bioline HIV-1/2 3.0. Thus the first RDT had missed 9 (22.5%) HIV reactive samples (also confirmed to be positive by western blot) and its sensitivity on comparison with ELISA was 77.5%. In addition, SD Bioline HIV-1/2 3.0 registered 5 false positive results (negative by ELISA and western blot) giving a specificity of 99.3%. The negative and positive predictive values of SD Bioline HIV-1/2 3.0 were 98.8% and 86.1%, respectively. The diagnostic performance of SD Bioline HIV-1/2 3.0 and its performance characteristics in comparison to Microlisa-HIV are summarized in Tables 2 and 3, respectively.

Since Pareekshak HIV-1/2 Triline card test and Pareekshak HIV 1/2 rapid test kit (Trispot) were used to evaluate only those samples that were reactive by the first test, their overall sensitivity and specificity could not be assessed though both the tests picked up all 31(100%) of ELISA reactive serum samples tested by them. Like SD Bioline HIV-1/2 3.0, both the tests also registered false positive results (5 false positives by Pareekshak HIV-1/2 Triline card test and 4 false positives by Pareekshak HIV 1/2 rapid test kit (Trispot)). An overview of the reactive results obtained by the 3 RDTs and their subsequent status as per Microlisa-HIV is provided in Table 4.

4. Discussion

Both ELISA and RDTs are widely employed immunological assays for serodiagnosis of HIV infection [9]. Discrepancy between results obtained by the two techniques is common [10]. Some studies suggest that the diagnostic performance of RDTs is comparable to that of ELISA [3]. However, in our evaluation RDT based algorithm employing SD Bioline HIV-1/2 3.0 as the initial test fared poorly compared to ELISA and missed a large proportion of HIV infections. Inferior performance of RDTs in comparison to ELISA has also been reported in another study from India where both the modalities were used to screen healthy blood donors for HIV infection and the RDT used missed 17 of 30 samples confirmed reactive by ELISA [2]. This discordance may possibly be due to low antibody titres especially in recent infections where the levels may well be below the detection limit of RDTs but are picked up by the more sensitive enzyme immunoassay and its spectrophotometric format of result analysis. Based on our findings we suggest that, with serial testing based algorithms wherein a negative result from a single initial RDT is considered sufficient to classify a sample as HIV nonreactive, false negative results may occur quite often leading to unknown silent transmission of HIV in the population.

Since the primary purpose of this study was not to compare the performance of different RDTs with each other and we have strictly adhered to the protocol of a serial testing algorithm, we cannot make recommendations regarding the use of any one RDT over others as the initial test. We also do not deny that the same RDT may perform differently under different field conditions, since on literature review we found studies that show the same rapid test brand as employed in our analysis to be 100% sensitive and equivalent in its diagnostic performance characteristics to Microlisa-HIV [11]. Thus while we cannot rule out the possibility that an RDT of the same or of a different test brand might perform better, as discussed above, the theoretical probability of an RDT approaching the sensitivity of an ELISA is meagre especially for low titre samples as seen in the diagnostic window period.

As with other studies, we also observed false positive results with RDTs [12]. False positive results with RDTs are a matter of concern since the relative ease of performance of these assays outside the laboratories increases the likelihood of HIV testing without proper counselling, which further leads to poor understanding on the part of the patients receiving a reactive report that they may or may not be positive [13]. In our study, the false positives with RDTs are definitely not due to cross-reactivity since all these samples were nonreactive by ELISA. While the cause of these false positives is not exactly known, the common reasons could be technical errors, mislabelling of samples, problems with components of the test devices, and subjective and ambiguous interpretation of faint bands as positive when the test sample is actually negative [14, 15]. A recent study has also pointed out the role of variation in specificity of HIV RDTs over time and geographic location as a possible cause of higher than previously encountered false positive HIV results [16].

A major constraint on the application of ELISA in VCT programs despite its high sensitivity has been its longer turnaround time and with studies revealing that a number of patients undergoing HIV testing do not return to the VCT centres to collect their reports [17, 18], RDTs seem to offer an excellent option with test results being available to the patients on the same visit. Though use of RDTs can increase

TABLE 4: Comparison of reactive results of rapid test kits with Microlisa-HIV (reference standard).

Test employed	Total number of tests performed	Number of samples positive	Number of samples reactive by Microlisa-HIV	Number of samples nonreactive by Microlisa-HIV
SD Bioline HIV-1/2 3.0	787	36	31	5
Pareekshak HIV-1/2 Triline card test	36	36	31	5
Pareekshak HIV 1/2 rapid test kit (Trispot)	36	35	31	4

HIV: human immunodeficiency virus.

the proportion of patients gaining access to HIV antibody test results [19], their use as the only screening test in VCT programs cannot be justified keeping in view the possibility of missing early infections as well as concerns regarding reporting false positive results.

A practical approach in the present scenario could be a serial RDT based testing algorithm to despatch a preliminary report to the patient followed by testing of all samples by ELISA to identify any false negative and false positive results. In resource limited settings like India, where serial testing algorithms are cost effective and putting up both RDTs and ELISA for all samples might not be economically feasible, efforts should be directed towards utilizing RDTs that simultaneously detect p24 antigen, so that early HIV infections are not missed, and confirming at least all the samples positive for anti-HIV antibodies by RDTs with a subsequent conventional ELISA and western blot to reduce the frequency of persons receiving false positive results.

5. Conclusion

Our study highlights that ELISA is a good screening assay for HIV infection. The performance of RDTs in comparison to ELISA is suboptimal and RDT based serial testing algorithm cannot parallel the testing accuracy of an ELISA based approach. While false negatives by RDTs increase the proportion of HIV reactive individuals receiving negative reports, false positives by RDTs are a matter of ethical concern. The diagnostic limitations of RDTs can be overcome by possible inclusion of ELISA as a second screening assay, employing RDTs additionally detecting p24 antigen as screening assays, and confirmation of reactive samples by western blot to reduce false negative and false positive results, respectively.

Conflict of Interests

The authors declare that there is no conflict of interests regarding the publication of this paper.

References

[1] "2013 UNAIDS report on the global AIDS epidemic," http://www.unaids.org/en/media/unaids/contentassets/documents/epidemiology/2013/gr2013/UNAIDS_Global_Report_2013_en.pdf.

[2] V. P. Torane and J. S. Shastri, "Comparison of ELISA and rapid screening tests for the diagnosis of HIV, hepatitis B and hepatitis C among healthy blood donors in a tertiary care hospital in Mumbai," *Indian Journal of Medical Microbiology*, vol. 26, no. 3, pp. 284–285, 2008.

[3] T. X. Lien, N. T. K. Tien, G. F. Chanpong et al., "Evaluation of rapid diagnostic tests for the detection of human immunodeficiency virus types 1 and 2, hepatitis B surface antigen, and syphilis in Ho Chi Minh City, Vietnam," *American Journal of Tropical Medicine and Hygiene*, vol. 62, no. 2, pp. 301–309, 2000.

[4] M. Claassen, G. U. van Zyl, S. N. J. Korsman, L. Smit, M. F. Cotton, and W. Preiser, "Pitfalls with rapid HIV antibody testing in HIV-infected children in the Western Cape, South Africa," *Journal of Clinical Virology*, vol. 37, no. 1, pp. 68–71, 2006.

[5] R. H. Gray, F. Makumbi, D. Serwadda et al., "Limitations of rapid HIV-1 tests during screening for trials in Uganda: diagnostic test accuracy study," *British Medical Journal*, vol. 335, no. 7612, article 188, 2007.

[6] B. Louie, E. Wong, J. D. Klausner et al., "Assessment of rapid tests for detection of human immunodeficiency virus-specific antibodies in recently infected individuals," *Journal of Clinical Microbiology*, vol. 46, no. 4, pp. 1494–1497, 2008.

[7] R. J. Wright and J. S. A. Stringer, "Rapid testing strategies for HIV-1 serodiagnosis in high-prevalence African settings," *American Journal of Preventive Medicine*, vol. 27, no. 1, pp. 42–48, 2004.

[8] "Guidelines for HIV testing," National AIDS Control Organisation, Ministry of Health and Family Welfare, http://naco.gov.in/upload/Policies%20&%20Guidelines/5-GUILDELINES%20FOR%20HIV%20TESTING.pdf.

[9] T. Hussain, K. K. Kulshreshtha, S. Sinha, V. S. Yadav, and V. M. Katoch, "HIV, HBV, HCV, and syphilis co-infections among patients attending the STD clinics of district hospitals in Northern India," *International Journal of Infectious Diseases*, vol. 10, no. 5, pp. 358–363, 2006.

[10] H. S. Iqbal, S. Solomon, K. G. Murugavel, S. S. Solomon, and P. Balakrishnan, "Evaluation and diagnostic usefulness of domestic and imported enzyme-linked immunosorbent assays for detection of human immunodeficiency virus type 1 antibody in India," *Clinical and Diagnostic Laboratory Immunology*, vol. 12, no. 12, pp. 1425–1428, 2005.

[11] S. Maity, S. Nandi, S. Biswas, S. K. Sadhukhan, and M. K. Saha, "Performance and diagnostic usefulness of commercially available enzyme linked immunosorbent assay and rapid kits for detection of HIV, HBV and HCV in India," *Virology Journal*, vol. 9, article 290, 2012.

[12] A. F. Aghokeng, E. Mpoudi-Ngole, H. Dimodi et al., "Inaccurate diagnosis of HIV-1 group M and O is a key challenge for ongoing universal access to antiretroviral treatment and HIV prevention in Cameroon," *PLoS ONE*, vol. 4, no. 11, Article ID e7702, 2009.

[13] B. Sibbald, "New rapid HIV test opens Pandora's box of ethical concerns," *Canadian Medical Association Journal*, vol. 162, no. 11, article 1600, 2000.

[14] D. B. Klarkowski, J. M. Wazome, K. M. Lokuge, L. Shanks, C. F. Mills, and D. P. O'Brien, "The evaluation of a rapid in situ HIV confirmation test in a programme with a high failure rate of the WHO HIV two-test diagnostic algorithm," *PLoS ONE*, vol. 4, no. 2, Article ID e4351, 2009.

[15] D. Klarkowski, D. P. O'Brien, L. Shanks, and K. P. Singh, "Causes of false-positive HIV rapid diagnostic test results," *Expert Review of Anti-Infective Therapy*, vol. 12, no. 1, pp. 49–62, 2014.

[16] D. Klarkowski, K. Glass, D. O'Brien, K. Lokuge, E. Piriou, and L. Shanks, "Variation in specificity of HIV rapid diagnostic tests over place and time: an analysis of discordancy data using a Bayesian approach," *PLoS ONE*, vol. 8, no. 11, Article ID e81656, 2013.

[17] R. O. Valdiserri, M. Moore, A. R. Gerber, C. H. Campbell Jr., B. A. Dillon, and G. R. West, "A study of clients returning for counseling after HIV testing: implications for improving rates of return," *Public Health Reports*, vol. 108, no. 1, pp. 12–18, 1993.

[18] G. Tao, B. M. Branson, W. J. Kassler, and R. A. Cohen, "Rates of receiving HIV test results: data from the U.S. National Health Interview Survey for 1994 and 1995," *Journal of Acquired Immune Deficiency Syndromes and Human Retrovirology*, vol. 22, no. 4, pp. 395–400, 1999.

[19] N. T. Constantine and H. Zink, "HIV testing technologies after two decades of evolution," *Indian Journal of Medical Research*, vol. 121, no. 4, pp. 519–538, 2005.

4

Emergence of Drug Resistance in Human Immunodeficiency Virus Type 1 Infected Patients from Pune, India, at the End of 12 Months of First Line Antiretroviral Therapy Initiation

Rajesh T. Patil,[1] Rajiv M. Gupta,[2] Sourav Sen,[3] Srikanth P. Tripathy,[4] Devidas N. Chaturbhuj,[5] Nitin K. Hingankar,[5] and Ramesh S. Paranjape[5]

[1] *Department of Microbiology, Azeezia Institute of Medical Sciences & Research, Kollam, Kerala, India*
[2] *DDGMS (IT) Office of Directorate General of Medical Services (Army) Integrated HQ of MoDAG's Branch, L Block, New Delhi, India*
[3] *Department of Microbiology, Army Hospital (Research & Referral), Delhi, India*
[4] *National JALMA Institute of Leprosy and other Mycobacterial Diseases (Indian Council of Medical Research), Agra, India*
[5] *National AIDS Research Institute (Indian Council of Medical Research), Pune, India*

Correspondence should be addressed to Rajesh T. Patil; drrajesh.patil@yahoo.co.in

Academic Editors: F. Krebs, C. Petrovas, J. Poudrier, F. Tuluc, and F. Vaida

Introduction. In India, 4,86,173 HIV infected patients are on first line antiretroviral therapy (ART) as of January 2012. HIV drug resistance (HIVDR) is drug and regimen-specific and should be balanced against the benefits of providing a given ART regimen. *Material & Methods.* The emergence of HIVDR mutations in a cohort of 100 consecutive HIV-1 infected individuals attending ART centre, on first line ART for 12 months, was studied. $CD4^+$ T-cell counts and plasma HIV-1 RNA level were determined. *Result.* Out of the 100 HIV-1 infected individuals, 81 showed HIVDR prevention (HIV-1 RNA level < 1000/mL), while the remaining 19 had HIV-1 viral RNA level > 1000/mL. HIVDR genotyping was carried out for individuals with evidence of virologic failure (HIV-1 RNA level > 1000/mL). The most frequent NRTI-associated mutation observed was M184V, while K103N/S was the commonest mutation at NNRTI resistance position. *Conclusion.* Our study has revealed the emergence of HIVDR in HIV-1 infected patients at the end of 12 months of first line ART initiation. For NRTIs, the prevalence of HIVDR mutations was 9% and 10% for NNRTIs. Our findings will contribute information in evidence-based decision making with reference to first and second line ART delivery and prevention of HIVDR emergence.

1. Introduction

Estimates place the number of people living with human immunodeficiency virus (HIV) in India in 2009 at 2.39 million with an estimated adult HIV prevalence of 0.31% [1]. Under National AIDS Control Programme (Phase III) of India 300743 patients are on antiretroviral therapy (ART) in 342 ART centers and 650 link ART centers as of January 2012 [1]. ART regimens in resource limited settings are usually selected at the national level following a public health approach. Generally only one first line regimen with alternative regimen(s) incorporating within class drug substitution is available in the public sector [2]. In India, the first line ART consists of zidovudine (AZT)/stavudine (d4T) + lamivudine (3TC) + nevirapine (NVP)/efavirenz (EFZ) [3, 4]. Because of the error-prone nature of HIV replication, its high mutation rate in the presence of drug selective pressure, and because of the need for lifelong treatment, it is anticipated that drug resistant (HIVDR) HIV strains will emerge among persons on treatment even if appropriate ART regimens are provided and optimal adherence to therapy is supported [5]. Emergence of HIVDR is drug and regimen-specific and should be balanced against the benefits of providing a given ART regimen. Studies have shown that the immunological failure can be delayed by 6 months to 2 years from the time of virologic failure [6]. HIV drug resistant mutations in patients on ART can occur before or after virologic failure and can continue to occur and get selected under drug pressure if the failed regimen is not replaced [7]. These drug resistant HIV not only exhibit resistance to several classes of antiretroviral drugs [8] but also cross-resistance within a class of antiretroviral drugs [9]. Due to the high cost of the plasma virus load determination, monitoring of HIV RNA levels in HIV infected patients on first line ART is still not offered as a standard of care test in resource limited settings. Studies have shown that the second line nucleoside reverse transcriptase inhibitor (NRTI) drugs like tenofovir, abacavir, and didanosine and nonnucleoside reverse transcriptase inhibitor (NNRTI) drugs like etravirine will be rendered ineffective if these PLHA harbouring HIVDR mutations are continued on a failing regimen [10]. ART prescription in resource limited settings is population based rather than based on the model of individual patient management utilized in resource-rich nations [2]. In a recent survey on prevalence of transmitted HIVDR among recently infected clients in Mumbai and among newly diagnosed HIV-1 primigravida women in Kakinada, the prevalence of transmitted HIVDR was classified as <5% to all relevant antiretroviral drug classes [11, 12]. This study was carried out to evaluate the emergence of HIVDR in 100 HIV-1 infected individuals at the end of 12 months of initiation of first line ART.

2. Material and Methods

2.1. Study Participants. This was a cross-sectional study wherein participants consisted of 100 consecutive HIV-1 infected individuals attending the ART centre from 2009 to 2011 who had completed 12-month duration from the time of initiation of first line ART. The first line ART regimen consisted of lamivudine (3TC) + Stavudine (d4T)/Zidovudine (AZT) + Nevirapine (NVP)/Efavirenz (EFZ). After taking written informed consent whole blood was collected in K_3EDTA. Plasma was separated by centrifugation at 1500 ×g for 10 min at room temperature. The plasma samples were aliquoted and stored in duplicate at −70°C. $CD4^+$ T lymphocyte counts were estimated in the whole blood collected in K_3EDTA by flow cytometry (FACS Count, BD Biosciences Immunocytometry Systems, San Jose, CA). Plasma HIV-1 RNA level was determined by Roche Amp Monitor test, version 1.5 (Roche Diagnostics, Branchburg, NJ).

2.2. HIV-1 Drug Resistance Genotyping and Phylogenetic Analysis. Plasma samples stored at −70°C were used for detection of HIVDR mutations by in-house assay described earlier after minor modifications [13]. HIV-1 RNA was extracted from plasma using QIAamp viral RNA Mini Kit (Qiagen, Valencia, CA). The HIV-1 *pol* gene region encoding protease (PR) and the 5′ end of reverse transcriptase (RT) was amplified by one tube reverse transcription — PCR using the RobusT I RT-PCR kit (Finnzymes Oy, Finland), followed by nested PCR, with outer primers: *Pol 2021F and Pol 4521R*. Two sets of inner primer were used to amplify HIV-1 pol region amplicons of 1–250 base pairs and 1–560 base pairs using *Pol 2135F and Pol 3338R* and *Pol 2135F and Pol 4470R, respectively*. The PCR amplicons were directly sequenced bidirectionally on an ABI PRISM 3100 genetic analyzer system (Applied Biosystems, Foster City, CA). The forward sequencing primers used were *Pol 2041F, Pol 2135F, Pol 2493F, Pol 3012F, Pol 3403F, Pol 3468* and the reverse sequencing primers were *Pol 2557R, Pol 3117R, Pol 3620R, Pol 3768R, Pol 3999R, Pol 4381R*. The regions sequenced by the in-house assay included PR (1–99) and RT (range: 1–250 to 1–560). The contig sequences were manually edited using SeqScape 2 software (Applied Biosystems) and were submitted to "HIVdb Program: Sequence Analysis" in the Stanford University HIV drug resistance database (http://sierra2.stanford.edu/sierra/servlet/JSierra) for drug resistance interpretation. The phylogenetic tree (Figure 1) was constructed using TreeMaker tool available on Los Alamos HIV sequence database, using general-time-reversible (GTR) distant model (available at http://www.hiv.lanl.gov/) with distance model GTR.

3. Results

Among the 100 HIV-1 infected study participants, 74 were males and 26 females. The age range was 21 to 70 years and heterosexual promiscuity was the most common mode of transmission (55%). The various first line ART combinations received by the study participants were (a) 3TC + AZT + NVP (n = 53), (b) 3TC + AZT + EFZ (n = 14), (c) D4T + 3TC + NVP (n = 13), (d) D4T + 3TC + EFZ (n = 8), (e) 3TC/D4T + AZT + NVP (n = 6), (f) 3TC + AZT + NVP/EFZ (n = 4), (g) 3TC/D4T + AZT + NVP/EFZ (n = 2).

3.1. HIV-1 RNA Levels and $CD4^+$ T-Cell Counts. Out of the 100 HIV-1 infected study participants, 81 showed HIVDR prevention (HIV-1 RNA level < 1000/mL), while the remaining 19 had HIV-1 viral RNA level > 1000/mL (range: 1,026–963,000) (median: 7,421). $CD4^+$ T-cell count in 10 study participants was >500 cells/μL, 200–499 cells/μL in 64, and 26 had <200 cells/μL. The details of $CD4^+$ T-cell counts, HIV-1 RNA level, the first line ART regimen for 19 study participants which had HIV-1 RNA level > 1000/mL are shown in Table 1. Based on the recommendations by WHO to monitor HIVDR prevention and associated factors in sentinel ART sites, individuals showing HIV RNA level (<1000 copies/mL after 12 months of initiation of first line ART) were considered to have "no effective HIVDR mutations" [2, 14] and emergence of HIVDR mutations was suspected in individuals with HIV RNA level ≥ 1000 copies/mL after 12 months of initiation of first line ART.

3.2. HIV-1 Drug Resistance Mutations and Subtyping. Of the 19 plasma samples which showed HIV-1 RNA level > 1000/mL, 16 could be amplified and sequenced. Out of these 16 study sequences, 10 displayed one or more HIVDR mutations out of which 9 sequences had NRTI and NNRTI associated resistance mutations and 1 NNRTI associated resistance mutations only (Table 1). No HIVDR mutation was observed in 6 study participants either to NRTI or to NNRTI.

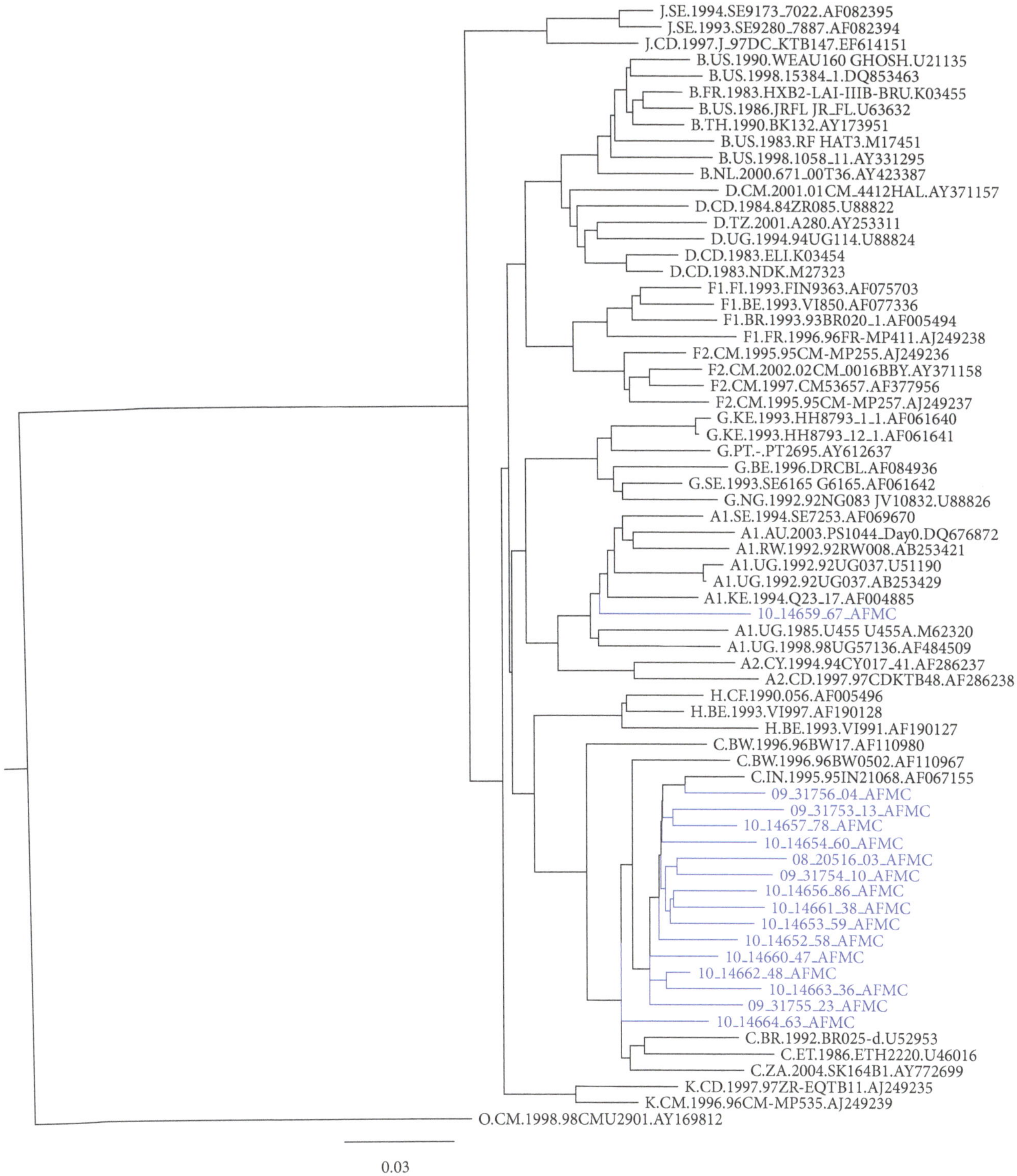

Figure 1: Phylogenetic tree of 16 HIV-1 pol sequences constructed using TreeMaker tool available on Los Alamos HIV sequence database, using general-time-reversible (GTR) distance model.

The commonest NRTI mutation observed was M184V (8/19) and the most common NNRTI was K103N/S (6/19). None of the study sequences showed any HIVDR mutations in protease region. Out of the 16 sequences 15 belonged to subtype C and 1 to subtype A1.

4. Discussion

According to WHO, in HIV-1 infected patients on first line ART for 12 months, the suggested standard to minimize the emergence of HIVDR is ≥70% [2]. In our study

TABLE 1: Details of GenBank accession number, first line ART regimen, CD4$^+$ T-cell counts, HIV-1 RNA level, and HIVDR mutations of 19 plasma specimens with HIV-1 RNA level >1000 copies/mL.

Serial number	GenBank accession number	ART Combination	CD4$^+$ T-cell counts (cells/μL) after 12 months of ART initiation	HIV-1 RNA level (copies/mL) after 12 months of ART initiation	HIVDR mutations	
					NRTI mutations	NNRTI mutations
1	HQ456679	3TC, AZT, NVP	312	9,63,000	M41L, M184V, T215Y, N348I	Y188L
2	HQ456669	3TC, AZT, NVP, EFZ	184	83,635	D67N, T69ADNT, K70R, M184V, T215F, K219Q	K103N, Y188, M230L
3	HQ456677	3TC, AZT, NVP, EFZ	95	33,668	D67N, K70R, M184V, T215F, K219EKQ	K103N, P225H, K238T
4	HQ456671	3TC, AZT, NVP, D4T	224	22,034	M184MV	K103N
5	HQ456667	3TC, AZT, NVP	<50	13,491	M41L, E44D, D67N, M184V, L210LS, T215Y	A98G, K101Q, Y181C
6	HQ456681	3TC, AZT, NVP, EFZ	240	7,421	M184V	K103N
7	HQ456680	3TC, AZT, EFZ	290	7,310	None	K103N, V106MV
8	HQ456672	D4T, 3TC, NVP	375	2,604	L74LV, M184V	K103S, M23OL, K238N
9	HQ456675	D4T, 3TC, NVP	275	1,397	M184V	G190A
10	HQ456668	3TC, AZT, NVP	368	1,335	M184V	K103N
11	HQ456673	3TC, AZT, NVP	143	4,12,721	None	None
12	HQ456678	3TC, AZT, NVP	280	58,243	None	None
13	HQ456674	3TC, AZT, NVP	264	39,916	None	None
14	HQ456676	3TC, AZT, NVP	278	2,526	None	None
15	HQ456670	D4T, 3TC, NVP	254	2,032	None	None
16	HQ456682	3TC, AZT, NVP	370	1,614	None	None
17	—	3TC, AZT, NVP	113	3,69,247	No amplification	
18	—	3TC, AZT, NVP, EFZ, D4T	390	2,030	No amplification	
19	—	3TC, AZT, NVP	240	1,026	No amplification	

the prevention of emergence of HIVDR was 81% while the prevalence of emergence of drug resistance in HIV-1 infected patients at virologic failure on first line ART after 12 months of treatment initiation was 19%. In a previous study, twelve months after ART initiations, 75% and 64.6% achieved viral load suppression of <1000 copies/mL were observed at the Chennai and Mumbai clinics, respectively [15]. Out of the 19 study participants with HIV RNA level > 1000 copies/mL, HIVDR mutations were observed in 10 (52.7%) study participants. No HIVDR mutations were observed in 6 study sequences. Amplification was not successful in 3 plasma samples which had HIV-1 RNA level > 1000 copies/mL. These 9 study participants were classified as having *potential HIVDR* that is specimens with a HIV-1 RNA level > 1000 copies/mL and no evidence of HIVDR on genotype testing [2]. The prevalence of NRTI-associated

HIVDR was 9% while it was 10% for NNRTIs. Of these 10 study sequences with HIVDR mutations, 9 exhibited one or more HIVDR mutations for NRTI as well as NNRTI, while the remaining 1 showed NNRTI-associated HIVDR mutation only. Lack of compliance to ART was recorded in 6 study participants. The commonest NRTI mutation observed was M184V (8/19), which was in agreement with previous Indian studies done on ART experienced individuals [13, 15–17]. This M184V HIVDR mutation which is the commonest and earliest HIVDR mutation to occur in lamivudine (3TC) treated individuals causes high-level resistance to lamivudine (3TC) and emtricitabine (FTC) and low-level resistance to didanosine (ddI) and abacavir (ABC) and increased susceptibility to zidovudine (AZT), stavudine (d4T), and tenofovir (TDF) [18]. Thymidine analog mutations (TAMs), selected by the thymidine analogs (AZT & d4T) which decrease susceptibility to these NRTIs, and to a lesser extent to ABC, ddI, and TDF [18], were seen in 4 study sequences. TAMs are common in low-income countries in which fixed-dose combinations containing thymidine analogs are the mainstay of therapy [18]. TAMs accumulate in two distinct but overlapping patterns [18]. The type I pattern includes the mutations M41L, L210W, and T215Y while type II pattern includes D67N, K70R, T215F, and K219Q/E. Type I TAMs were seen in 2 study sequences in our study out of which in 1 study sequence all the three type I TAMs were seen along with D67N. Type II TAMs were seen in 2 study sequences. E44D, an accessory mutation that generally occurs with type I pattern TAM, was seen in 1 study participant. This mutation occurs in about 1% of viruses from untreated patients and in a significantly higher proportion of viruses from patients receiving NRTI [18]. A62V a multinucleoside HIVDR mutation was seen in 1 study sequence. The Q151M complex was not seen in any of the study sequences in our study. N348I a nonpolymorphic HIVDR mutation was seen in 1 study sequence which occurs in about 10% of NRTI-treated patients [18]. N348I causes a twofold reduction in AZT susceptibility when it occurs in combination with multiple TAM [18]. The most common primary NNRTI resistance mutation was K103N/S which was observed in 6 study participants (K103N-5; K103S-1), which is also the most common mutation documented in another Indian study [17], whereas two other Indian studies [13, 16] found Y181C/V & G190A and V106M & Y181C, respectively, as the commonest NNRTI mutations. The other primary NNRTI resistance mutations that were seen in our study were V106M (2/19), Y181C (1/19), Y188L (2/19), and G190A (1/19). All of them cause high-level resistance to nevirapine and variable resistance to efavirenz, ranging from about twofold for V106A and Y181C, sixfold for G190A, 20-fold for K103N, and more than 50-fold for Y188L [18]. L100I, K101P, P225H, F227L, M230L, and K238T are secondary mutations that usually occur in combination with one of the primary NNRTI resistance mutations [18]. Of these secondary mutations P225H (1/19) & K238T/N (2/19) were the secondary NNRTI mutation seen in our study. They usually occur in combination with K103N as observed in our study. These HIVDR mutations synergistically reduce nevirapine and efavirenz susceptibility [18]. M230L, seen in 1 study sequence, may occur alone which decreases the susceptibility of all NNRTI including etravirine by 20-fold or more [18]. V90I was observed in 1 study sequence which is associated with decreased virologic response to etravirine in the DUET clinical trial [18]. This mutation was also documented in earlier Indian studies [13, 19, 20]. Among the study participants with evidence of virologic failure high-level resistance was seen to nevirapine (10/19), lamivudine (8/19), efavirenz (8/19), emtricitabine (8/19), and didanosine (8/19), intermediate resistance to abacavir (4/19), didanosine (4/19), etravirine (3/19), and stavudine (3/19), and low-level resistance to tenofovir (3/19).

In previous HIVDR mutation studies from India on ARV experienced individuals, the median duration of therapy has ranged from 2.15 to 3 years [10, 13, 16, 17, 20]. Almost all ART centers in India monitor HIV infected individuals on first line ART only with $CD4^+$ T-cell count which may not give the true picture of response to therapy. This is the first Indian study that has evaluated HIVDR prevention on a population level, 12 months after initiation of first line ART, which can be addressed, if necessary, by changes in ART regimen protocols. Based on the distribution of HIVDR mutations detected in such HIVDR prevention monitoring studies conducted at multiple sites, suitable action can be planned to initiate alternative as well as second line ART protocols. Early recognition of emergence of HIVDR mutations in HIV-1 infected patients on first line ARV for 12 months with HIV-1 RNA level testing followed by HIVDR testing will help in preserving second line drugs and can also delay the need for newer class of antiretroviral drugs which will be costly for resource limited countries like India. In addition, emergence of HIVDR in HIV-1 infected individuals on first line ART can be further reduced if issues like patient related factors and ART site factors are identified and addressed.

In conclusion, to the best of our knowledge, this is the first Indian study carried out to monitor HIVDR mutations in HIV-1 infected individuals after 12 months of first line ART initiation. In India, multicentric monitoring of HIVDR prevention in sentinel ART sites in HIV-1 infected individuals after initiation of first line ART will be an essential component of national ART program, so as to provide necessary data for national working groups in evidence-based decision making with reference to first and second line ART delivery and prevention of HIVDR emergence.

5. Sequence Data

GenBank accession numbers for the 16 study sequences reported in our study were from HQ456667 to HQ456682.

Conflict of Interests

The authors declare that there is no conflict of interests regarding the publication of this paper.

Acknowledgments

The authors acknowledge Department of Microbiology, Armed Forces Medical College, Pune, for the study and

National AIDS Research Organization (Indian Council of Medical Research), Pune, India, for conducting the HIV-1 drug resistance genotyping. They are grateful to the HIV-1 infected patients who participated in this study.

References

[1] National AIDS Control Organisation: Annual report 2009-10, Department of AIDS Control Ministry of Health & Family Welfare, Government of India, 2011, http://www.nacoonline.org/ .

[2] M. R. Jordan, D. E. Bennett, S. Bertagnolio, C. F. Gilks, and D. Sutherland, "World Health Organization surveys to monitor HIV drug resistance prevention and associated factors in sentinel antiretroviral treatment sites," *Antiviral Therapy*, vol. 13, supplement 2, pp. 15–23, 2008.

[3] Antiretroviral Therapy Guidelines for HIV-Infected Adults and Adolescents: May 2013, http://www.naco.gov.in/NACO /About_NACO/.

[4] "Department of Human Health Services (DHHS) guidelines," Contentfiles/Adult and Adolescents Guidelines, http://www .aidsinfo.nih.gov/.

[5] J. M. Coffin, "HIV population dynamics in vivo: implications for genetic variation, pathogenesis, and therapy," *Science*, vol. 267, no. 5197, pp. 483–489, 1995.

[6] S. G. Deeks, J. N. Martin, E. Sinclair et al., "Strong cell-mediated immune responses are associated with the maintenance of low-level viremia in antiretroviral-treated individuals with drug-resistant human immunodeficiency virus type 1," *Journal of Infectious Diseases*, vol. 189, no. 2, pp. 312–321, 2004.

[7] C. A. Sabin, T. Hill, F. Lampe et al., "UK Collaborative HIV Cohort, (UK CHIC) study Group. Treament exhaustion of HAART among individuals infected with HIV in UK: multicentre cohort study," *BMJ*, vol. 49, pp. 306–309, 2005.

[8] R. W. Shafer, M. A. Winters, S. Palmer, and T. C. Merigan, "Multiple concurrent reverse transcriptase and protease mutations and multidrug resistance of HIV-1 isolates from heavily treated patients," *Annals of Internal Medicine*, vol. 128, no. 11, pp. 906–911, 1998.

[9] V. Miller and B. A. Larder, "Mutational patterns in the HIV genome and cross-resistance following nucleoside and nucleotide analogue drug exposure," *Antiviral Therapy*, vol. 6, supplement 3, pp. 25–44, 2001.

[10] N. Kumarasamy, V. Madhavan, K. K. Venkatesh et al., "High frequency of clinically significant mutations after first-line generic highly active antiretroviral therapy failure: implications for second-line options in resource-limited settings," *Clinical Infectious Diseases*, vol. 49, no. 2, pp. 306–309, 2009.

[11] D. N. Chaturbhuj, N. K. Hingankar, P. Srikantiah et al., "Transmitted HIV drug resistance among HIV-infected Voluntary Counseling and Testing Centers (VCTC) clients in Mumbai, India," *AIDS Research and Human Retroviruses*, vol. 26, no. 8, pp. 927–932, 2010.

[12] S. R. Thorat, D. N. Chaturbhuj, N. K. Hingankar et al., "Surveillance of transmitted HIV type 1 drug resistance among HIV type 1-positive women attending an antenatal clinic in Kakinada, India," *AIDS Res Hum Retroviruses*, vol. 27, no. 12, pp. 1291–1297, 2011.

[13] L. Rajesh, R. Karunaianantham, P. R. Narayanan, and S. Swaminathan, "Antiretroviral drug-resistant mutations at baseline and at time of failure of antiretroviral therapy in HIV type 1-coinfected TB patients," *AIDS Research and Human Retroviruses*, vol. 25, no. 11, pp. 1179–1185, 2009.

[14] P. K. Lee, T. L. Kieffer, R. F. Siliciano, and R. E. Nettles, "HIV-1 viral load blips are of limited clinical significance," *Journal of Antimicrobial Chemotherapy*, vol. 57, no. 5, pp. 803–805, 2006.

[15] N. K. Hingankar, S. R. Thorat, A. Deshpande et al., "Initial virologic response and HIV drug resistance among HIV-Infected individuals initiating first-line antiretroviral therapy at 2 clinics in Chennai and Mumbai, India," *Clinical Infectious Diseases*, vol. 54, supplement 4, pp. S348–S354, 2012.

[16] S. Sen, S. P. Tripathy, A. A. Patil, V. M. Chimanpure, and R. S. Paranjape, "High prevalence of human immunodeficiency virus type 1 drug resistance mutations in antiretroviral treatment-experienced patients from Pune, India," *AIDS Research and Human Retroviruses*, vol. 23, no. 10, pp. 1303–1308, 2007.

[17] A. Gupta, D. G. Saple, G. Nadkarni et al., "One-, two-, and three-class resistance among HIV-infected patients on antiretroviral therapy in private care clinics: Mumbai, India," *AIDS Research and Human Retroviruses*, vol. 26, no. 1, pp. 25–31, 2010.

[18] R. W. Shafer and J. M. Schapiro, "HIV-1 drug resistance mutations: an updated framework for the second decade of HAART," *AIDS Reviews*, vol. 10, no. 2, pp. 67–84, 2008.

[19] A. Deshpande, A. C. Jeannot, M. H. Schrive, L. Wittkop, P. Pinson, and H. J. Fleury, "Analysis of RT sequences of subtype C HIV-type 1 isolates from indian patients at failure of a first-line treatment according to clinical and/or immunological WHO guidelines," *AIDS Research and Human Retroviruses*, vol. 26, no. 3, pp. 343–350, 2010.

[20] S. Sen, S. P. Tripathy, V. M. Chimanpure, A. A. Patil, R. D. Bagul, and R. S. Paranjape, "Human immunodeficiency virus type 1 drug resistance mutations in peripheral blood mononuclear cell proviral DNA among antiretroviral treatment-naive and treatment-experienced patients from Pune, India," *AIDS Research and Human Retroviruses*, vol. 23, no. 4, pp. 489–497, 2007.

Factors Determining Survival and Retention among HIV-Infected Children and Adolescents in a Community Home-Based Care and a Facility-Based Family-Centred Approach in Kampala, Uganda: A Cohort Study

W. Massavon,[1,2] L. Barlow-Mosha,[3] L. Mugenyi,[4] W. McFarland,[5] G. Gray,[6] R. Lundin,[1] P. Costenaro,[1] M. M. Nannyonga,[2] M. Penazzato,[1] D. Bagenda,[3,7] C. P. Namisi,[2] D. Wabwire,[3] M. Mubiru,[3] S. Kironde,[2] D. Bilardi,[1] A. Mazza,[8] M. G. Fowler,[3,9] P. Musoke,[3,10] and C. Giaquinto[1]

[1] *Department of Paediatrics, University of Padua, Via Giustiniani 3, 35128 Padua, Italy*
[2] *St. Raphael of St. Francis Hospital (Nsambya Hospital), Kampala, Uganda*
[3] *Makerere University, Johns Hopkins University Research Collaboration, Kampala, Uganda*
[4] *Infectious Diseases Research Collaboration, Mulago Hospital Complex, Kampala, Uganda*
[5] *Department of Global Health Sciences, University of California San Francisco, 50 Beale Street, 12th Floor, San Francisco, CA 94105, USA*
[6] *University of Witwatersrand, 1 Jan Smuts Avenue, Braamfontein 2000, Johannesburg, South Africa*
[7] *Department of Global Heath and Population, Harvard University School of Public Health, Boston, MA, USA*
[8] *Santa Chiara Hospital, Via Largo Gold Medals 9, 38122 Trento, Italy*
[9] *Department of Pathology, Johns Hopkins School of Medicine 600 N. Wolfe Street/Carnegie 43 Baltimore, MD 21287, USA*
[10] *Department of Paediatrics and Child Health, Makerere University, Kampala, Uganda*

Correspondence should be addressed to W. Massavon; wmassavon@gmail.com

Academic Editors: R. Ansari and L. Sarmati

We describe factors determining retention and survival among HIV-infected children and adolescents engaged in two health care delivery models in Kampala, Uganda: one is a community home-based care (CHBC) and the other is a facility-based family-centred approach (FBFCA). This retrospective cohort study reviewed records from children aged from 0 to 18 years engaged in the two models from 2003 to 2010 focussing on retention/loss to follow-up, mortality, use of antiretroviral therapy (ART), and clinical characteristics. Kaplan Meier survival curves with log rank tests were used to describe and compare retention and survival. Overall, 1,623 children were included, 90.0% (1460/1623) from the CHBC. Children completed an average of 4.2 years of follow-up (maximum 7.7 years). Median age was 53 (IQR: 11–109) months at enrolment. In the CHBC, retention differed significantly between patients on ART and those not (log-rank test, adjusted, $P < 0.001$). Comparing ART patients in both models, there was no significant difference in long-term survival (log-rank test, $P = 0.308$, adjusted, $P = 0.489$), while retention was higher in the CHBC: 94.8% versus 84.7% in the FBFCA (log-rank test, $P < 0.001$, adjusted $P = 0.006$). Irrespective of model of care, children receiving ART had better retention in care and survival.

1. Background

Sub-Saharan Africa (SSA) is home to the vast majority of infants, children, and adolescents living with HIV and morbidity and mortality remain high [1–3]. For example, mortality among HIV-infected children has been measured at 4.3% per year in East Africa and 8.3% in West Africa [4, 5]. A recent meta-analysis conducted in SSA reported a higher risk of early death among perinatally infected children [6]. Studies have also shown that substantial proportions of children and adolescents initiate treatment in SSA with advanced disease (46.3%–72.0%) and comorbidities such as tuberculosis (TB) (5.7%–34.0%) and malnutrition (33%–54%) that tend to be associated with early mortality and poor clinical outcomes [7–10].

Significant child mortality can be averted if antiretroviral therapy (ART) is started early [11–14]. However, despite overwhelming evidence demonstrating the benefits of ART, in practice high mortality and poor retention persist among HIV-infected children and adolescents in care in the resource-limited settings of SSA. In addition to scarce resources for programmes for children, the situation is compounded by a combination of factors including late HIV diagnosis, missed opportunities to initiate ART, health care programmes not tailored to the needs of the infected child and their family, and logistic bottlenecks in implementation of care and treatment programmes [15, 16]. Initiation of ART even among children known to be eligible may be missed. For instance, in a study of ART-eligible children in The Gambia, only 32.7% started ART, 47.1% were lost to follow-up, and 13.5% died before initiating ART [17].

Retention in care while awaiting ART eligibility can also be a challenge. As an illustration, retention varied from 71% to 95% and 62% to 93% at 12 and 24 months, respectively, among children and adolescents in ART programmes in several countries of SSA [18]. A prior study in Uganda showed that even with frequent CD4 monitoring, HIV-infected children experienced significant clinical events while ineligible for ART according to the 2006 WHO guidelines [19]. Another study in Uganda showed that mortality was highest among HIV-infected children under two years [20]. Given this situation, it is important to assess factors that determine survival and retention in care among HIV-infected children and adolescents in care in resource-limited settings.

The present study focuses on retention and survival in two different ART delivery models for HIV-infected children and adolescents in Kampala, Uganda. One is a facility-based, family-centred approach (FBFCA) adopted by the mother to child transmission (MTCT)-Plus programme of the Makerere University-Johns Hopkins University (MU-JHU) Research Collaboration. The other is a community home-based care (CHBC) implemented by the children's HIV programme of the Home Care Department of Nsambya Hospital. The American Academy of Paediatrics defined family-centred care as based on the understanding that the family is the child's primary source of strength and support [21]. Beyond that, the family provides an enabling environment for using index HIV patients to reach other infected and affected family members, build family support for therapy and chronic care, integrate other medical needs for the family, and thus enhance uptake of services for HIV and other medical conditions for the family as a unit [22]. In general, CHBC includes any form of care (physical, psychosocial, palliative, and spiritual) given to the sick and the affected in their own homes and care extended from the hospital or health facility to their homes through family participation and community involvement [23, 24].

Factors that determine retention and survival of HIV-infected children and adolescents in these health care models are not well understood. The present study therefore aims at identifying factors that determine these outcomes for the CHBC of Nsambya Hospital and the FBFCA of MU-JHU. We also examine pre-ART deaths among children and adolescents in the CHBC to compare mortality rates prior to and after ART initiation and to ascertain whether children experiencing mortality prior to initiating ART had met the 2010 WHO [25] or the 2011 updated United States (US) [26] treatment guidelines for initiating ART or not.

2. Methods

2.1. Study Design, Setting, and Population. This retrospective cohort study covered eight years of records review (2003 to 2010) from two facilities implementing HIV paediatric programmes in Kampala, Uganda. They included the children's HIV programme of the Home Care Department of Nsambya Hospital, which uses community home-based care (CHBC) and the MTCT-plus programme of MU-JHU Research Collaboration, which adopts a facility-based family-centred approach (FBFCA). Prior to the study, all children in the FBFCA had been initiated on ART; thus, the record review at the FBFCA involved only children on ART. The facilities are both private-not-for-profit but differ in service delivery approaches, including catchment areas and enrolment practices. The study population included all HIV positive infants, children, and adolescents aged 0–18 years, enrolled in both programmes over the study period. Services are generally free of charge under both models.

2.2. Description of Health Care Models. The FBFCA of MU-JHU Collaboration was established in 2003 with funding from Columbia University. Its catchment area includes Kampala and Wakiso districts and covers approximately 20 km radius from Mulago hospital in Kampala. Enrolment into the FBFCA occurred between 2003 and 2005 and targeted all HIV-infected family members as a unit. However, HIV-infected pregnant women in PMTCT served as the starting point for identifying other infected family members such as infants, children, and spouses or partners to be enrolled into care. Eligibility of the women included being pregnant, testing HIV positive, attendance of PMTCT clinic, disclosure of HIV status to spouse or partner, willingness to be home visited, and living within 20 km radius from Mulago Hospital. The FBFCA offered comprehensive HIV care, including early infant diagnosis (EID), treatment and psychosocial support services, other medical services, and routine follow-up to eligible women and their families. All children enrolled in the study had been initiated on ART prior to the study start date, in contrast to the CHBC. The programme has a uniform design that has been implemented in many countries. Although funding ended in December 2011, the families continue to be followed in a family care approach with funding from the US President's Emergency Plan for AIDS Relief (PEPFAR).

The CHBC also started in 2003 and it integrates facility-based care with home-based care using community involvements as important linkages to decentralize HIV services. It has a catchment area covering four districts: Kampala, Wakiso, Mukono, and Mpigi within 21 km radius from Nsambya hospital. In contrast to the FBFCA, children and adolescents in the CHBC were identified directly for participation. The components of the CHBC, details of enrolment practice, pre-ART care, and ART care packages, as well as patient tracking system, have been described in an earlier work [27]. The CHBC was funded by international donors and partners and indirectly supported by PEPFAR.

Both health care models share some common elements such as providing additional support including nutritional supplements, patient education, and counselling of patients and their caregivers. Additionally, peer support groups for both adults and children have been developed to promote emotional support. Other components of psychosocial support include financial assistance for income generating activities, a music, dance, and drama group, and home visiting to track defaulting patients. Furthermore, the FBFCA trains peer-educators to provide support and help in the clinics.

2.3. Clinical and Laboratory Follow-Up. Patients were followed up routinely using similar appointment systems, standard guidelines, and procedures. Generally, children on ART had monthly clinic visits under both models, while visits for pre-ART patients depended on their clinical conditions and varied between one month under the CHBC and 3–6 months under the FBFCA. Initiation of ART was based on the Ugandan National ART guidelines that are adopted from the WHO guidelines [25, 28–30], which have changed over time, especially with the more recent move in 2013 to initiate treatment in all children under 5 years of age, irrespective of clinical or immune status [11]. During visits, patients were evaluated clinically using WHO clinical staging, age, weight, height, ART status, and laboratory investigations like haemoglobin levels and 6-monthly CD4 cell counts to monitor response to therapy. Adherence to clinical appointments was assessed using appointment schedules, while adherence to medication was assessed by caregivers and self-reports in addition to pill counts. Apart from ART, patients in care received universal Cotrimoxazole prophylaxis for opportunistic infections and secondary prophylaxis for cryptococcal meningitis.

2.4. Study Outcomes. The main study outcomes were (a) retention in care, (b) deaths among patients on ART, and (c) pre-ART deaths (deaths before ART initiation) among patients in the CHBC programme. Death was ascertained through medical records and verbal autopsies carried out by trained community volunteers and counsellors. Retention was defined as the proportion of patients known to be alive (either by patient record review or by telephone calls or home visits) and in care at the end of the follow-up period. We defined loss to follow-up (LTFU) as 90 days or more (if on ART) and 180 days or more (if not on ART) without contact since the last clinic appointment. Attrition included deaths and LTFU. Known transfers to continue ART or care at other facilities were not considered as attrition.

2.5. Statistical Analysis. We analysed factors that determined retention and mortality among children and adolescents enrolled in the two HIV service delivery models described above. We used frequency distributions, medians, and interquartile range (IQR) to describe baseline characteristics and compared these using Chi-square and Wilcoxon Rank-Sum tests, respectively. The baseline characteristics included age groups (at enrolment), gender, CD4 cell counts, CD4 percent, growth responses (weight-for-age and height-for-age z-scores), WHO disease stages, ART status, and age at ART initiation. Because of differences in baseline characteristics in the two study groups, all analyses were adjusted for age at ART initiation, CD4 percent, CD4 cell counts, proportions on ART, nutritional status, and WHO clinical staging using Cox regression. In addition, Cox regression was used to determine factors associated with attrition among patients on ART in both models and among patients in the CHBC separately, in unadjusted and adjusted analyses. Kaplan Meier curves with log rank tests were used to describe and compare retention and survival, stratified by model of care as well as by age groups. Data on CD4 cell count and CD4 percent were log transformed because of skewed distribution. Finally, we used Chi-square test to examine the number and proportions of children dying prior to ART initiation in terms of whether they met or did not meet the 2011 US or 2010 WHO guidelines for initiating ART. All statistical testing was two-sided and conducted at the 5% significance level. Data from both programmes were extracted from databases, merged, and analysed with Intercooled STATA software version 12.

Ethical clearance was approved by the MildMay Institutional Review Board and Ethics Committee, and the study was registered by the Uganda National Council for Science and Technology (UNCST, ref. no. HS 1021). The relevant committees waived informed consent. The study was funded by the University of Padua and supported by Casa Accoglienza alla vita padre Angelo and PENTA Foundation.

3. Results

3.1. Baseline Characteristics. Overall, 1,623 infants, children, and adolescents were included in the analyses, 90.0% (1460/1623) were in the CHBC (Table 1). There were slightly but not significantly more females compared to males. At enrolment, 47.1% in the CHBC and 38.9% in the FBFCA were over 60 months of age ($P = 0.097$). Baseline median CD4 cell counts were 393 cells/mm^3 in the CHBC versus 727 cells/mm^3 in FBFCA ($P < 0.001$) and median CD4 percents were 5.8% in CHBC versus 17.0% in FBFCA ($P < 0.001$). By WHO clinical staging, 86.4% and 96.9% were in stages I-II in the CHBC and FBFCA, respectively, versus 13.6% and 3.1% in stages III-IV in the CHBC and FBFCA, respectively ($P < 0.001$). ART was initiated among 30.2% in the CHBC model compared to 100% in the FBFCA ($P < 0.0001$). Median age at ART initiation was 91.0 months for children in the CHBC versus 45.9 months in the FBFCA

TABLE 1: Baseline characteristics of HIV-infected children and adolescents in a community home-based care model and a facility-based family-centred approach, Kampala, Uganda, 2003–2010.

Characteristics	Community home-based care approach N = 1,460 n (%)	Facility-based family-centred approach N = 163 n (%)	Total N = 1,623 n (%)	P values
Age (months)				
<12	371 (25.4)	54 (33.1)	425 (26.2)	0.097
12–35	228 (15.6)	21 (12.9)	249 (15.3)	
36–59	173 (11.9)	23 (14.1)	196 (12.1)	
60+	688 (47.1)	65 (38.9)	753 (46.4)	
Gender				
Female	746 (51.1)	87 (53.4)	833 (51.3)	0.581
Male	714 (48.9)	77 (46.6)	790 (48.7)	
Cd4 count and percent				
Median CD4 (IQR)	393 (51–762)	727 (442–1348)	438 (78–824)	<0.001
Median CD4% (IQR)	5.8 (0.1–16.9)	17.0 (10.0–25.0)	8.1 (0.2–18.1)	<0.001
Level of immunosuppression by CD4				
Not significant	273 (24.4)	39 (25.0)	312 (24.4)	0.424
Mild	122 (10.8)	21 (13.5)	143 (11.1)	
Advanced	131 (11.6)	12 (7.7)	143 (11.1)	
Severe	605 (53.5)	84 (53.8)	689 (53.5)	
On ART				
Yes	441 (30.2)	163 (100)	604 (37.2)	<0.001
No	1019 (69.8)	0 (0.0)	1019 (62.8)	
Age at ART initiation (months)				
Median (IQR)	91.0 (48.9–135.5)	45.9 (6.5–85.0)	78.6 (34.0–124.6)	<0.001
WHO clinical staging				
I-II	1258 (86.4)	157 (96.9)	1415 (87.5)	<0.001
III-IV	198 (13.6)	5 (3.1)	203 (12.5)	
Growth response weight-for-age				
≤ −2SD	430 (37.4)	24 (16.9)	454 (35.2)	<0.001
> −2SD	719 (62.6)	118 (83.1)	837 (64.8)	
Height-for-age				
≤ −2SD	508 (44.3)	43 (30.3)	551 (42.8)	0.001
> −2SD	639 (55.7)	99 (69.7)	738 (57.2)	

($P < 0.001$). In terms of growth response, 37.4% in the CHBC versus 16.9% in the FBFCA had weight-for-age z-scores of ≤ -2SD ($P < 0.001$), while 55.7% in the CHBC versus 69.7% in the FBFCA had height-for-age z-scores of > -2SD ($P = 0.001$).

3.2. Retention in Care. An overall average of 4.2 years of follow-up was observed (maximum 7.7 years). Retention in care was substantially and significantly higher among children on ART compared to those not on ART within the CHBC model ($P < 0.001$, before and after adjustment). A total of 266 children were lost to follow-up, all were within the CHBC model (18.2%) with only two (0.5%) on ART lost to follow-up. Among children on ART, retention was higher in the CHBC (94.8%, 95% CI: 92.7%–96.8%) compared to (84.7%, 95% CI: 79.1%–90.2%; $P = 0.001$, adjusted $P = 0.006$) in the FBFCA (Figures 1(a) and 1(b)).

3.3. Factors Associated with Attrition among Children and Adolescents on ART in Both Models. In univariate analysis, attrition was significantly associated with model of care (HR: 0.40, 95% CI: 0.23–0.70, $P = 0.002$), mild immunosuppression (HR: 4.17, 95% CI: 1.31–13.31, $P = 0.016$), severe immunosuppression (HR: 3.14, 95% CI: 1.10–8.94, $P = 0.032$), age at ART initiation (HR: 0.74, 95% CI: 0.61–0.90, $P = 0.003$), and weight-for-age z-scores of >-2SD (HR: 0.40, 95% CI: 0.21–0.77, $P = 0.006$).

At multivariate modelling, the risk of attrition was significantly associated with model of care (HR: 0.29, 95% CI: 0.12–0.70, $P = 0.006$) with the CHBC model promoting

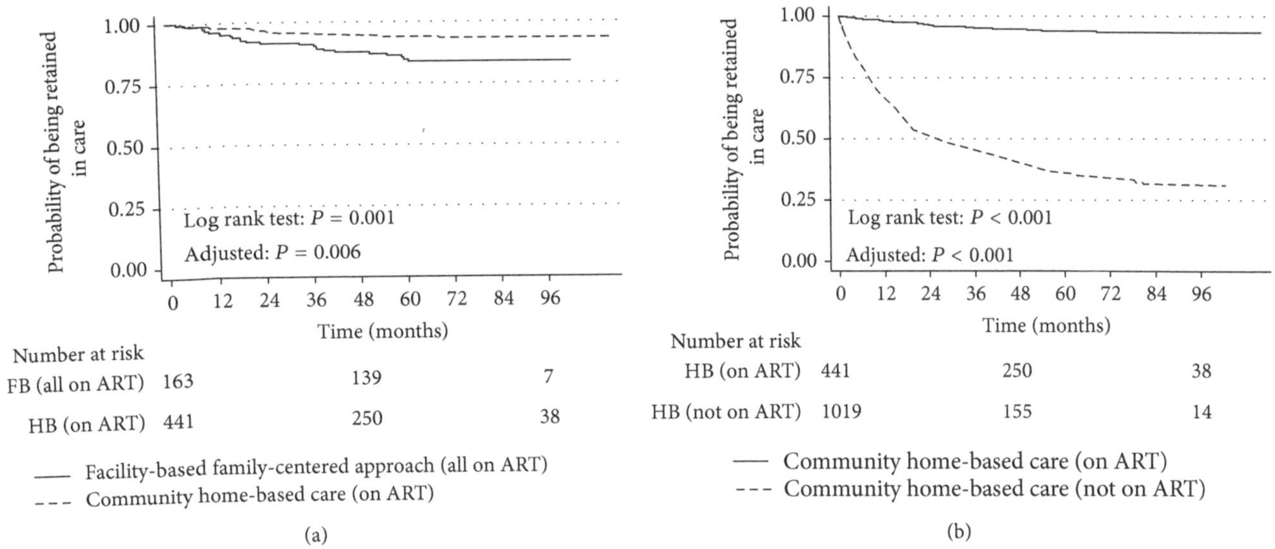

Figure 1: Retention in care, HIV-infected children and adolescents in a facility-based family centred approach (FBFCA) and a community home-based care (CHBC) model, on and not on ART, Kampala, Uganda, 2003–2010. It compares retention among patients on ART in the two models, and it was higher in the CHBC.

retention, mild immunosuppression (HR: 4.66, 95% CI: 1.21–17.98, $P = 0.026$), and weight-for-age z-scores of >–2SD (HR: 0.31, 95% CI: 0.15–0.65, $P = 0.002$, Table 2).

3.4. Factors Associated with Attrition among Children and Adolescents in the CHBC (30% on ART). At univariate analysis, the risk of attrition in the CHBC was significantly associated with age group 36–59 months (HR: 0.46, 95% CI: 0.33–0.64, $P < 0.001$), age group 60+ months (HR: 0.44, 95% CI: 0.35–0.56, $P < 0.001$), CD4 cell count (HR: 0.85, 95% CI: 0.78–0.93, $P < 0.001$), CD4 percent (HR: 0.80, 95% CI: 0.66–0.96, $P = 0.016$), and severe immunosuppression (HR: 1.87, 95% CI: 1.44–2.43, $P < 0.001$). The risk of attrition was also significantly associated with WHO clinical stages III-IV (HR: 1.84, 95% CI: 1.47–2.29, $P < 0.001$), weight-for-age z-scores of > −2SD (HR: 0.76, 95% CI: 0.62–0.93, $P = 0.007$), height-for-age z-scores of > −2SD (HR: 0.69, 95% CI: 0.56–0.84, $P < 0.001$), and receipt of ART (HR: 0.06, 95% CI: 0.04–0.09, $P < 0.001$).

At multivariate analysis, the risk of attrition was significantly associated with CD4 cell count (HR: 0.84, 95% CI: 0.74–0.95, $P = 0.006$), WHO clinical stages III-IV (HR: 1.94, 95% CI: 1.34–2.80, $P < 0.001$), and receipt of ART (HR: 0.04, 95% CI: 0.02–0.08, $P < 0.001$, Table 3).

3.5. Retention Stratified by Age Groups. When retention was stratified by age groups among children and adolescents in the two models, the difference was only significant in the age group 12–35 months ($P = 0.015$) and borderline in age group 36–59 months ($P = 0.060$). This means that age has a confounding effect on retention in care (Figure 2).

3.6. Mortality on ART. There was no significant difference in survival of children and adolescents receiving ART between the two models (Figure 3(a), $P = 0.308$, adjusted $P = 0.489$). However, there was a significant difference between pre-ART deaths (deaths that occurred before ART initiation) and deaths among ART patients in the CHBC (Figure 3(b), log rank test: $P = 0.001$, before and after adjustment). Overall, 34 children died while on ART, 4.8% (21/441) within the CHBC and 8.0% (13/163) within the FBFCA. The estimated time-point mortality for ART patients in the CHBC were 1.9% at 12 months, 5.9% at 60 months, and 5.9% at 96 months. For the FBFCA, estimated time-point mortality at 12, 60, and 96 months were 1.2%, 8.3%, and 9.3%, respectively.

3.7. Survival Stratified by Age Groups. When survival was stratified by age groups in the two models, there was no significant difference, except a borderline effect for age group 36–59 months (log rank test: $P = 0.060$, Figure 4). Thus, there was not enough evidence to suggest that age had a confounding effect on survival.

3.8. Pre-ART Mortality. Sixty deaths were recorded among children in the CHBC who were not on ART (Table 4). Most were known to have met the 2011 US (81.7%) and the 2010 WHO (80.0%) treatment initiation guidelines. All recorded infant deaths (under 12 months) were among those who had met both US and WHO treatment guidelines before they died but had not been initiated on ART related to factors including delayed infant HIV diagnosis, availability of ARVs, and loss to follow-up. In addition, about 20% of deaths occurred in children and adolescents who had not yet met either guideline for initiation.

4. Discussion

We found that by far the most significant factor determining retention in care among infants, children, and adolescents

TABLE 2: Factors associated with *attrition* among HIV-infected children and adolescents *on ART* in a community home-based care model and a facility-based family-centred approach, Kampala, Uganda, (2003–2010) using Cox regression.

Characteristics	Unadjusted (univariate analysis)		Adjusted* (multivariate analysis)	
	HR‡ (95% CI)	*P*	HR‡ (95% CI)	*P*
Model of care				
FBFCA	1	0.002	1	0.006
CHBC	0.40 (0.23–0.70)		0.29 (0.12–0.70)	
Age (months)				
<12	1		1	
12–35	0.73 (0.31–0.70)	0.465	1.95 (0.39–9.89)	0.419
36–59	0.29 (0.09–0.87)	0.028	1.63 (0.18–15.17)	0.664
60+	0.43 (0.22–0.85)	0.015	3.19 (0.27–37.03)	0.354
Gender				
Female	1	0.675		
Male	1.13 (0.64–1.99)			
Cd4 count and percent				
CD4†	0.86 (0.69–1.06)	0.162		
CD4%†	1.00 (0.57–1.77)	0.992		
Level of immunosuppression by CD4				
Not significant	1		1	
Mild	4.17 (1.31–13.31)	0.016	4.66 (1.21–17.98)	0.026
Advanced	0.87 (0.16–4.73)	0.868	0.89 (0.09–9.12)	0.921
Severe	3.14 (1.10–8.94)	0.032	3.16 (0.81–12.39)	0.099
Age at ART initiation				
Months†	0.74 (0.61–0.90)	0.003	0.67 (0.31–1.44)	0.309
WHO clinical staging				
I-II	1	0.309		
III-IV	1.52 (0.68–3.38)			
Growth response				
Weight-for-age				
≤ −2SD	1	0.006	1	0.002
> −2SD	0.40 (0.21–0.77)		0.31 (0.15–0.65)	
Height-for-age				
≤ −2SD	1	0.060		
> −2SD	0.54 (0.28–1.03)			

‡Hazard of attrition; †log transformed due to skewed data;
*only factors significant at univariate or borderline were considered into multivariate.

with HIV was being on ART. Once on ART, there was no difference in survival between the CHBC and FBFCA. In addition to ART initiation directly promoting survival [31–33], we observed a substantial indirect survival effect by ART dramatically enhancing retention (Figure 1(b)). The CHBC model therefore stands to improve child survival greatly if ART is initiated early. Furthermore, patients can benefit from ancillary interventions to promote health and well-being such as food supplements, adherence counselling, and psychosocial support also effective only if retained in the programmes [34–36]. Of note, the CHBC and FBFCA models reach two different populations of HIV-infected children (Table 1). The FBFCA engages the children at or nearer to birth, whereas the CHBC attempts to find them in the communities and thus complementing each other. Operational synergies between the two models could result in a wider reach and greater ART coverage among HIV-infected children and adolescents.

We also observed that the majority of the pre-ART deaths occurred in children and adolescents who had met the 2011 US and the 2010 WHO treatment guidelines but did not initiate therapy for various reasons. This finding illustrates the failure of timely initiation of ART, which in turn may be linked to programmes that are not tailored to meet the needs of the infected child and family. For instance, at the time of this study, there were no PMTCT/EID services within the CHBC. That scenario, coupled with delayed HIV diagnosis, drug stock-outs, logistic challenges, and fragile linkages to ART initiation and psychosocial support services may have

TABLE 3: Factors associated with *attrition* among HIV-infected children and adolescents in the CHBC model, Kampala, Uganda (2003–2010) using Cox regression.

Characteristics	Unadjusted (univariate analysis) HR‡ (95% CI)	P	Adjusted* (multivariate analysis) HR‡ (95% CI)	P
ART				
No	1	<0.001	1	<0.001
Yes	0.06 (0.04–0.09)		0.04 (0.02–0.08)	
Age (months)				
<12	1		1	
12–35	0.85 (0.65–1.10)	0.218	2.18 (0.97–4.92)	0.060
36–59	0.46 (0.33–0.64)	<0.001	1.65 (0.74–3.69)	0.225
60+	0.44 (0.35–0.56)	<0.001	1.38 (0.63–3.01)	0.418
Gender				
Female	1	0.243		
Male	1.11 (0.93–1.33)			
Cd4 count and percent				
CD4†	0.85 (0.78–0.93)	<0.001	0.84 (0.74–0.95)	0.006
CD4%†	0.80 (0.66–0.96)	0.016		
Level of immunosuppression by CD4				
Not significant	1			
Mild	0.99 (0.66–1.49)	0.968		
Advanced	0.89 (0.59–1.34)	0.590		
Severe	1.87 (1.44–2.43)	<0.001		
Age at ART initiation				
Months†	0.85 (0.66–1.10)	0.209		
WHO clinical staging				
I-II	1	<0.001	1.94 (1.34–2.80)	<0.001
III-IV	1.84 (1.47–2.29)			
Growth response weight-for-age				
≤ −2SD	1	0.007		
> −2SD	0.76 (0.62–0.93)			
Height-for-age				
≤ −2SD	1	<0.001	0.81 (0.60–1.09)	0.162
> −2SD	0.69 (0.56–0.84)			

‡Hazard of attrition; †Log transformed due to skewed data;
*only factors significant at univariate or borderline were considered into multivariate.

TABLE 4: Deaths among children and adolescents in community home-based care who were not on ART classified according to whether the US 2011 or WHO 2010 initiation guidelines were met or not, Kampala, Uganda, 2003–2010.

Age group for US (months)	N	US CDC guidelines[1] for ART met	Age group for WHO (months)	N	WHO guidelines[2] for ART met
<12	11	11 (100%)	<12	11	11 (100%)
12–35	13	10 (76.9%)	12–24	9	9 (100%)
36–59	4	3 (75.0%)	24–59	8	5 (62.5%)
60+	32	25 (78.1%)	>60	32	23 (71.9%)
Overall	60	49 (81.7%)	Overall	60	48 (80.0%)

Source: WHO and US treatment guidelines.
[1]US CDC 2011 criteria for ART initiation: <12 months all should be on ART; 12–35 months if CD4 < 1000 or <25%; 36–59 months if CD4 < 750 or <25%; 60+ months if CD4 < 500.
[2]WHO 2010 criteria for ART initiation: <12 months all should be on ART; 12–24 months all should be ART; 24–59 months if CD4 < 750 or <25%; 60+ months if CD4 < 350.

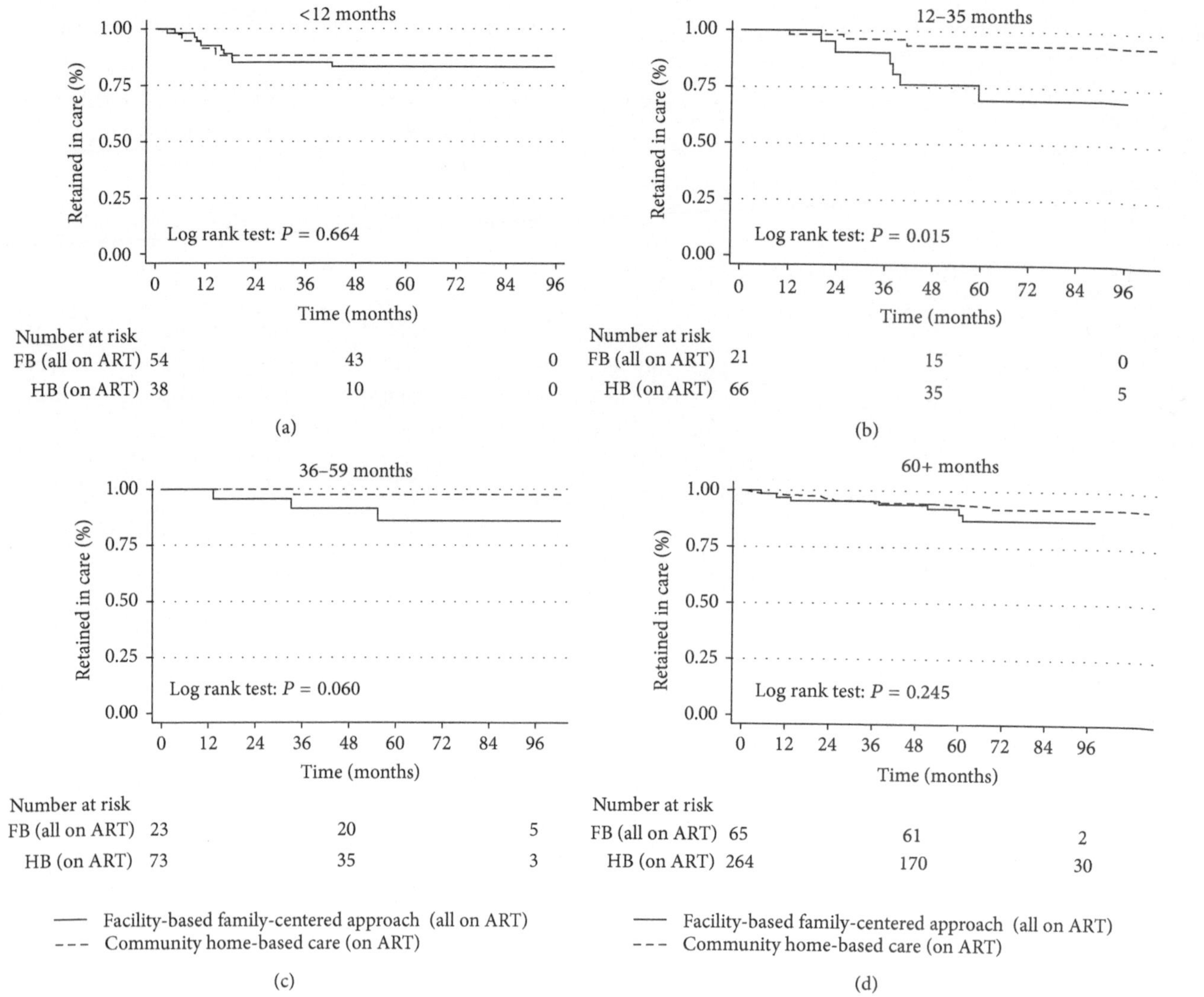

Figure 2: Retention stratified by age group among HIV-infected children and adolescents in a CHBC and a FBFCA in Kampala, Uganda (2003–2010). It stratifies retention by age groups in the two models. Age groups 12–35 months and 36–59 months appear to be confounders for retention.

resulted in considerable LTFU and deaths (Figures 1(b) and 3(b)) between testing and initiating care and treatment [37–40] in the CHBC. There is an urgent need for concerted efforts to ensure timely initiation of ART in children and adolescents in the CHBC. To that effect, simplification of treatment guidelines to universal treatment regardless of disease stage would not only help such efforts but also eliminate missed opportunities to initiate ART, while awaiting eligibility criteria to be met [3].

We also saw that nearly one out of every five deaths occurred in children and adolescents who had not yet met eligibility for initiation according to local guidelines. As shown by the literature, significant clinical events do occur in HIV-infected children and adolescents even before meeting the previous guidelines [19, 20]. Our data therefore support the 2013 WHO consolidated guidelines recommending early ART initiation for children less than five years old regardless of CD4 cell count [41]. However, the new guidelines may not address substantial mortality for children over five. Given the number of deaths we observed in children over five who had not met the guidelines, coupled with substantial LTFU when not on ART, we believe the benefits of early ART outweigh the risk of delayed ART for this older group as well. We therefore endorse extending initiation of ART to all HIV-infected children and adolescents irrespective of their CD4 cell counts as a means to avert child deaths.

Among patients on ART in both models, retention was higher in the CHBC. Factors that may explain this observation include decentralized voluntary counselling and testing and ART refills involving outreach clinics within the communities. In addition, ART patients in the CHBC have a "priority" tracking system within the clinics compared to patients not receiving ART, due to scanty resources [27]. However, the "priority" tracking may not have promoted retention of children not on ART. This disparity calls for an integrated approach towards patients tracking. Although all

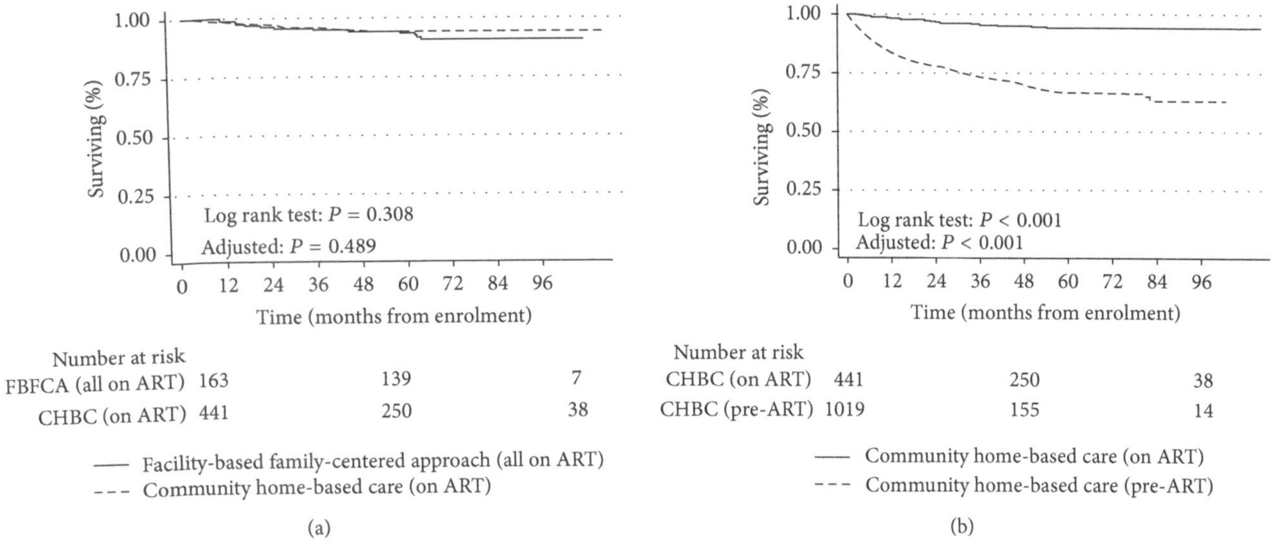

FIGURE 3: Survival on antiretroviral therapy (ART) among HIV-infected children and adolescents in a facility-based family-centred approach (FBFCA) and a community home-based care (CHBC) model, Kampala, Uganda, 2003–2010. (a) compares survival trends among children and adolescents on ART in both models and shows that they were not significantly different. On the other hand, (b) shows that survival trends differed significantly between patients on ART in the CHBC and those not receiving ART (pre-ART).

the children were on ART in the FBFCA and retention was relatively stable, the services were not decentralized. Hence, we believe that geographical access may have been a barrier to retention over time. We also think that socioeconomic factors and education level of caretakers may have contributed to the differences in retention.

We also noted that age was a confounder for retention but not survival (Figures 2 and 4). Indeed, when retention was stratified by age groups, more children in the CHBC than in the FBFCA were retained in the age groups 12–35 months and 36–59 months. Many of the children in the FBFCA in those age groups were "graduates" of the PMTCT programme and were exposed to single dose Nevirapine (sd NVP) for PMTCT and were on NVP-based first line ART regimens. Studies from Uganda and elsewhere have shown that exposure to sd NVP during PMTCT and initiating NVP-based first line ART regimens in HIV-infected children was associated with suboptimal clinical outcomes [42–45] and may partly explain this observation. Additionally, maternal health issues could be contributory factors. On the contrary, the CHBC had no PMTCT programme and most probably had more non-NVP-exposed children for those age groups and thus better outcomes on ART. For the age group 5 years plus, retention was not different between the two models, as they were either far removed from exposure or were never exposed to sd NVP.

Additionally, we found that among patients receiving ART, attrition was significantly associated with model of care, mild immunosuppression, and being more underweight (Table 2), whereas in the CHBC, the risk of attrition was significantly associated with CD4 cell count, WHO clinical stages III-IV, and absence of ART (Table 3). These findings have been described consistently in the literature [10, 13, 27].

In terms of growth responses, we saw that children in the CHBC were significantly more underweight, whereas those in the FBFCA were significantly more stunted with some overlap. Although it is well recognized that HIV infection in children compromises growth responses, in Uganda, 39% and 16% of all children less than 5 years are stunted and underweight, respectively, demonstrating that important non-HIV contributors to stunting and wasting exist in particular high background rates of TB and other coinfections, food insecurity, and malnutrition [46, 47]. Children in the FBFCA were relatively younger, mainly enrolled through PMTCT/EID programmes and were all on ART. Thus, the observed growth responses could be related to complications of perinatal HIV infection, younger age, and background factors. In contrast, children in the CHBC were older and only 30% were on ART. In an earlier study [27], we noted that about 46% of the patients in the CHBC were orphans and the majority were malnourished, older, and less likely to receive ART. We therefore think that these factors could be contributing to the observed growth responses in that cohort.

We note potential limitations to our data and conclusions. First, the data were observational and based on programmatic information. Second, the two programmes should be interpreted in the context of reaching different populations of children and the direct comparisons are cautious. Patients were not randomized for one or the other model, but rather circumstances (such as distance to facilities) dictated what options were available. Third, some aspects of the interventions were shared by both models, such as guidelines for initiating ART and nutritional support and could be potentially confounding. Fourth, the high level of loss to follow-up among patients not on ART in the CHBC leaves

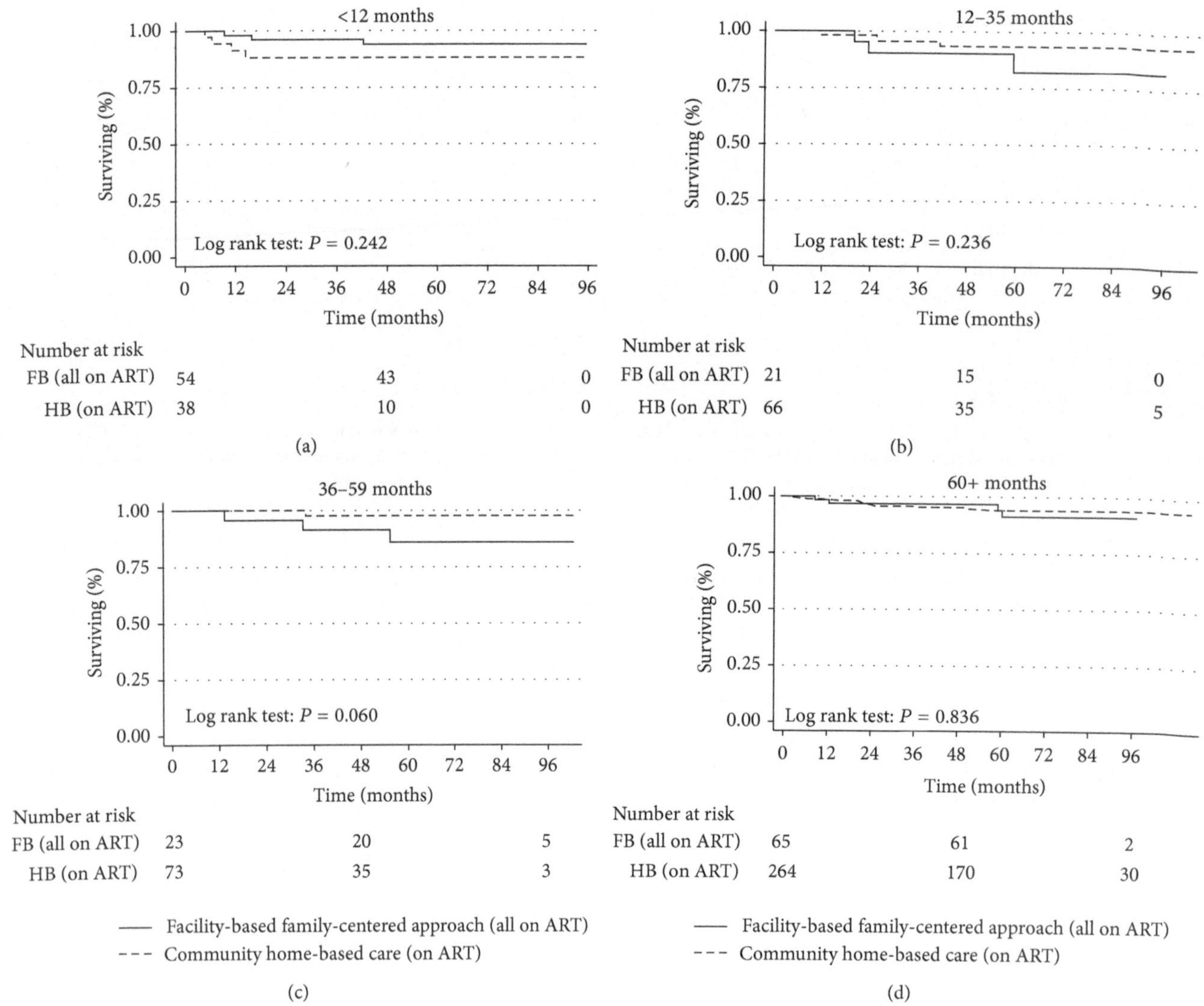

FIGURE 4: Survival stratified by age group among HIV-infected children and adolescents in a CHBC and a FBFCA in Kampala, Uganda (2003–2010). It stratifies survival by age groups in the two models. Apart from a borderline effect for age group 36–59 months ($P = 0.060$), there was not enough evidence to suggest that age had a confounding effect on survival in the two models.

much doubt on the final disposition of the children in that programme. We expect that many of the children lost to care may have died; however, the characteristics of those who died and those who may have accessed care elsewhere are not known [48–50]. Additionally, there were differences in the study population sizes, proportions in age groups, and baseline characteristics, all of which could be potential confounders. Consequently, the analyses were adjusted, including stratification of retention and survival by model of care and age groups, in order to minimize any potentially confounding effects.

We also acknowledge that our findings reflect data from programmes in one urban setting in East Africa and therefore may not be generalizable to family-centred approach and community home-based care models in other settings. Despite the limitations, we firmly believe that our findings remain valid and relevant.

5. Conclusion

We conclude that, irrespective of model of care, children receiving ART had better retention in care and therefore long-term survival. Encouragingly, if children were on ART, then their survival was as good, if not slightly better, in the CHBC compared to the FBFCA. Based on our observations, substantial improvement in child survival can be achieved in either a community-based or a family-care model as long as HIV-infected children are identified early and begun on ART. To ensure this occurs, early identification of HIV-infected children requires strong linkages of pregnant HIV-infected women to PMTCT services and active tracking to ensure all HIV exposed infants receive Polymerase Chain Reaction-based early infant diagnosis. Additionally, rapid early initiation of ART among HIV-infected infants and children is essential. We anticipate the move to early initiation of ART in all HIV-infected children and adolescents in resource-limited settings, irrespective of their CD4 cell counts, will improve survival.

Among ART patients in both models, attrition was significantly associated with model of care, mild immunosuppression, and being underweight. In the CHBC, attrition was significantly associated with CD4 cell count, WHO clinical stages III-IV, and absence of ART.

Conflict of Interests

The authors declare that they have no conflict of interests.

Authors' Contribution

W. Massavon conceived the study and participated in the drafting and editing of the paper, data analysis, and interpretation of the findings. L. Barlow-Mosha, L. Mugenyi, W. McFarland, and G. Gray participated in the data analysis, editing of the paper, and interpretation of findings. R. Lundin, P. Costenaro, M. M. Nannyonga, P. C. Namisi, and D. Wabwire participated in the drafting and editing of the paper. D. Bagenda and M. Mubiru participated in the data analysis. A. Mazza, S. Kironde, and D. Bilardi participated in editing the paper. M. Penazzato, P. Musoke, M. G. Fowler, and C. Giaquinto participated in editing of the paper and interpretation of findings. All authors read and approved the final paper.

Acknowledgments

This paper was developed through a Manuscript Writing Workshop organized by the NIH Office of AIDS Research-funded OCTAVE Project, NIMH-funded UCSF ITAPS Programme (R25MH064712-08), and the Fogarty International Centre AITRP Programme (D43TW00003). The authors are grateful to all the children and families enrolled in both programmes. The authors appreciate the support offered by the management of both institutions. The authors thank Peter Mudiope and Tobias Chirwa for assisting with data analysis. The authors thank the *Provincia Autonoma di Trento and Regione Trentino Alto Adige* for funding NHC since 2006 through *Casa Accoglienza alla Vita Padre Angelo*, and the PENTA Foundation for supporting the interventions.

References

[1] WHO/UNAIDS/UNICEF, "Global HIV/AIDS response: epidemic update and health sector progress towards universal access: progress report 2011," 2011, http://whqlibdoc.who.int/publications/2011/9789241502986_eng.pdf.

[2] UNAIDS, "Getting to zero: 2011–2015 strategy Joint United Nations Programme on HIV/AIDS (UNAIDS)," 2011, http://www.unaids.org/en/media/unaids/contentassets/documents/unaidspublication/2010/JC2034_UNAIDS_Strategy_en.pdf.

[3] UNAIDS, "Global report: UNAIDS report on the global AIDS epidemic 2013," 2013, http://www.unaids.org/en/media/unaids/contentassets/documents/epidemiology/2013/gr2013/UNAIDS_Global_Report_2013_en.pdf.

[4] V. Leroy, K. Malateste, H. Rabie, P. Lumbiganon, and S. Ayaya, "Outcomes of antiretroviral therapy in children in Asia and Africa: a comparative analysis of the IeDEA pediatric multiregional collaboration," *Journal of Acquired Immune Deficiency Syndromes*, vol. 62, pp. 208–219, 2013.

[5] D. K. Ekouevi, A. Azondekon, F. Dicko et al., "12-month mortality and loss-to-program in antiretroviral-treated children: the IeDEA pediatric West African database to evaluate AIDS (pWADA), 2000–2008," *BMC Public Health*, vol. 11, article 519, 2011.

[6] R. Becquet, M. Marston, F. Dabis et al., "Children who acquire hiv infection perinatally are at higher risk of early death than those acquiring infection through breastmilk: a meta-analysis," *PLoS ONE*, vol. 7, no. 2, Article ID e28510, 2012.

[7] G. Y. Asfawesen, J. Solomie, T. Bisirat, G. M. Berhanu, B. Mebratu, and S. Rahlenbeck, "Outcome in a paediatric cohort receiving ART in Addis Abeba, Ethiopia," *Acta Paediatrica*, vol. 100, no. 8, pp. 1164–1167, 2011.

[8] J. Ben-Farhat, M. Gale, E. Szumilin, S. Balkan, and E. Poulet, "Paediatric HIV care in sub-Saharan Africa: clinical presentation and 2-year outcomes stratified by age group," *Tropical Medicine and International Health*, 2013.

[9] C. Bolton-Moore, M. Mubiana-Mbewe, R. A. Cantrell et al., "Clinical outcomes and CD4 cell response in children receiving antiretroviral therapy at primary health care facilities in Zambia," *Journal of the American Medical Association*, vol. 298, no. 16, pp. 1888–1899, 2007.

[10] J. K. Leyenaar, P. M. Novosad, K. T. Ferrer et al., "Early clinical outcomes in children enrolled in human immunodeficiency virus infection care and treatment in lesotho," *Pediatric Infectious Disease Journal*, vol. 29, no. 4, pp. 340–345, 2010.

[11] WHO, "Consolidated guidelines on the use of antiretroviral drugs for treating and preventing HIV infection: recommendations for a public health approach," 2013.

[12] A. D. Harries, S. D. Lawn, H. Getahun, R. Zachariah, and D. V. Havlir, "HIV and tuberculosis—science and implementation to turn the tide and reduce deaths," *Journal of the International AIDS Society*, vol. 15, no. 2, Article ID 17396, 2012.

[13] M. C. Marazzi, S. de Luca, L. Palombi, P. Scarcella, and F. Ciccacci, "Predictors of adverse outcomes in HIV-1 infected children receiving combination antiretroviral treatment: results from a DREAM cohort in Sub-Saharan Africa," *Pediatric Infectious Disease Journal*, vol. 33, no. 3, pp. 295–300, 2014.

[14] G. Tene, M. Lahuerta, C. Teasdale, V. Mugisha, and L. Kayonde, "High retention among HIV-infected children in Rwanda during scale-up and decentralization of HIV care and treatment programs, 2004 to 2010," *Pediatric Infectious Disease Journal*, vol. 32, pp. e341–e347, 2013.

[15] C. Mugglin, G. Wandeler, J. Estill, M. Egger, and N. Bender, "Retention in care of HIV-infected children from HIV test to start of antiretroviral therapy: systematic review," *PLoS ONE*, vol. 8, Article ID e56446, 2013.

[16] J. B. Nachega, E. J. Mills, and M. Schechter, "Antiretroviral therapy adherence and retention in care in middle-income and low-income countries: current status of knowledge and research priorities," *Current Opinion in HIV and AIDS*, vol. 5, no. 1, pp. 70–77, 2010.

[17] U. Okomo, T. Togun, F. Oko, K. Peterson, and A. Jaye, "Mortality and loss to programme before antiretroviral therapy among HIV-infected children eligible for treatment in The Gambia, West Africa," *AIDS Research and Therapy*, vol. 9, article 28, 2012.

[18] M. L. McNairy, M. R. Lamb, R. J. Carter, R. Fayorsey, and G. Tene, "Retention of HIV-infected children on antiretroviral treatment in HIV care and treatment programs in Kenya, Mozambique, Rwanda and Tanzania," *Journal of Acquired Immune Deficiency Syndromes*, vol. 62, no. 3, pp. e70–e81, 2012.

[19] E. D. Charlebois, T. D. Ruel, A. F. Gasasira et al., "Short-term risk of HIV disease progression and death in Ugandan children not eligible for antiretroviral therapy," *Journal of Acquired Immune Deficiency Syndromes*, vol. 55, no. 3, pp. 330–335, 2010.

[20] M. Munyagwa, K. Baisley, J. Levin, M. Brian, and H. Grosskurth, "Mortality of HIV-infected and uninfected children in a longitudinal cohort in rural south-west Uganda during 8 years of follow-up," *Tropical Medicine and International Health*, vol. 17, pp. 836–843, 2012.

[21] Committee on Hospital Care, "Family-centered care and the pediatrician's role," *Pediatrics*, vol. 112, pp. 691–696, 2003.

[22] E. Luyirika, M. S. Towle, J. Achan, J. Muhangi, and C. Senyimba, "Scaling up paediatric HIV care with an integrated, family-centred approach: an observational case study from Uganda," *PLoS ONE*, vol. 8, Article ID e69548, 2013.

[23] WHO, "Community home-based care in resource-limited settings: a framework for action," 2002, http://www.who.int/chp/knowledge/publications/comm_home_based_care/en/index.html.

[24] N. Mohammad and J. Gikonyo, "Operational Challenges Community Home Based Care (CHBC) for PLWHA in Multi-Country Aids Programs (MAP) in Africa," Africa Region Working Paper Series No. 88, 2005, http://www.worldbank.org/afr/wps/wp88.pdf.

[25] WHO, "Antiretroviral therapy for HIV infection in infants and children: towards universal access," Recommendations for a public health approach, 2010, http://www.who.int/hiv/pub/paediatric/infants2010/en/index.html.

[26] "Panel on Antiretroviral Therapy and Medical Management of HIV-Infected Children. Guidelines for the Use of Antiretroviral Agents in Pediatric HIV Infection," 2011, http://aidsinfo.nih.gov/contentfiles/lvguidelines/pediatricguidelines.pdf.

[27] W. Massavon, R. Lundin, P. Costenaro et al., "Attrition and loss to follow-up among children and adolescents in a community home-based care HIV programme in Uganda," *Pediat Therapeut*, vol. 3, article 183, 2013.

[28] WHO, "Scaling Up Antiretroviral Therapy in Resource-Limited Settings: Treatment Guidelines for a Public Health Approach 2003 Revision," 2004, http://www.who.int/hiv/pub/prev_care/en/arvrevision2003en.pdf.

[29] WHO, "Antiretroviral Therapy of HIV Infection In Infants and Children: Towards Universal Access," Recommendations for a public health approach, 2006, http://www.who.int/hiv/pub/guidelines/paediatric020907.pdf.

[30] WHO, "Antiretroviral Therapy for HIV Infection in Adults and Adolescents," Recommendations for a public health approach, 2006, http://www.who.int/hiv/pub/guidelines/artadultguidelines.pdf.

[31] P. Piot and T. C. Quinn, "Response to the AIDS pandemic—a global health model," *New England Journal of Medicine*, vol. 368, pp. 2210–2218, 2013.

[32] A. Saez-Cirion, C. Bacchus, L. Hocqueloux, V. Avettand-Fenoel, and I. Girault, "Post-treatment HIV-1 controllers with a long-term virological remission after the interruption of early initiated antiretroviral therapy ANRS VISCONTI Study," *PLOS Pathogens*, vol. 9, Article ID e1003211, 2013.

[33] B. S. Taylor, T. J. Wilkin, N. Shalev, and S. M. Hammer, "CROI 2013: advances in antiretroviral therapy," *Topics in Antiviral Medicine*, vol. 21, no. 2, pp. 75–89, 2013.

[34] J. van Griensven, L. de Naeyer, J. Uwera, A. Asiimwe, C. Gazille, and T. Reid, "Success with antiretroviral treatment for children in Kigali, Rwanda: experience with health center/nurse-based care," *BMC Pediatrics*, vol. 8, article 39, 2008.

[35] T. H. Boyles, L. S. Wilkinson, R. Leisegang, and G. Maartens, "Factors influencing retention in care after starting antiretroviral therapy in a rural South African programme," *PLoS ONE*, vol. 6, no. 5, Article ID e19201, 2011.

[36] M. R. Lamb, W. M. El-Sadr, E. Geng, and D. Nash, "Association of adherence support and outreach services with total attrition, loss to follow-up, and death among ART patients in sub-Saharan Africa," *PLoS ONE*, vol. 7, Article ID e38443, 2012.

[37] A. D. Harries, R. Zachariah, S. D. Lawn, and S. Rosen, "Strategies to improve patient retention on antiretroviral therapy in sub-Saharan Africa," *Tropical Medicine and International Health*, vol. 15, no. 1, pp. 70–75, 2010.

[38] S. Rosen and M. P. Fox, "Retention in HIV care between testing and treatment in sub-Saharan Africa: a systematic review," *PLoS Medicine*, vol. 8, no. 7, Article ID e1001056, 2011.

[39] R. Pati, M. Lahuerta, B. Elul et al., "Factors associated with loss to clinic among HIV patients not yet known to be eligible for antiretroviral therapy (ART) in Mozambique," *Journal of the International AIDS Society*, vol. 16, Article ID 18490, 2013.

[40] M. Penazzato, S. Crowley, L. Mofenson et al., "Programmatic impact of the evolution of WHO pediatric antiretroviral treatment guidelines for resource-limited countries (Tukula Fenna Project, Uganda)," *Journal of Acquired Immune Deficiency Syndromes*, vol. 61, pp. 522–525, 2012.

[41] G. Hirnschall, A. D. Harries, P. J. Easterbrook, M. C. Doherty, and A. Ball, "The next generation of the World Health Organization's global antiretroviral guidance," *Journal of the International AIDS Society*, vol. 16, Article ID 18757, 2013.

[42] M. Penazzato, A. Prendergast, J. Tierney, M. Cotton, and D. Gibb, "Effectiveness of antiretroviral therapy in HIV-infected children under 2 years of age," *Cochrane Database of Systematic Reviews*, vol. 7, Article ID CD004772, 2012.

[43] J. Kay, H. Wanzira, and T. Sandison, "Virologic suppression in nevirapine-exposed HIV-infected infants initiating antiretroviral therapy in rural Uganda," *Journal of Tropical Pediatrics*, vol. 58, pp. 194–199.

[44] V. Musiime, F. Ssali, J. Kayiwa et al., "Response to nonnucleoside reverse transcriptase inhibitor-based therapy in HIV-infected children with perinatal exposure to single-dose nevirapine," *AIDS Research and Human Retroviruses*, vol. 25, no. 10, pp. 989–996, 2009.

[45] P. Palumbo, J. C. Lindsey, M. D. Hughes et al., "Antiretroviral treatment for children with peripartum nevirapine exposure," *New England Journal of Medicine*, vol. 363, no. 16, pp. 1510–1520, 2010.

[46] P. M. Musoke, P. Mudiope, L. N. Barlow-Mosha et al., "Growth, immune and viral responses in HIV infected African children receiving highly active antiretroviral therapy: a prospective cohort study," *BMC Pediatrics*, vol. 10, article 56, 2010.

[47] A. Kekitiinwa, K. J. Lee, A. S. Walker et al., "Differences in factors associated with initial growth, CD4, and viral load responses to ART in HIV-infected children in Kampala, Uganda, and the United Kingdom/Ireland," *Journal of Acquired Immune Deficiency Syndromes*, vol. 49, no. 4, pp. 384–392, 2008.

[48] J. K. L. Yu, S. C. C. Chen, K. Y. Wang et al., "True outcomes for patients on antiretroviral therapy who are "lost to follow-up" in Malawi," *Bulletin of the World Health Organization*, vol. 85, no. 7, pp. 550–554, 2007.

[49] M. W. G. Brinkhof, M. Pujades-Rodriguez, and M. Egger, "Mortality of patients lost to follow-up in antiretroviral treatment programmes in resource-limited settings: Systematic review and meta-analysis," *PLoS ONE*, vol. 4, no. 6, Article ID e5790, 2009.

[50] WHO, "Retention in HIV programmes: defining the challenges and identifying solutions: meeting report," Geneva, Switzerland, 2012, http://www.who.int/hiv/pub/meetingreports/programmes/en/.

Missed Doses and Missed Appointments: Adherence to ART among Adult Patients in Uganda

C. Shumba, L. Atuhaire, R. Imakit, R. Atukunda, and P. Memiah

Uganda Program, Institute of Human Virology, University of Maryland, 124 Luthuli Avenue, Bugolobi, Kampala, Uganda

Correspondence should be addressed to C. Shumba; konstansezw@googlemail.com

Academic Editors: F. Krebs and H. C. Mwandumba

Background. Missed doses and appointments are predictors of incomplete adherence among patients on ART. The AIDSRelief model emphasizes treatment preparation and continuous treatment support for ART patients including community followup. *Methods.* In August 2008, a survey was conducted among patients on antiretroviral therapy (ART) (interquartile range for duration of ART = 29–46 months, median = 33 months, $n = 763$, age >16 years), in 15 health facilities in Uganda. Missed doses and appointments among adult patients on ART and the factors most associated with these were identified. Reasons for missed doses were also explored. *Results.* The survey revealed that 97% of the patients had not missed their doses in the last week while 93% had not missed their appointments in the last three months. For those who had missed their doses, the most common reasons were travel (48%) and forgetfulness (28%). There was a significant association between missing doses and missing appointments ($P = 0.0004$) and between alcohol use and missed doses ($P < 0.005$). *Conclusions.* The level of adherence to medication and clinic appointments for patients on ART in the study population was very high. It is important to strengthen adherence strategies at both facility and community levels to assist patients that are likely to miss their doses or appointments.

1. Background

Uganda has more than 1.2 million people living with HIV infection and in 2010 more than 120,000 got infected with HIV [1]. Although there are various efforts to scale up AIDS treatment, many HIV-infected people are unable to access treatment and the increasing new HIV infections still exceed the government's capacity to provide treatment [2]. While attempts are being made to reduce new infections and to scale up antiretroviral therapy (ART), it is equally important to improve adherence to regimens among the few who are already accessing ART for successful treatment [3]. ART delays progression to AIDS and death, hence, improved the quality of life for people living with HIV [4, 5]. Maintaining good adherence has been found to be difficult to achieve and sustained by both patients and health care providers [6, 7]. A major concern with the use of ART is the emergence of viral resistance, which is mainly due to insufficient compliance [8].

Different tools have been used to determine ART adherence rates and on average the rate of adherence to ART is about 70% [9]. A meta-analysis found adherence rates for African patients to be approximately 77% [10]. A study by Oyugi et al., that assessed correspondence between multiple measures of adherence and viral load suppression, found that the mean adherence was 91–94% by all measures [11]. Patients' adherence is dynamic either improving or declining over time. A prospective study conducted in southwest Ethiopia showed that adherence had declined by 3% by the third month of follow-up visit compared to the results of the baseline study at month zero [6]. ART is a long-term treatment, and sustaining acceptable level of drug adherence poses a challenge for both the patient and health care workers [12]. Therefore, the benefits of ART can only be achieved if health providers realize that adherence is a dynamic process, complex, and cannot be predicted by only patient characteristics, but continuous monitoring and integration into regular clinic followup [6, 12]. Different studies have revealed predictors of adherence success. These are a combination of patient demographic and behavioral factors and disease characteristics, medication factors and health systems factors [6, 13–15].

The aim of this study is to describe the factors associated with incomplete adherence among adult patients on ART in 15 health facilities in Uganda.

2. Study Setting and Methods

The study was conducted in 15 faith-based and stand-alone HIV clinics that provide high-quality HIV care and treatment to rural and underserved communities in the northern, southern, central, eastern, and western regions of Uganda. The study setting is described in detail in another paper [16].

2.1. Data Collection. Data was collected using the AIDSRelief Adherence Survey that has been piloted, validated, and used in six African countries. The survey was designed to identify specific indicators that influence the adherence to antiretroviral therapy and the increase in quality of life. The study assessed missed clinic appointments, missed doses, and whether patients had ever run out of medication as the measures of adherence. A sample of 763 patient adherence surveys were done to assess disease, treatment knowledge and services received between August 2008 and March 2009. In August 2008, we conducted a survey of patients having been on ART (interquartile range for duration of ART = 29–46 months, median=33 months, n = 763, >16 years), in 15 facilities in Uganda.

This survey was done as a part of a routine quality improvement program. The adherence survey questionnaire was administered by trained health staff. Informed consent forms were provided to the patients after full explanation from the health staff about the survey. The patients appended their signature indicating consent to participate in the survey. Each patient had the right to withdraw at anytime in the course of the survey.

2.2. Data Analysis. Data were entered, cleaned, and coded in to a computer and analyzed using Stata version 11. Bivariate analysis was carried out to determine the statistical significant association between explanatory variables and the outcome variable. Chi-square tests and their P values at the level of significance of 5%, as well as confidence intervals (CI), were used to define statistical associations between explanatory variables and outcomes.

3. Results

Out of the 763 patients who participated in this study, 50.5% were in the age group of 16–39 years. About 70% of the total study participants were females. Most (66.6%) of the patients were engaged in an income generating activity before starting on ART. Over half (54%) of the patients owned a home, and 31.6% were renting at the time of the survey. Many of the patients (42.1%) had primary education and 38.4% had secondary education, while only 7.7% had attained university education. The 763 patients who participated in this study varied in age, gender, socioeconomic status, and education (Table 1).

Table 1: Demographic characteristics of the study population.

Demographic characteristics	Frequency (percentage)
Age	
16–39	384 (50.53)
40–50	281 (36.97)
>50	95 (12.50)
Gender	
Female	528 (69.5%)
Male	232 (30.5%)
Socioeconomic status	
Engaged in any income generating activity before starting ART	
No	258 (33.4)
Yes	514 (66.6)
Living situation	
Own home	417 (54.02)
Rent	244 (31.60)
Living with friends	1 (0.13)
Living with relatives	71 (9.20)
Others	39 (5.05)
Education status	
Primary	295 (42.1)
Secondary	269 (38.4)
University	54 (7.7)
Below primary school	83 (11.8)

The survey revealed that 97% of the patients had not missed their doses in the last week and 93% of patients had not missed appointments in the past three months. There was no significant association between the measures of adherence in this study (missed doses, missed appointments, and ever run out of medication) and the sociodemographic factors namely age, gender, and education level (Table 2).

Out of the patients who reported ever missing their doses for the period on ART, the most common reasons were travelled, forgot, work conflict, and felt unwell (Table 3).

This study found that patients on ART that missed their appointments (29.2%) were more likely to miss their doses compared to those that did not (5.7%). The findings are depicted in Table 4: P value = 0.0004, OR = 6.80, 95% CI (2.41–18.66).

Patients on ART who used alcohol were more likely to miss a dose during the course of their treatment compared to those who did not use alcohol (Table 5: P value < 0.005 with CI 2.40–27.83).

TABLE 2: Factors linked to the three measures of adherence in this study.

Adherence measure	Independent variables	No Freq. (%)	Yes Freq. (%)	OR (95% CI limits)	P value
(1) Ever run out of medication(N = 444)		418 (94.1)	26 (5.9)		
	Gender (N = 439)				
	Male	122 (92.4)	10 (7.6)	0.58 (0.24–1.46)	0.296
	Female	239 (95.4)	14 (4.6)		
	Age (N = 43)				
	16–39	205 (96.61)	14 (6.39)		0.656
	40–50	157 (95.15)	8 (4.85)		
	>50	53 (96.36)	2 (3.64)		
	Educational level (N = 419)				
	Below primary	56 (94.92)	3 (5.08)		0.629
	Primary	167 (95.98)	7 (4.02)		
	Secondary	145 (94.16)	9 (5.84)		
	University	29 (90.63)	3 (9.38)		
(2) Doses missed in the last week (N = 763)		739 (96.9)	24 (3.1)		
	Gender (N = 760)				
	Male	222 (95.7)	10 (4.3)	0.60 (0.25–1.49)	0.228
	Female	514 (97.3)	14 (2.7)		
	Age (N = 760)				
	16–39	370 (96.4)	14 (3.6)		0.694
	40–50	273 (97.2)	8 (2.8)		
	>50	93 (97.9)	2 (2.1)		
	Disclosed HIV status to sexual partner (N = 714)				
	No	426 (96.4)	16 (3.6)	0.60 (0.21–1.66)	0.402
	Yes	266 (97.8)	6 (2.2)		
	Educational level (N = 419)				
	Below primary	55 (93.22)	4 (6.78)		0.450
	Primary	170 (97.70)	4 (2.30)		
	Secondary	148 (96.10)	6 (3.90)		
	University	31 (96.88)	1 (3.13)		
(3) Appointments missed in the past 3 months (N = 763)		706 (92.5)	57 (7.5)		
	Gender (N = 760)				
	Male	217 (93.5)	15 (6.5)	1.00 (0.51–1.96)	0.989
	Female	494 (93.6)	34 (6.4)		
	Disclosed HIV status to sexual partner (N = 717)				
	No	415 (93.0)	31 (7.0)	0.95 (0.50–1.80)	0.995
	Yes	253 (93.4)	18 (6.6)		
	Age (N = 760)				
	16–39	363 (94.5)	21 (5.5)		0.540
	40–50	260 (92.5)	21 (7.5)		
	>50	88 (92.6)	7 (7.4)		

TABLE 2: Continued.

Adherence measure	Independent variables	No Freq. (%)	Yes Freq. (%)	OR (95% CI limits)	P value
	Educational level ($N = 419$)				
	Below Primary school	56 (94.92)	3 (5.08)		0.079
	Primary	163 (93.68)	11 (6.32)		
	Secondary	143 (92.86)	11 (7.14)		
	University	26 (81.25)	6 (18.75)		

*The differences in N are due to nonresponse.

TABLE 3: Reasons for missed doses.

Reasons for missing doses	No Freq. (%)	Yes Freq. (%)
Travelled ($N = 58$)	30 (50.8)	29 (49.2)
Forgot ($N = 60$)	43 (71.7)	17 (28.3)
Work conflict ($N = 59$)	57 (96.6)	2 (3.4)
Felt unwell (59)	57 (96.6)	2 (3.4)
Side effects (59)	58 (98.3)	1 (1.7)
Tired of taking medication (59)	58 (98.3)	1 (1.7)

TABLE 4: Relationship between missed appointments and missed doses.

Missed appointment	Missed doses		Total
	No	Yes	
No	694 (94.3)	42 (5.7)	736
Yes	17 (70.8)	7 (29.2)	24

4. Discussion

This study found that patients on ART that missed their appointments were more likely to miss their doses compared to those that did not. While we explored the reasons for missed doses, we did not do the same for missed appointments, therefore, it is difficult to understand the reasons for missed appointments. However, what was clear is that missing a scheduled appointment is associated with missing ART doses. Other authors reported other common reasons responsible for nonadherence that are related to income and they include failure to get transport to reach ART clinics hence missing pharmacy refills, missed clinic appointments and missed doses [10, 17]. However, another study found that patients in developing countries can achieve good adherence despite limited resources [6]. A study by Byakika-Tusiime et al. [18] showed that in ART centers, where patients were required to pay user fees, their adherence levels were low while Orrell et al.found that low socioeconomic status was not a predictor of adherence for patients with fully subsidized therapy [19]. This clearly applies to this study context where all the patients despite their low income have good access to fully subsidized therapy and exhibited high adherence comparable to high income settings. Notwithstanding, it is important to consider the fact that some patients may lack the means to access the fully subsidized therapy due to poverty. In this way, poverty acts as an intervening variable in hindering access to the much needed lifesaving therapy. Regardless, there would be need to further understand the experiences of the patients who miss appointments in order to tailor interventions that best suit them.

Our study was unique as it looked at patients who had been on treatment for a considerable amount of time. The study by Oyugi et al. followed up patients from baseline to 12 weeks [11] while in our study patient duration of ART was more than 2 years at least. Most studies have not considered patient adherence beyond 2 years after ART initiation [4, 12, 15].

Our study is also the first of its kind that has explored the risk factors associated with incomplete adherence among elderly HIV patients. We found that there was no difference in adherence between the elderly who made up 12.5% of the study population and other age groups. However, this could be due to the small number of patients with nonadherence events to allow for risk factor analysis across all age groups including the elderly.

In our study, gender and disclosure were not associated with adherence. In contrast, another study found that women were more likely than men to forget to refill medications and not to know how to take the medications correctly [20]. A few studies have reported age as an influencing factor to adherence especially in infancy and adolescents [7, 18]. Generally however, it has been reported that sociodemographic factors seem not to predict adherence [6], although there are a few factors which have been reported to hinder adherence such as low income which has been cited as a strong predictor of failure to adhere to ART [4, 7, 10].

In general, patient self-reported adherence in this survey was very high (97%). Although self-reported outcomes of adherence may have a weakness of reliability, a study by Oyugi et al. found no significant difference between patient-reported and objective measures of adherence [11]. Our findings are higher than the average adherence rates for African patients [10] but consistent with those in a prospective observational cohort study conducted in Dakar, Senegal, where adherence was estimated to be over 91% and similar to the study by Oyugi et al. [11]. Our findings are consistent

Table 5: Relationship between alcohol use and adherence.

	Adherence measure	Yes Freq.	No Freq.	OR 95% CI limits	P value
Alcohol use	Missing doses (N = 417)				
	Yes	9	6	OR = 7.92	**<0.01**
	No	64	338	CI (2.40–27.83)	
	Missing appointment (N = 417)				
	Yes	8	23	OR = 1.72	0.206
	No	65	321	CI (0.63–4.19)	
	Ever run out off medication (N = 417)				
	Yes	6	16	OR = 1.84	0.215
	No	67	328	CI (0.57–5.16)	

with follow-up cohorts that were done in developed countries such as the APROCO cohort study and the Ciel Bleu trial [4]. The high levels of adherence in this patient-population can be attributed to the model of HIV care and treatment that is used. The model emphasizes adherence as a therapeutic intervention with intensive treatment preparation, patient specific care and treatment plan, community-based treatment services with home-based followup during ART startup. Disclosure is highly encouraged and all clinics have well-defined catchment area as well as longitudinal medical records for all patients.

This study found an association between alcohol use and missed doses. This is similar to other studies where alcohol consumption has also been reported to affect adherence [21–23]. Alcohol use is known to be a proxy for loss of control, thus, affecting adherence. In a study done in Botswana, around 40% of the patients surveyed admitted missing a dose because of alcohol consumption [24]. Related studies also show that alcohol is greatly related to the reduced adherence [25, 26]. A systematic review conducted in 2009 revealed that HIV/AIDS patients that used alcohol were 50–60% not likely to adhere to their medications [27].

There was some association between the educational status and missed appointments in the last three months in this study ($P < 0.1$) although the population educational levels were generally very low. A systematic review conducted in 2006, revealed that education and literacy levels are important predictors of adherence [28]. This paper found out that patient understanding of their medication regimen and their knowledge of the relationship between nonadherence and buildup of resistance to medication also predict better adherence. A patient's belief and self-determination to therapy influence adherence to medication. It is not clear however, what the optimal educational level would be to get better adherence but perhaps what is more important is the patient understanding of adherence on the disease mechanism.

While many studies have shown that disclosure is associated with adherence [7, 28, 29], we did not find this association. The rate of disclosure to a friend or a relative in our patient pool for this study was quite high (99%) since patients are encouraged to disclose their HIV status to a treatment buddy before starting ART in order to improve the social support [16]. It is very important for health workers to find out the patients' disclosure before administering ART, while continuing to support those who would not have disclosed [28].

Different studies have also revealed that when patients experience side effects of prescribed medication, they tend to stop treatment or take it irregularly [6, 18]. In this study, only one patient out of those who missed their doses reported missing medication due to side effects and another due to pill fatigue. Similarly, patients have reported taking drug holidays as a result of pill fatigue [28]. Additionally, pill burden has been found to contribute to poor adherence [4, 7, 28]. However, pill burden was not mentioned as a problem for the patients in our study.

A number of studies have reported on irregular drug supply as an important predictor of adherence to ART [28, 30]. As far as the researchers know, drug stockouts in this study's patient population have never occurred but it is definitely appreciated that erratic drug supply can interrupt patient adherence. Some researchers have even argued that health care-related challenges could be the most important barriers to ART adherence in resource-limited settings [31]. Patient-provider relationships, the time spent at health facility, and opening hours can influence adherence to ART [17, 31]. Future research will need to study how these factors may be viewed as affecting adherence in this setting.

5. Conclusion

While the level of good patient adherence to ART in this study was generally high, it is important to continue to reinforce the importance of adherence. High adherence rates can be achieved if HIV clinics and providers reduce the number of missed appointments as this study has shown that this is an important predictor of adherence. The model of treatment and care used in this population group is worth emulating. The reasons for missed appointments need to be explored to target interventions appropriately. Most patients reported that travelling and forgetfulness were important predictors of missed doses in this study. Thus, creativity in collaboration with the patients is required to design strategies to reduce this. Additionally, treatment and care providers need to strengthen patient education and counseling on the negative impact of alcohol use on adherence.

Conflict of Interests

The authors declare that they have no conflict of interests.

Authors' Contribution

C. Shumba participated in the coordination of the study and drafted the paper. L. Atuhaire participated in the coordination of the study and drafting of the paper. R. Atukunda participated in the coordination of the study and drafting of the paper. P. Memiah conceived of the study and designed the study and helped to draft the paper. R. Imakit performed statistical analysis. All authors read and approved the final paper.

References

[1] WHO, UNAIDS, and UNICEF. Global HIV/AIDS Response—Epidemic Update and Health Sector Progress Towards Universal Access—Progress Report, 2011.

[2] MOH, Uganda UNGASS Progress Report, January 2008-December 2009, Uganda, 2010.

[3] J. Knodel, J. Kespichayawattana, C. Saengtienchai, and S. Wiwatwanich, "The role of parents and family members in ART treatment adherence: evidence from Thailand," *Research on Aging*, vol. 32, no. 1, pp. 19–39, 2010.

[4] I. Lanièce, M. Ciss, A. Desclaux et al., "Adherence to HAART and its principal determinants in a cohort of Senegalese adults," *AIDS*, vol. 17, supplement 3, pp. S103–S108, 2003.

[5] A. M. Abaasa, J. Todd, K. Ekoru et al., "Good adherence to HAART and improved survival in a community HIV/AIDS treatment and care programme: the experience of the AIDS Support Organization (TASO), Kampala, Uganda," *BMC Health Services Research*, vol. 8, article 241, 2008.

[6] A. Amberbir, K. Woldemichael, S. Getachew, B. Girma, and K. Deribe, "Predictors of adherence to antiretroviral therapy among HIV-infected persons: a prospective study in Southwest Ethiopia," *BMC Public Health*, vol. 8, article 265, 2008.

[7] A. R. Ayalu and B. Sibhatu, Determinants of Adherence to Antiretroviral Therapy among HIV Infected Patients in Africa, 2011.

[8] A. N. Soe, S. Tansuphasawadikul, B. Phonrat et al., "Early viral suppression predicting long-term treatment success among HIV patients commencing NNRTI-based antiretroviral therapy," *Journal of Antivirals and Antiretrovirals*, vol. 2, no. 2, pp. 33–37, 2010.

[9] S. Low-Beer, B. Yip, M. V. O'Shaughnessy, R. S. Hogg, and J. S. G. Montaner, "Adherence to triple therapy and viral load response," *Journal of Acquired Immune Deficiency Syndromes*, vol. 23, no. 4, pp. 360-361, 2000.

[10] E. J. Mills, J. B. Nachega, I. Buchan et al., "Adherence to antiretroviral therapy in sub-Saharan Africa and North America: a meta-analysis," *JAMA*, vol. 296, no. 6, pp. 679–690, 2006.

[11] J. H. Oyugi, J. Byakika-Tusiime, E. D. Charlebois et al., "Multiple validated measures of adherence indicate high levels of adherence to generic HIV antiretroviral therapy in a resource-limited setting," *Journal of Acquired Immune Deficiency Syndromes*, vol. 36, no. 5, pp. 1100–1102, 2004.

[12] O. W. Fong, C. F. Ho, L. Y. Fung et al., "Determinants of adherence to highly active antiretroviral therapy (HAART) in Chinese HIV/AIDS patients," *HIV Medicine*, vol. 4, no. 2, pp. 133–138, 2003.

[13] G. S. Reiter, L. Wojtusik, R. Hewitt et al., "Elements of success in HIV clinical care," *Topics in HIV Medicine*, vol. 8, article 67, 2000.

[14] J. R. Ickovics and C. S. Meade, "Adherence to HAART among patients with HIV: breakthroughs and barriers," *AIDS Care*, vol. 14, no. 3, pp. 309–318, 2002.

[15] M. Etienne, M. Hossain, R. Redfield, K. Stafford, and A. Amoroso, "Indicators of adherence to antiretroviral therapy treatment among HIV/AIDS patients in 5 African countries," *Journal of the International Association of Physicians in AIDS Care*, vol. 9, no. 2, pp. 98–103, 2010.

[16] C. Shumba, "Behavioral characteristics of adult patients on ART in Uganda," *Global Journal of Medicine and Public Health*, vol. 1, no. 1, 2012.

[17] T. L. Freeman, K. E. Steward, R. DeMasi, and M. S. Saag, "Adherence in the age of highly active anti-retroviral therapy (ART): racial and gender differences," in *National HIV Prevention Conference*, Atlanta, Ga, USA, August 1999.

[18] J. Byakika-Tusiime, J. H. Oyugi, W. A. Tumwikirize, E. T. Katabira, P. N. Mugyenyi, and D. R. Bangsberg, "Adherence to HIV antiretroviral therapy in HIV+ Ugandan patients purchasing therapy," *International Journal of STD and AIDS*, vol. 16, no. 1, pp. 38–41, 2005.

[19] C. Orrell, D. R. Bangsberg, M. Badri, and R. Wood, "Adherence is not a barrier to successful antiretroviral therapy in South Africa," *AIDS*, vol. 17, no. 9, pp. 1369–1375, 2003.

[20] D. A. Murphy, M. Sarr, S. J. Durako, A. B. Moscicki, C. M. Wilson, and L. R. Muenz, "Barriers to HAART adherence among human immunodeficiency virus—infected adolescents," *Archives of Pediatrics and Adolescent Medicine*, vol. 157, no. 3, pp. 249–255, 2003.

[21] S. D. Weiser, K. Leiter, M. Heisler et al., "A population-based study on alcohol and high-risk sexual behaviors in Botswana," *PLoS Medicine*, vol. 3, no. 10, article e392, 2006.

[22] G. Chander, B. Lau, and R. D. Moore, "Hazardous alcohol use: a risk factor for non-adherence and lack of suppression in HIV infection," *Journal of Acquired Immune Deficiency Syndromes*, vol. 43, no. 4, pp. 411–417, 2006.

[23] M. J. Stirratt, R. H. Remien, A. Smith, O. Q. Copeland, C. Dolezal, and D. Krieger, "The role of HIV serostatus disclosure in antiretroviral medication adherence," *AIDS and Behavior*, vol. 10, no. 5, pp. 483–493, 2006.

[24] E. Kip, V. J. Ehlers, and D. M. Van Der Wal, "Patients adherence to anti-retroviral therapy in Botswana," *Journal of Nursing Scholarship*, vol. 41, no. 2, pp. 149–157, 2009.

[25] C. J. Gill, D. H. Hamer, J. L. Simon, D. M. Thea, and L. L. Sabin, "No room for complacency about adherence to antiretroviral therapy," *AIDS Behavior*, vol. 14, pp. 778–784, 2005.

[26] C. S. Hendershot, S. A. Stoner, D. W. Pantalone, and J. M. Simoni, "Alcohol use and antiretroviral adherence: review and meta-analysis," *Journal of Acquired Immune Deficiency Syndromes*, vol. 52, no. 2, pp. 180–202, 2009.

[27] E. J. Mills, J. B. Nachega, D. R. Bangsberg et al., "Adherence to ART: A systematic review of developed and developing nation patient reported barriers and facilitators," no. 11, article 438, 2006.

[28] L. Li, S. J. Lee, Y. Wen, C. Lin, D. Wan, and C. Jiraphongsa, "Antiretroviral therapy adherence among patients living with HIV/AIDS in Thailand," *Nursing and Health Sciences*, vol. 12, no. 2, pp. 212–220, 2010.

[29] S. Weiser, W. Wolfe, D. Bangsberg et al., "Barriers to antiretroviral adherence for patients living with HIV infection and AIDS in Botswana," *Journal of Acquired Immune Deficiency Syndromes*, vol. 34, no. 3, pp. 281–288, 2003.

[30] J. B. Nachega, E. J. Mills, and M. Schechter, "Antiretroviral therapy adherence and retention in care in middle-income and low-income countries: current status of knowledge and research priorities," *Current Opinion in HIV and AIDS*, vol. 5, no. 1, pp. 70–77, 2010.

[31] S. Biadgilign, A. A. Reda, A. Deribew et al., "Knowledge and attitudes of caregivers of HIV-infected children toward antiretroviral treatment in Ethiopia," *Patient Education and Counseling*, vol. 85, no. 2, pp. e89–e94, 2011.

Determinants of Mortality among HIV Positives after Initiating Antiretroviral Therapy in Western Ethiopia: A Hospital-Based Retrospective Cohort Study

Mitiku Teshome Hambisa,[1] Ahmed Ali,[2] and Yadeta Dessie[1]

[1] *Department of Public Health, College of Health and Medical Sciences, Haramaya University, P.O. Box 235, Harar, Ethiopia*
[2] *Department of Epidemiology and Biostatistics, School of Public Health, Addis Ababa University, P.O. Box 25819/1000, Addis Ababa, Ethiopia*

Correspondence should be addressed to Mitiku Teshome Hambisa; mitikkuuf@gmail.com

Academic Editors: V. C. Bond and V. Venketaraman

Studies revealed that there are various determinants of mortality among HIV positives after ART initiation. These determinants are so variable with context and dynamic across time with the advancement of cares and treatments. In this study we tried to identify determinants of mortality among HIV positives after initiating ART. A retrospective cohort study was conducted among 416 ART attendees enrolled between July 2005 to January 2012 in Nekemte Referral Hospital, Western Ethiopia. Actuarial table was used to estimate survival of patients after ART initiation and log rank test was used to compare the survival curves. Cox proportional-hazard regression was applied to determine the independent determinants of time to death. The estimated mortality was 4%, 5%, 6%, 7%, and 7% at 6, 12, 24, 36 and 48 months respectively with mortality incidence density of 1.89 deaths per 100 person years (95% CI 1.74, 3.62). Forty years and above AHR = 3.055 (95% CI 1.292, 7.223), low baseline hemoglobin level (AHR = 0.523 (95% CI .335, 0.816)), and poor ART adherence (AHR 27.848 (95% CI 8.928, 86.8)) were found to be an independent determinants of mortality. These determinants of mortality have to be taken into account to enhance better clinical outcomes of ART attendees.

1. Introduction

HIV/AIDS remains one of the leading causes of death globally. It is projected to continue as a significant cause of premature mortality [1]. According to the joint 2011 HIV/AIDS report of WHO, UNAIDS, and UNICEF, an estimated 34 million people were living with HIV/AIDS globally with 2.7 million new HIV infections in 2010. Of these, 68% were residing in sub-Saharan Africa [2]. Ethiopia is one of the seriously affected countries in sub-Saharan Africa with a large number of people (approximately 800,000) that are living with HIV/AIDS and 44,751 AIDS-related deaths. An estimated number of 249,174 adults (86% of eligible) are on ART treatment [3–5]. The average life expectancy at birth is low, 51 years for males and 53 years for females. It is expected to further decline if the present HIV infection rates continue [3].

Different studies from different countries reported that WHO clinical staging, viral load, age, gender, CD4 cell count, total lymphocyte count (TLC), body mass index (BMI), ART adherence, and baseline hemoglobin level were determinants of mortality [6–10]. Even though studies had identified these determinants of mortality, they are so variable with context and dynamic across time with advancement of care and treatments as many years are being spent on highly active antiretroviral therapy (HAART) [11]. Thus, it is needed to generate locally consumable data to provide evidence for organizations working on HIV/AIDS and ART at national, regional, and district levels on factors determining the mortality of HIV positives attending ART. Therefore, the objective of this study was to identify independent determinants of mortality in PLWHA after initiation of ART and to estimate the time of death of PLWHA who are on ART. Important baseline variables like BMI, CD4 count, and TLC were included in this study to address the limitations of the previous cohort studies done in Ethiopia.

2. Methods

2.1. Study Setting. The study was conducted at Nekemte Referral Hospital, East Wollega, from December 1, 2011, to January 1, 2012. Nekemte is an administrative capital of the East Wollega Zone. It is 331 km to the west of Addis Ababa, the capital of Ethiopia. There was one public referral hospital in Nekemte. The hospital provides preventive, curative, and rehabilitative services for populations of more than 1.5 million. It also provides patient care and treatment for HIV/AIDS. ART service program was initiated in 2005 in the hospital. A total of 6056 patients had been enrolled of which 3,200 had ever started ART and 1,711 were on ART at the time of the study [12].

2.2. Participants. The study participants were PLWHA who had been on ART in the hospital from July, 2005, to January 1, 2012, who have complete registration, intake, and followup forms. To be included, the patient has to be older than fourteen years and started ART at same hospital. Patients who get diagnosed outside of the hospital (transfer in), transfer out, loss to followup (drop, lost), women who were pregnant at the time of ART initiation, lactating mothers in WHO stage I or II who started ART exclusively to prevent vertical transmission, and patients with competing causes of death (cause of death other than HIV like accident, patients with immune-compromising chronic diseases such as diabetes, thyroid disease, or any non-AIDS malignancies) were excluded.

The study subjects were randomly selected based on the inclusion criteria. Profiles of all patients on ART between July, 2005, and January 1, 2012, were evaluated, and exposure status was first identified as stages I-II (unexposed) versus stages III-IV (exposed). Then, after loss to follow up, drop out, PMTCT, deaths with competing causes, and transfer out or patients started on ART since January 2009 or subjects with incomplete data were excluded. Finally those who fulfill inclusion criteria, unique ID number were given in increasing order for both exposed and unexposed ART groups separately. Then, simple random sampling technique was employed separately to select 416 samples from both groups (138 from stages I-II and 278 from stages III-IV) using computer-generated random number table.

2.3. Data Collection. The data collection tool was developed from ART entry and followup forms being used in the ART clinic of the Hospital. The data were collected by reviewing pre-ART register, lab request, monthly cohort and follow up form, ART intake form, patients' card, and death certificate complemented by home visitors registration and phone calls done by drug adherence supporters to confirm death when patients were absent from their appointment. The most recent laboratory results before starting ART were used as a baseline value. When there was no pretreatment laboratory test, result obtained within one month of ART initiation was used. A total of three days training was given for one supervisor and two data collectors. Overall, data collection process was controlled by the principal investigator. Data quality was ensured by designing proper data collection materials, by checking the collected data daily for completeness, and thorough continuous supervision. All the completed data collection forms were examined again for completeness and consistency during data management, storage, and analysis by principal investigator.

2.4. Variables. The main outcome measure was cumulative survival rates from the initiation of ART to January 01, 2012. The independent variables were sociodemographic characteristics (age, sex, religion, marital status, employment, educational status and dependent children at home), baseline clinical, laboratory and ART information (opportunistic illness, WHO clinical staging, TB test and treatment, ART treatment, chemoprophylaxis, drug allergies, hemoglobin, T-cell lymphocyte count, CD4 count, and side effects), and ART treatment.

2.5. Data Analysis. The data were entered into Epi-Info 3.5.3 for windows and analyzed using SPSS version 16.0. We described the patient cohort characteristics in terms of mean/median value for continuous data and percentage for categorical data. The end point in this study was death from all AIDS-related causes which was confirmed by reviewing medical registration in the Hospital, registration by ART adherence supporters, or by calling using the registered phone number. Individuals alive and on ART were censored at the end of the study period. At the end, the outcome of each subject was dichotomized in to censored or death. Finally, survival analysis and Kaplan-Meier test were used to measure the association of patient's characteristics with time from ART initiation to death. Life table was used to estimate survival after initiation of ART, and logrank test was used to compare survival curves. Cox proportional-hazard regression was used to calculate the bivariate and adjusted hazard rate to determine independent determinants of time to death.

2.6. Ethical Considerations. Ethical approval was obtained from Research Ethics Committee of the School of Public Health at Addis Ababa University, College of Health Sciences for approval. Following the approval, Official letter of cooperation was written to the concerned bodies: Nekemte Referral Hospital and East Wollega Zone Health Bureau by the School of Public Health, Addis Ababa University. As the study was conducted through review of medical records, the individual patients were not subjected to any harm as long as the confidentiality is kept. To keep the confidentiality, ART clinic health officer and nurse of Nekemte Referral Hospital extracted the data from the medical records. In addition to that, no name or personal identifications were used on data collection form. The recorded data were not accessed by a third person, except the principal investigators, and was kept confidentially.

3. Results

3.1. Sociodemographic Characteristics of the Study Subjects. A total of 416 HIV-infected patients' records were reviewed for initial and repeated measurements, but repeated values are excluded from the analysis due to the incompleteness of records. Four hundred sixteen (386 alive and 30 death) adult patients were included in the study. One hundred and seventy four (41.8%) were males, and the mean age was 33.6 (SD = 9.04). Three hundred thirty (79.3%) were of age less than 40 years. Most of them (54.8%) followed Orthodox Christian. One hundred thirty five (32.5%) had primary education, and 39.4% had no formal education. Most of them (64.4%) were married (Table 1).

3.2. Baseline Clinical and Laboratory Information of the Cohort. The median weight at ART initiation was 51 kg (interquartile range (IQR, 45 kg–58 kg)). The mean hemoglobin level was 12.99 g/dL (IQR, 12.4–13.6). The median CD4 count was 141 cells/μL (IQR, 73–199). Almost all (99.5%) were given cotrimoxzazole prophylaxis (CPT) at the time of ART initiation, and 9.9% had TB coinfection. Majorities (61.3%) were in WHO stage III, 28.4% were in WHO stage II, 5.5% were in WHO stage IV, and 4.8% in WHO stage I at ART initiation. Baseline ART regimens were d4t (30)-3TC-NVP for 242 patients (58.2%), d4t (30)-3TC-EFV for 82 patients (19.7%), AZT-3TC-EFV for 44 patients (10.6%), AZT-3TC-NVP for 37 patients (8.9%), d4t (40)-3TC NVP for 8 patients (1.9%), and d4t (40)-3TC-EFV for 3 patients (0.7%). Majority of them (95.9%) had good ART adherence, while 4.1% poorly adhered (not shown). Majority of the patients (83.7%) were initiated ART at CD4 < 200 cells/μL which indicates the most of them were in severe immune depression at baseline, while only small portion (5%) of the patients started ART at WHO stage IV (see Table 1).

3.3. Survival Analysis and Bivariate Cox Regression Analysis. The median followup was 47 months with minimum follow up time of 14 days and the maximum of 97 months. Thirty (7.2%) subjects were died, of which 18 (60%) were within the first 6 months. The rest (92.8%) were alive up to the end of the last censored date (January 1, 2012). The estimated mortality was 4%, 5%, 6%, 7%, and 7% at 6, 12, 24, 36, and 48 months, respectively, with mortality incidence density of 1.89 deaths per 100 person-years (95% CI 1.74, 3.62) (Figure 2, Table 2). In bivariate Cox regression analysis, age, sex, educational status, occupation, and WHO clinical staging were not associated with mortality. Functional status, dependent children at home, marital status, baseline hemoglobin, CD4 count, TLC (total lymphocyte count), BMI (body mass index), and ART adherence were all associated with mortality at P value less than 0.05 (Figure 1, Table 2).

3.4. Multivariable Analysis Using Cox-Proportional Hazard Model. In multivariable Cox regression analysis, variables that showed significance in bivariate (except marital status which was dropped as it was highly correlated with age) were entered in to the multivariable model. Age and sex of the patients were included in the multivariable model irrespective of their association with mortality as they are the most common confounding variables in epidemiology. Finally, age ≥40 years AHR = 3.055 (95% CI 1.292, 7.223), lower baseline hemoglobin level AHR = 0.523 (95% CI 0.335, 0.816), and poor ART adherence AHR = 27.848 (95% CI 8.928, 86.863) were indicated as significant independent

Table 1: Baseline sociodemographic characteristics of HIV patients upon initiation of antiretroviral therapy in Nekemte Referral Hospital, 2012.

Baseline variables	Frequency (n = 416)	Percentage
Gender		
Male	174	41.8
Female	242	58.2
Age		
Age 14–40	330	79.3
Age ≥ 40	86	20.7
Ethnicity		
Oromo	285	68.5
Amhara	105	25.2
Tigre	17	4.1
Gurage	9	2.2
Religion		
Protestant	149	35.8
Orthodox	228	54.8
Adventist	2	0.5
Catholic	2	0.5
Muslim	35	8.4
Occupation		
Farmer	59	14.2
Merchant	41	9.9
Government employee	73	17.5
NGO employee	11	2.6
Daily laborer	112	26.9
Jobless	104	25
Driver	10	2.4
Student	6	1.4
Educational status		
No education	164	39.4
Primary	135	32.5
Secondary	80	19.2
Tertiary and above	37	8.9
Dependent children		
Yes	309	74.3
No	107	25.7
Marital status		
Never married	40	9.6
Married	268	64.4
Separated	3	0.7
Divorced	29	7.0
Widowed	76	18.3
Employment status		
Working	278	66.8
Unemployed	9	2.2
Not working due to ill health	129	31.0
ARV eligibility criteria used to initiate ART		
CD4 below 200	348	83.7
WHO stage IV	21	5
WHO stage I, II, and III with TLC < 1200	47	11.3

TABLE 2: Actuarial table estimates of the cumulative progression to death for 416 study subjects starting ART between 2005 and 2012 in Nekemte Referral Hospital.

Life table				
Interval start time in months	Number entering interval	Number of deaths	Cumulative proportion of survival at the end of interval	Hazard rate
0	416	18	**0.96**	0.01
6	395	0	**0.96**	0.00
12	395	4	**0.95**	0.00
18	391	2	**0.94**	0.00
24	388	0	**0.94**	0.00
30	388	1	**0.94**	0.00
36	386	2	**0.93**	0.00
42	306	1	**0.93**	0.00
48	205	1	**0.93**	0.00
54	154	0	**0.93**	0.00
60	148	0	**0.93**	0.00
66	138	1	**0.92**	0.00
72	66	0	**0.92**	0.00
78	10	0	**0.92**	0.00
84	4	0	**0.92**	0.00
90	2	0	**0.92**	0.00

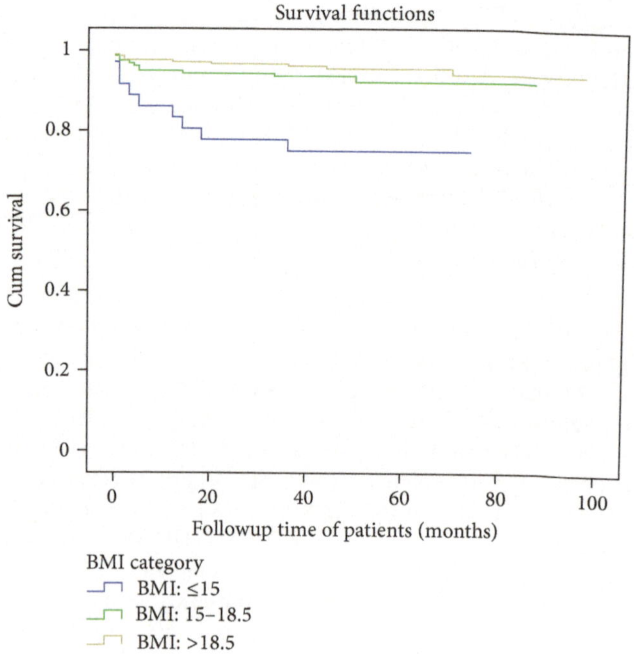

FIGURE 1: Survival functions of HIV patients by BMI category upon initiation of antiretroviral therapy between 2005 and 2012 in Nekemte Referral Hospital.

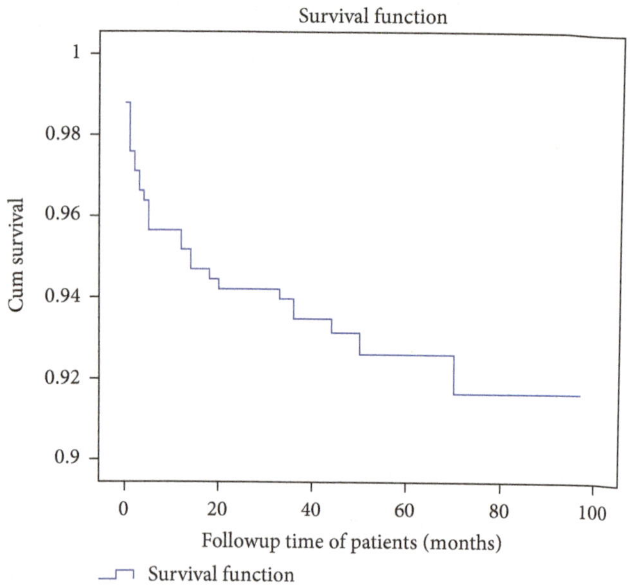

FIGURE 2: Overall survival curve of the cohort ($n = 416$) starting ART between 2005 and 2012 in Nekemte Referral Hospital, 2012.

determinants of mortality. Of those, patients with poor ART adherence and older age had the highest risk of death with HR of 27.848 (95% CI 8.928, 86.863) and 3.055 (95% CI 1.292, 7.223), respectively, while one unit increase in hemoglobin level reduces HIV mortality by 48% [HR 0.523 (95% CI 0.335, 0.816)] (Table 3).

4. Discussions

In this cohort study, we identified 7.2% mortality rate. This was less when compared with the finding reported from Assela and Shashamane Hospitals in Ethiopia (10.3%) [8]. This lower percentage could be attributed to the fact that the real-case scenario (only confirmed dead cases) was used as events in this study which might underestimate mortality. In addition, the decline could reflect the increased care and support given to PLWHA. Most of the deaths (60%) were within the first 6 months. Similar findings were reported from different African countries including Ethiopia that attributed most of the late initiation of ART with the advanced clinical condition [9, 10, 13]. These facts were also revealed in our study in which most of the patients (84.4%) had an advanced disease as evidenced by a baseline CD4 < 150 cells/mL and advanced WHO clinical stage, in which 66.8% of patients were in WHO stage III and IV. Furthermore, about half of the patients (47.6%) were malnourished at baseline (BMI < 18.5 kg/m^2), and a considerable proportion (15.6%) of them were in severe immune depression (CD4 count < 50 cells/mm^3).

Pertaining to serial months mortality at 6, 12, 18, 30, and 48 moths, our study found a low level of mortality when compared with study done in Zewditu Hospital in Ethiopia [14] and Malawi [15]. This survival difference might be attributed to the large proportion of the patients started ART at WHO stage I and II (33.2%), and there was a good follow up as a result of default tracers recruited by ICAP-Ethiopia program which supported the patients, high drug accessibility, and changing pattern of types of drug regimen at different time.

Previous studies reported that age of the patient was found to be the predictor of mortality, where most of the patients in older age were more likely to die [7, 16]. Similar scenario had happened in our case age 40 years and above AHR = 3.364 (95% CI 1.211, 9.348 were 3 times at higher risk of mortality than in which patients aged less than 40 years. This could be due to the fact that individuals are at higher risk of complications and respond poorly to ART as a result of combined effect of aging, HIV infection, and antiretroviral treatment [16]. It is known that as age increases immune status becomes incompetent which is consisered to be a risk for many chronic diseases which results in death.

Patients with poor ART adherence had the highest risk of death with 27 times more likely to die than adherent patients AHR 27.848 (95% CI 8.928, 86.8). Similarly, a study conducted in Kampala, Uganda, nonadherent participants had a mortality of 42.5 deaths per 100 person-years and were two times as likely to die as adherent participants [17]. The non-adherence to HAART leads to virologic, immunologic, clinical failure, and failure to suppress viral replication, thus increasing the likelihood of developing HIV mutations that could lead to the development of drug-resistant viral strains [18]. Non-adherence to HAART also leads to failure to prevent further viral destruction of the cellular immune system with consequent reduction in the level of CD4+ cells and the development of opportunistic infections [19]. Adherence to HAART is critical to the survival of HIV/AIDS-infected people as low adherence is the main reason for poor treatment outcomes among people receiving antiretroviral therapy [18]. Other point that need attention in our study is that the hazard rate of poor ART adherence is inflated (27 times than adherent patients) and the CI is wide showing low precision and lower frequency in this category, even though it was highly significant which necessitates a large-scale study with large sample size.

Lower baseline hemoglobin level at ART initiation (moderate and/or severe anemia) is one of the independent predictor of mortality in HIV-infected patients in several previous studies conducted in the world including Ethiopia [6, 8, 9, 14]. Our study also revealed similar scenario. In this study, in contrast to other studies, in which the WHO clinical stage was found to be stronger predictor of mortality [8–10], it was not found to be associated with mortality in similar aspect of a study reported from South Western Uganda [20]. This might be due to the fact that majority of the patients (95.9%) have good ARV adherence, large proportion (33.2%) started ART early at WHO stage I and II, and very large proportion (91.4%) of patients in WHO stage III and IV were alive up to the last censored date which indicates low number of events in this category. It might also be attributed with the possibility of misclassification of WHO clinical staging as it is determined by clinical judgment of health care providers which is a common problem in developing countries with limited diagnostic capacities.

There was no significant gender difference in our study which is in agreement with the study done in Assela and Shashemane Hospitals in Ethiopia [8], though it contrasted with the study reported from Arba minch Hospital, Ethiopia, which revealed that men had a higher risk of death AOR = 1.78 (95% CI 1.47, 2.16) [7]; however, some other studies

Table 3: Multivariate Cox regression analysis and model fit of the cohort studied ($N = 416$) between 2005 and 2012 in Nekemte Referral Hospital, Ethiopia.

Determinants	Crude HR (95% CI)	Adjusted HR (95% CI)
Gender		
Male	1.233 (0.602, 2.527)	1.607 (0.686, 3.762)
Female	1	1
Age		
14–40	1	1
≥40	1.977 (0.925, 4.224)	3.055 (1.292, 7.223)*
Functional status at baseline		
Working	1	1
Ambulatory	2.460 (1.129, 5.360)*	1.531 (0.676, 3.470)
Bedridden	10.634 (3.373, 33.520)*	0.891 (0.205, 3.883)
Dependent children at home		
No	4.013 (1.948, 8.266)*	1.521 (0.651, 3.554)
Yes	1	1
Baseline hemoglobin level	0.597 (0.431, 0.827)*	0.523 (0.335, 0.816)*
CD4 count category at baseline		
CD4 count: >150	6.287 (2.318, 17.051)*	2.940 (0.750, 7.909)
CD4 count: 100–149	4.340 (1.542, 12.217)*	2.049 (0.597, 7.038)
CD4 count: 50–99	1.499 (0.423, 5.314)	0.676 (0.168, 2.724)
CD4 count: <50	1	1
Baseline TLC category		
TLC: >1200	8.183 (1.831, 36.576)*	2.656 (0.414, 17.022)
TLC: 600–1200	4.655 (1.397, 15.518)*	3.342 (0.891, 12.535)
TLC: <600	1	1
BMI category		
BMI: >18.5	6.426 (2.599, 15.890)*	1.586 (0.540, 4.662)
BMI: 15–18.5	1.553 (0.659, 3.658)	0.954 (0.361, 2.518)
BMI: ≤15	1	1
ART adherence		
Poor	52.672 (24.393, 113.735)*	27.848 (8.928, 86.863)*
Good	1	1

Note: *Statistically significant at $P < 0.05$.

reported that females have significantly higher survival rate than males [3, 9, 21]. It had been reasoned as males were poorly adhering than females. However, in our study, there was no association between gender and ART adherence, rather majority of the patients (95.9%) have good ART adherence.

Johanssen et al. reported CD4 count < 50 Cells/μL at baseline, moderate and severe anemia, thrombocytopenia, and severe malnutrition as predictors of mortality [9]. Further, Ojikutu and his colleagues indicated that low BMI both in ART+ and ART− groups strongly predicts the mortality [6]. Though it can be considered as our strength to include BMI which was missed from the previous studies done in the country, base line BMI was not associated with mortality in our study which may be due to the recent nutritional intervention for severely malnourished patients in this specific hospital.

This study has the following limitations. Selection bias is possibly introduced due to the fact that patients with incomplete records of major variables were excluded. Lack of data on viral load (HIV-RNA) during the course of ART which could have been more suitable to serve as immunological or virological marker is one limitation. Narrow scope of the study setting, study population being only from one hospital set up and population from specific area is another limitation. Missing data and limited diagnostic tests which could confirm the presence of certain opportunistic infections prevented us from analyzing the role of past opportunistic infections on survival time, though several studies report this as an important mortality determinant.

5. Conclusions

This study has revealed an overall lower mortality rate, but a high mortality of the cohort in the first 6 months of ART initiation; older age, low baseline hemoglobin level, and poor ART adherence were independent determinants of mortality. These determinants should be taken into account by health care providers to enhance better clinical outcomes of ART attendees.

Conflict of Interests

The authors have no any conflict of interests.

Authors' Contribution

M. T. Hambisa participated in designing the study, supervised data collection, performed the statistical analysis, and served as the main author of the paper. A. Ali participated in the designing of the study, has involved in the interpretation of data, and has participated in drafting the paper. Y. Dessie prepared and revised the manuscript critically for publication. All authors approved the final manuscript.

Acknowledgments

The authors are grateful to the Addis Ababa University, School of Public Health for financially supporting this research. Our special thanks also go to all supervisors and data collectors for their cooperation during data collection.

References

[1] *AIDS Epidemic Update*, UNAIDS, Geneva, Switzerland, 2009.

[2] WHO, UNAIDS and UNICEF, "GLOBAL HIV/AIDS response epidemic update and health sector progress towards universal access," Progress Report, 2011.

[3] *Guide for Implementation of the Antiretroviral Therapy Program in Ethiopia*, Federal HIV/AIDS Prevention and Control Office Federal Ministry of Health Ethiopia, Addis Ababa, Ethiopia, 2007.

[4] *Country Progress Report on HIV/AIDS Response*, FHAPCO, Addis Ababa, Ethiopia, 2012.

[5] *Report on Progress towards Implementation of the UN Declaration of Commitment on HIV/AIDS*, Federal HIV/AIDS Prevention and Control Office Federal Ministry of Health Ethiopia, Addis Ababa, Ethiopia, 2010.

[6] B. O. Ojikutu, H. Zheng, R. P. Walensky et al., "Predictors of mortality in patients initiating antiretroviral therapy in Durban, South Africa," *South African Medical Journal*, vol. 98, no. 3, pp. 204–208, 2008.

[7] Z. Mulissa, D. Jerene, and B. Lindtjørn, "Patients present earlier and survival has improved, but pre-ART attrition is high in a six-year HIV cohort data from Ethiopia," *PLoS ONE*, vol. 5, no. 10, Article ID e13268, 2010.

[8] A. Worku and M. San Sebastián, "Determinants of survival in adult HIV patients on antiretroviral therapy in Oromiyaa, Ethiopia," *Global Health Action*, vol. 3, article 5398, 2010.

[9] A. Johannessen, E. Naman, B. J. Ngowi et al., "Predictors of mortality in HIV-infected patients starting antiretroviral therapy in a rural hospital in Tanzania," *BMC Infectious Diseases*, vol. 8, article 52, 2008.

[10] I. Sieleunou, M. Souleymanou, A. M. Schönenberger, J. Menten, and M. Boelaert, "Determinants of survival in AIDS patients on antiretroviral therapy in a rural centre in the Far-North Province, Cameroon," *Tropical Medicine and International Health*, vol. 14, no. 1, pp. 36–43, 2009.

[11] A. G. Pacheco, S. H. Tuboi, S. B. May et al., "Temporal changes in causes of death among HIV-infected patients in the HAART era in Rio de Janeiro, Brazil," *Journal of Acquired Immune Deficiency Syndromes*, vol. 51, no. 5, pp. 624–630, 2009.

[12] *Nekemte Referral Hospital Annual ART Report 2005–2012*, Nekemte Referral Hospital, Nekemte, Ethiopia, 2012.

[13] D. Jerene, A. Næss, and B. Lindtjørn, "Antiretroviral therapy at a district hospital in Ethiopia prevents death and tuberculosis in a cohort of HIV patients," *AIDS Research and Therapy*, vol. 3, no. 1, article 10, 2006.

[14] A. Bedru, *Assessment of predictors of survival in patients living with HIV/AIDS after the advent of highly active antiretroviral therapy in Addis Ababa Ethiopia [MPH thesis]*, School of Public Health, Addis Ababa University, 2009.

[15] R. Zachariah, M. Fitzgerald, M. Massaquoi et al., "Risk factors for high early mortality in patients on antiretroviral treatment in a rural district of Malawi," *AIDS*, vol. 20, no. 18, pp. 2355–2360, 2006.

[16] S. Grabar, L. Weiss, and D. Costagliola, "HIV infection in older patients in the HAART era," *Journal of Antimicrobial Chemotherapy*, vol. 57, no. 1, pp. 4–7, 2006.

[17] A. M. Abaasa, J. Todd, K. Ekoru et al., "Good adherence to HAART and improved survival in a community HIV/AIDS treatment and care programme: the experience of the AIDS Support Organization (TASO), Kampala, Uganda," *BMC Health Services Research*, vol. 8, article 241, 2008.

[18] WHO/UNAIDS/UNICEF, "Towards universal access: scaling-up priority HIV/AIDS intervention in the health sector," Progress Report, pp. 122–132, 2009.

[19] F. Maggiolo, M. Airoldi, H. D. Kleinloog et al., "Effect of adherence to HAART on virologic outcome and on the selection of resistance-conferring mutations in NNRTI- or PI-treated patients," *HIV Clinical Trials*, vol. 8, no. 5, pp. 282–292, 2007.

[20] E. H. Geng, D. V. Glidden, N. Emenyonu et al., "Tracking a sample of patients lost to follow-up has a major impact on understanding determinants of survival in HIV-infected patients on antiretroviral therapy in Africa," *Tropical Medicine and International Health*, vol. 15, no. 1, pp. 63–69, 2010.

[21] S. C. C. Chen, J. K. L. Yu, A. D. Harries et al., "Increased mortality of male adults with AIDS related to poor compliance to antiretroviral therapy in Malawi," *Tropical Medicine and International Health*, vol. 13, no. 4, pp. 513–519, 2008.

8

New Insights into HIV/AIDS-Associated Cryptococcosis

Spinello Antinori

Department of Biomedical and Clinical Sciences Lvigi Sacco, Università degli Studi di Milano, Via GB Grassi 74, 20157 Milano, Italy

Correspondence should be addressed to Spinello Antinori; spinello.antinori@unimi.it

Academic Editors: C. A. Hughes and B. Joos

Cryptococcal meningitis is a life-threatening opportunistic fungal infection in both HIV-infected and HIV-uninfected patients. According to the most recent taxonomy, the responsible fungus is classified into a complex that contains two species (*Cryptococcus neoformans* and *C. gattii*), with eight major molecular types. HIV infection is recognized worldwide as the main underlying disease responsible for the development of cryptococcal meningitis (accounting for 80–90% of cases). In several areas of sub-Saharan Africa with the highest HIV prevalence despite the recent expansion of antiretroviral (ARV) therapy programme, cryptococcal meningitis is the leading cause of community-acquired meningitis with a high mortality burden. Although cryptococcal meningitis should be considered a neglected disease, a large body of knowledge has been developed by several studies performed in recent years. This paper will focus especially on new clinical aspects such as immune reconstitution inflammatory syndrome, advances on management, and strategies for the prevention of clinical disease.

1. Introduction

The encapsulated yeast, *Cryptococcus* spp., is a major cause of fungal meningitis and meningoencephalitis especially in immunocompromised patients [1, 2]. This basidiomycete fungus was first isolated in 1894 by Sanfelice in fruit juices and subsequently recovered from the tibial lesion of a patient by Busse and Buschke [3–5]. The genus has been named from the Greek words, *kryptos* (hidden) and *kokkos* (berry) but a long lists of names and synonyms have been generated until the adoption of the actual nomenclature [6].

However, although *C. neoformans* has been recognized for more than 100 years, the worldwide spread of HIV infection as well as the increasing number of patients with impaired immunity were responsible for the dramatic surge of this life-threatening infection only in the 80's [7–9]. Although effective treatment for HIV disease has decreased significantly incidence of cryptococcal meningitis (CM) in western countries, it remains a common cause of infectious morbidity and mortality especially among HIV-positive patients living in sub-Saharan Africa and South-east Asia [10–16]. This paper will focus on main aspects of AIDS-associated cryptococcal meningitis with special attention on recent findings on immune reconstitution inflammatory syndrome, diagnosis, treatment, and prevention. Data were identified by searches on PubMed and Scopus using a combination of search terms including "cryptococcosis," "AIDS," "immune reconstitution inflammatory syndrome," "cryptococcal antigen," "cryptococcal meningitis," "cryptococcal diagnosis," "antifungal treatment," "primary prophylaxis," and "prophylaxis discontinuation." Moreover references from relevant key articles and from my own files were included. The final search date was October 2012.

2. Biology, Microbiology, and Serotypes Distribution

More than 30 species of the genus *Cryptococcus* exist but only two are considered important human pathogens. The fungus is actually classified into the *Cryptococcus neoformans* complex that consists of two species: *C. neoformans* and *C. gattii* [17–19]. *C. neoformans* var. *grubii* (serotype A), C.

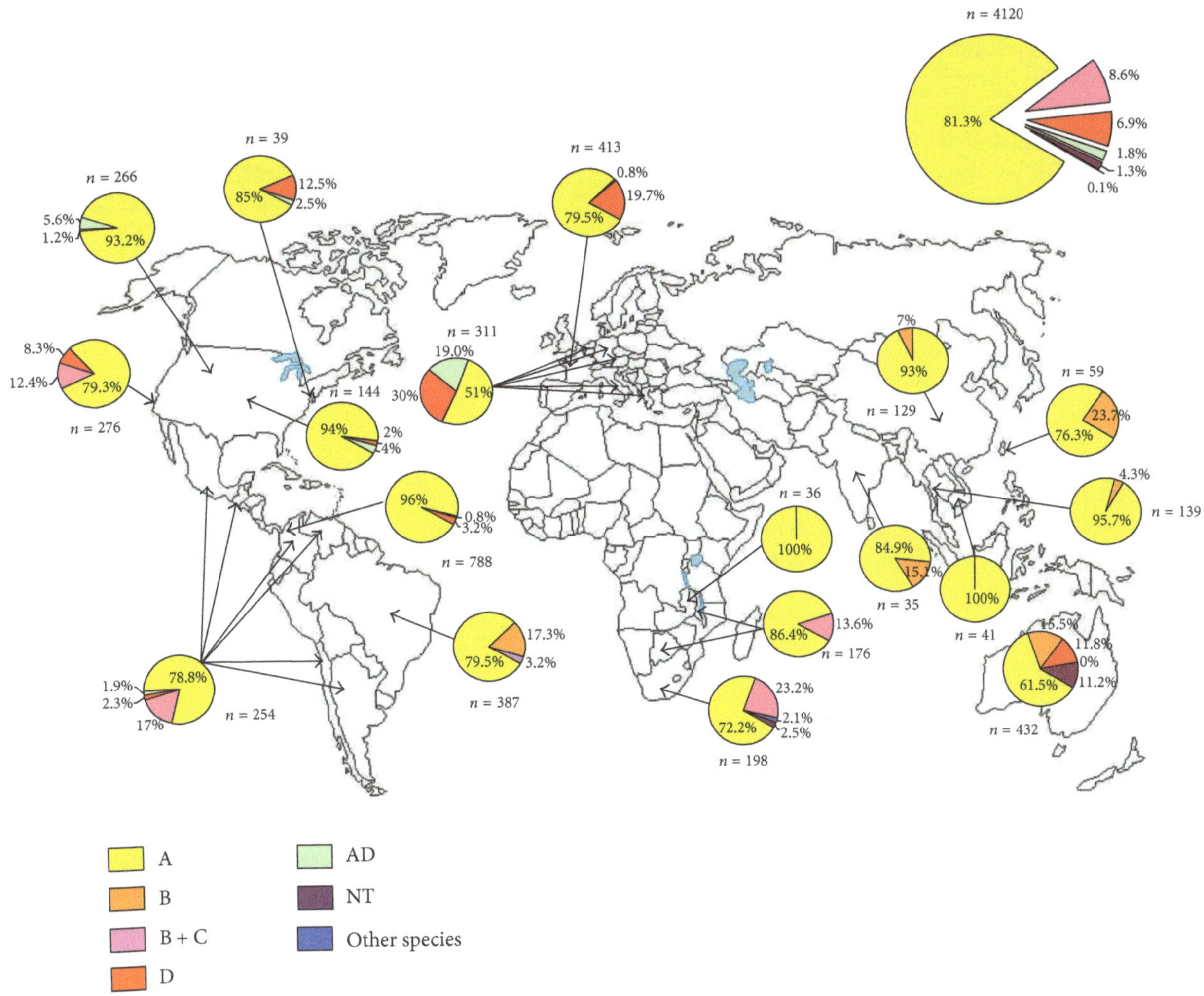

FIGURE 1: Worldwide geographic diffusion of different serotypes of *Cryptococcus neoformans* complex (based on [25–48]).

neoformans var. *neoformans* (serotype D), and AD hybrids generally cause disease in immunocompromised patients whereas *C.gatti* (serotype B and C) can cause disease also in immunocompetent patients [9, 20–22].

Molecular typing has identified eight major molecular types within the 2 species: VNI/AFLP1, VNII/AFLP1A (*C.* neoformans var. *grubii*), VNIII/AFLP3 (AD hybrid), VNIV/AFLP2 (*C. neoformans* var. *neoformans*), and VGI/AFLP4, VGII/AFLP6, VGIII/AFLP5, VGIV/AFLP7 (*C. gattii*) [23].

Non-*neoformans* cryptococcal infections are rarely encountered and have been recently reviewed [24].

C. neoformans var. *grubii* has a worldwide distribution and is the most prevalent species (Figure 1) whereas *C. neoformans* var. *neoformans* is found predominantly in Western Europe [25–37]. *Cryptococcus gattii* was originally known to be geographically restricted to tropical and subtropical regions [38–40] but, since 1999, an unprecedented emergence of *C. gattii* was observed in the east coast of Vancouver Island, British Columbia where the organism is now endemic and where the incidence is the highest ever reported (37 times greater than reported in Australia) [41, 42]. Moreover, there is recent evidence that the *C. gattii* strain of the Vancouver outbreak has spread to the Pacific Northwest of the United States [43]. Finally, in recent years *C. gattii* has been isolated also in temperate regions of Europe (Austria, Italy, Spain, The Netherlands) as well as of Asia (Japan, South Korea) [44–47].

3. Epidemiology and Risk Factors

The analysis of the risk factors associated with development of cryptococcosis employed in several studies clearly demonstrates that HIV infection is the major underlying condition predisposing to the development of this disease [8, 33, 48]. Several studies have underscored the profound impact that the emergence of HIV/AIDS epidemic has had on the epidemiology of cryptococcal infection [8, 12, 13, 49, 50]; in fact, it has been reported that there were 1264 proven cases of cryptococcosis in the United States during the 12-year period from 1965 to 1977 [51]. In contrast a 1500% increase was observed in the period from 1981 to 1990 due to the AIDS epidemic; because of the introduction of azoles therapy and, by the mid-90s, of the highly active antiretroviral therapy (HAART), a declining incidence was observed in all Western countries [10–13, 52]. A completely different situation is registered in sub-Saharan Africa: worth noting an increasing numbers of cases of CM were observed among young Congolese adults starting from the early 60s possibly as the beginning of the HIV epidemic [53]. In a large part of sub-Saharan Africa as demonstrated by a recent controlled clinical trial conducted on bacterial meningitis, as well as in other studies, *C. neoformans* is now emerged as the leading cause of meningitis accounting for 26 to 45% of cases in several series [54–57].

It has been estimated that in 2006 at least 957,900 cases of CM had occurred worldwide with the highest burden from sub-Saharan Africa (720,000 cases with 504,000 deaths) [1] Moreover, despite the fact that also in sub-Saharan Africa, an increasing number of HIV-positive patients are now receiving HAART, a study conducted in South Africa which showed that the number of new India ink positive cases of CM was not falling [58]. However, in Burkina Faso where the incidence of HIV infection was lower and probably where better ART programs are employed, a steady decline of CM was observed during an 8-year period in parallel with the increased use of HAART [59]. Both studies are a reminder of the importance of more huge implementation of ART in Africa with a more widespread and earlier access to these life-saving therapies.

4. Pathogenesis

The portal of entry of *Cryptococcus* is usually through inhalation of spores or desiccated yeast cells from the environment. Deposition in the alveoli produces an asymptomatic infection that is either cleared or controlled by a strong cell-mediated immune response leading to a dormant latent infection with development of granuloma in the lungs or hilar lymph nodes [60, 61]. In immunocompromised individuals, the fungus can spread from the lungs to the central nervous system to cause meningoencephalitis that is fatal if left untreated.Once *C. neoformans* enters the circulatory system it must survive for dissemination to occur and macrophage can be a vehicle either for dissemination and distribution through the host; crossing the blood brain barrier (BBB) is probably mediated by transcytosis (i.e., transcellular penetration through microvascular endothelial cells) and there is evidence that the capsule is involved [62, 63].

Macrophages probably play also an important role in the BBB crossing by *C. neoformans* with a mechanism of "Trojan horse"; it has been shown *in vitro* that active macrophage phagosomal extrusion is a possible escape strategy allowing continued propagation and dissemination of the fungus [64]. Recently, Charlier et al. presented proofs of concept for the hypothesis of the Trojan horse in a mouse model comparing intravenous inoculation of the yeast in a free form and after ingestion by cultured monocytes [65].

5. Clinical Manifestations

The fungus *Cryptococcus* can infect any organ in the body but showing a predilection for the lung and the central nervous system (CNS). The lung is the usual portal of entry of the microorganism and the infection can run either an asymptomatic course, especially among immunocompetent subjects, or progress to a life-threatening pneumonia with respiratory failure as observed in patients with AIDS [66].

In the pre-HAART era, cryptococcal infection was identified as the only cause of acute respiratory failure in 9% of a cohort of 210 patients with AIDS [66]; black race, lactate dehydrogenase, lactate dehydrogenase level >500 IU/L, presence of skin lesions, and interstitial infiltrates were the variables independently predictive of developing acute respiratory failure [66]. In a case series of 18 HIV-positive patients diagnosed with cryptococcal meningitis, Driver et al. found that 78% had respiratory symptoms during the 4-month period before meningitis appeared as compared with 50% at the time of diagnosis [67]. More recently,in Uganda among HIV-infected subjects hospitalized with pneumonia and undergoing bronchoscopy, the diagnosis of pulmonary cryptococcosis was made in 11% of cases [68]. Worth noting the diagnosis of pulmonary cryptococcosis was unsuspected in all these cases before diagnostic testing, thus confirming a lack of awareness of this pulmonary pathogen, as described in an autopsy study conducted on south African miners [69]. Among HIV-infected hospitalized patients with acute respiratory infections in rural Thailand, *Cryptococcus* species was found to be the second leading infection (after tuberculosis), and in 43% of all cryptococcal antigen positive, there was no evidence of past or concomitant meningitis nor any alternative etiology was identified [70].

C. neoformans shows a predilection to invade the central nervous system causing meningitis or meningoencephalitis in about 77–86% of patients [2, 71–89]; usually CM presents itself with a subacute or chronic course but occasionally may be fulminant [71]. Signs and symptoms of presentation may vary according to the host with fever and headache more frequently observed in the HIV-positive subjects (Table 1) and altered mental status among HIV-negative people [2, 7, 20, 27, 28, 55–57, 72–90]. In the HIV-positive patient CM is a late opportunistic infection usually observed when the T lymphocyte CD4+ cell count falls below 50–100/μL; two-thirds of patients had less than 50 CD4+ cells/μL and the median value reported in several series is below 30/μL [2, 77, 79].

Meningismus or neck stiffness is observed globally in about 61% of cases but more frequently in HIV-positive patients in Africa [28, 55–57, 80–85] compared to HIV-positive patients in Western countries [7, 20, 71–77] or HIV-uninfected patients [2, 20, 27, 79, 87, 89, 91]. However, this finding may reflect a delayed presentation in sub-Saharan Africa in comparison with patients observed in western countries. Altered mental status, which is the most important predictor of poor outcome of patients with CM, is present in 18–28% of patients with AIDS and in half of those without HIV infection (Table 1) [72–90]. Fungemia, expression of disseminated disease is observed in 47–71% of HIV-positive patients but only in 27% of HIV-negative subjects affected by cryptococcosis. Ocular involvement with visual changes is reported in near one-third of HIV-infected patients. Several manifestations can occur such as oculomotor palsies, retinal hemorrhages, and endophthalmitis [91–94]. Vision loss may be due to yeasts infiltration of optic nerve or may be caused

TABLE 1: Clinical and mycological features of cryptococcal meningitis.

Signs and symptoms	HIV-positive patients, $n = 1366^*$	HIV-positive patients, Africa, $n = 4149^\dagger$	HIV-negative patients, $n = 675^\#$	Total, $n = 6190$	HIV-positive children, $n = 160^\wedge$
Headache	839/1014 (82.7)	2646/3324 (79.6)	292/500 (58.4)	3777/4838 (78.1)	40/60 (66.7)
Fever	812/1080 (75.2)	1914/3322 (57.6)	352/500 (70.4)	3078/4902 (62.8)	31/60 (51.7)
Cough	267/994 (26.9)	16/67 (23.9)	78/324 (24.1)	361/1385 (26.1)	NR
Dyspnea	119/872 (13.6)	NR	56/292 (19.2)	175/1164 (15.1)	7/47 (14.9)
Meningismus or neck stiffness	342/889 (38.5)	2240/3330 (67.3)	181/453 (39.9)	2763/4672 (59.1)	14/56 (25)
Visual changes	171/593 (28.8)	NR	2/16 (12.5)	173/609 (28.4)	1/40 (2.5)
Altered mental status	203/1080 (18.8)	937/3347 (27.9)	236/451 (52.3)	1378/4878 (28.2)	15/60 (25)
Seizures	28/456 (6.1)	304/3323 (9.1)	48/458 (10.5)	380/4237 (8.9)	9/60 (15)
Skin lesions	19/321 (5.9)	NR	6/32 (18.7)	25/343 (7.3)	1/60 (1.6)
AIDS-defining illness	540/1101 (49)	484/568 (85.2)	—	1024/1669 (61.3)	8/30 (27)
		Mycology			
Positive CSF culture	1200/1274 (94.2)	3030/3364 (90.1)	381/464 (82.1)	4611/5102 (90.4)	97/110 (88.2)
Positive CSF antigen	489/530 (92.3)	1693/1757 (96.3)	432/447 (96.6)	2614/2734 (95.6)	38/62 (61.3)
Positive India ink	886/1132 (78.3)	3075/3360 (91.5)	269/456 (58.9)	4230/4948 (85.5)	44/50 (88)
Positive serum antigen	292/305 (95.7)	NR	121/141 (85. 8)	413/446 (92.6)	10/34 (29.4)
Positive blood cultures	645/1369 (47.1)	371/524 (70.8)	106/395 (26.8)	1122/3991 (28.1)	22/43 (51.2)

NR: not reported.
*References [7, 20, 72–80].
†References [28, 55–57, 81–86].
#References [20, 79–81, 87–91].
^References [100–103, 105].

by increased intracranial pressure [95]. Permanent blindness was associated with visual loss within the first week of hospital admission [94].

Skin lesions due to *C. neoformans* are found in 6% of AIDS patients with CM but the frequency is higher in patients infected with serotype D due to the seemingly higher skin tropism of this serotype [96–98]. Skin lesions are usually expression of the haematogenous dissemination of the fungus and can be single or multiple and present with a wide variety of pictures (papules, pustules, vesicles, nodules, ulcers) although a molluscum contagiosum-like appearance is the most frequently reported (Figure 2).

6. Cryptococcosis in Children

Cryptococcal disease seems to occur less frequently in AIDS children than in adults with a prevalence of 0.8 to 1.4% [99–101]. However, in Thailand a 2.97% point prevalence was observed during an eight-year study among hospitalized HIV-infected patients [102]. In South Africa, in the largest study so far conducted, the incidence of cryptococcosis among HIV-positive children was 47 cases per 100.000 persons [103]. Median age at time of diagnosis was 7 years that is similar to the figures (7.8 and 9.8 years) previously reported in the literature [103–105]. In the South Africa experience, there was the demonstration of the highest incidence among children with less than 1 year of age with a second peak among children in the 5-through 10-year age group [103].

Older studies suggested that children with HIV infection acquired by vertical transmission may be less likely to develop *C. neoformans* infection than children infected by other routes [100, 117]. However, these observations were not confirmed in those studies conducted in Africa and may reflect the fact that the predominant risk for pediatric AIDS at the beginning of epidemic was transfusion [101, 102].

Clinical features in children were similar to those observed in adults but those diagnosed in Africa showed higher frequency of headache (86% versus 53%), nuchal rigidity (69% versus 7%), seizures (38% versus 13%), and focal neurologic signs (23% versus 7%) in comparison with patients observed in USA [100, 101].

7. Elevated Intracranial Pressure

Elevated intracranial pressure (ICP) is a common complication of AIDS-associated CM. The pathophysiology of elevated ICP in patients with CM is poorly understood and it is likely caused by several convergent factors. It has been postulated that it may be due to the outflow obstruction precipitated by aggregation of fungal polysaccharide accumulating in arachnoid villi and subarachnoid spaces thus providing the blockage of the channels for CSF drainage [118]. This picture is consistent with communicating hydrocephalus. Moreover, another possible important factor is cerebral oedema resulting from cytokine-induced inflammation and possibly osmotic effect by fungus-derived mannitol [119].

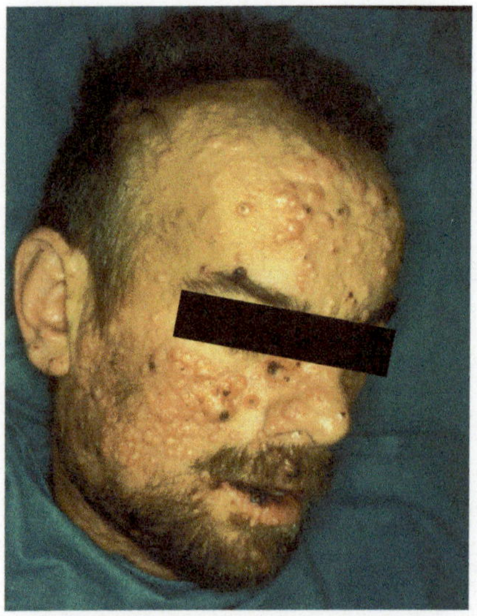

Figure 2: Patients with cryptococcal meningitis and disseminated infection with multiple papular and molluscum-like lesions on the face.

In an old observational study about 60% of the patients had an intracranial pressure of ≥250 mm H_2O, 30% of whom showed an intracranial pressure of ≥350 mm H_2O [119]. Similar results were subsequently confirmed in two large studies showing that 19–27% of patients with CM have a CSF pressure of ≥350 mm H_2O [120, 121]. The highest value of CSF opening pressure is consistently associated with higher fungal burden, significantly more frequent observation of papilledema, hearing loss, meningismus and increased risk of early mortality [119, 120]. However this latter finding was not confirmed in the study of Bicanic and coworkers [121].

A recent autopsy study elegantly demonstrated a correlation between high concentration of viable and dead organisms in the arachnoid granulations and raised cerebrospinal fluid pressure with the consequence of the obstruction of CSF resorption [122].

The optimal management of elevated ICP without hydrocephalus in the setting of CM is still uncertain and debated. The updated guidelines by the Infectious Diseases Society of America on the basis of the study by Graybill and coworkers recommend, after appropriate brain imaging to exclude hydrocephalus or space-occupying lesions, CSF drainage by lumbar puncture (with a BII evidence) [123]; if symptoms persist with concomitant high CSF pressure (>250 mm H_2O) daily drainage by repeated lumbar puncture or positioning of temporary percutaneous lumbar drains is recommended (with a BIII evidence). However, daily lumbar punctures although associated with immediate relief of headache may be associated with the risk of brain herniation [124].

The placement of lumbar drains has been proposed for control of raised ICP when the more conservative measures have failed; this technique allows the removal of more cerebrospinal fluid than can be safely removed by daily lumbar puncture [125, 126]. The use of temporary lumbar drainage has been used also in resource-poor setting without significant increase of bacterial infections [127]. Finally, the use of permanent ventriculoperitoneal shunts can be reserved for patients with true hydrocephalus or raised ICP refractory to all other measures employed [128].

8. Cryptococcal Immune Reconstitution Inflammatory Syndrome (IRIS)

Cryptococcal immune reconstitution inflammatory syndrome (IRIS) can be associated with a clinical deterioration of the disease or with a new presentation of cryptococcal disease after reversal of the immune deficiency state [129, 130]. Cryptococcal IRIS has been initially described in HIV-infected patients after starting highly active antiretroviral therapy (HAART) but it has been subsequently recognized also in the transplantation setting and following treatment with adalimumab and alemntuzumab [131–133]. Recently a group of experts on behalf of the International Network for the Study of HIV-associated IRIS (INSHI) proposed the adoption of two clinical case definitions of IRIS associated with cryptococcosis among HIV-infected patients: (1) paradoxical cryptococcal IRIS involving patients who had a diagnosis of cryptococcal disease before starting ART; (2) ART-associated cryptococcosis characterized by incident or unmasking cryptococcosis after starting antiretroviral treatment [134].

The incidence of paradoxical IRIS associated with cryptococcosis in AIDS patients was reported to be 15.9 events/100 patient-years of follow-up (95% CI 8.5–22.9) in one study from USA, 4.2/100 person-years(PY) of follow-up (95% CI 2.2–7.8) in another study conducted in France, and 25/100 PY in South Africa [135–137].

On the other hand, the incidence of unmasking (or ART-associated) IRIS is lower ranging from 0.2% to 1.6% as reported in two retrospective and three prospective studies [110, 137–140].

A meta-analysis of 54 cohort studies comprising more than 13.000 patients starting HAART indicated that CM was associated with the development of IRIS in 19.5% of cases (95% CrI 6.7–44.8%). It ranked second among the opportunistic infections more frequently associated with IRIS but, more notably, had the highest mortality attributed to the syndrome (20.8%) [141]. However, the study by Muller et al. was criticized because it failed to distinguish paradoxical from unmasking IRIS with the possible underestimate of the true frequency of paradoxical-cryptococcal IRIS [142]. The differences in the incidence of cryptococcal IRIS reported across different studies probably reflect the typology of the study (retrospective versus prospective), different clinical definitions employed, and different settings (resource-limited countries versus high-income countries). However, what is undoubted is the fact that cryptococcal IRIS is a true problem with an high expected burden especially in sub-Saharan Africa, Southeast Asia and Latin America [143]. The pathogenesis of cryptococcal IRIS is complex and not fully understood but is mainly attributable to the severe immunodeficiency that is unable to clear the foreign antigens and the subsequent cytokine storm induced by the restored inflammatory response [144].

Another controversial point is the establishment of the period of time during which the patients are at risk of developing cryptococcal IRIS. In fact, the time of appearance of IRIS varied quite widely among the different studies with the shortest interval after the start of HAART reported to be few days and the longest 22–27 months [145–148]. However, in four studies (two retrospective and two prospective) performed on patients affected by cryptococcosis the median time elapsing between initiation of HAART and onset of IRIS was reported to be 30 days (range 3–330 days) [135], 44 days (range 36–62 days) [149], 63 days (range 12–129 days) [150], and 8 months (range 2–37 months) [136]. It is plausible that the observed discrepancy can be explained by differences in the clinical pictures presented with less central nervous system involvement in the study reporting the longest interval [135]. This finding is in keeping with the results of a review of 25 episodes of IRIS-associated cryptococcosis showing a median time interval of 3.5 months for patients with CNS manifestations compared to 7 months for those with lymphadenitis [151].

In the case definition elaborated by the experts of INSHI, they proposed a maximum time of 12 months for the development of paradoxical IRIS after ART initiation; although acknowledging that the cut-off chosen was largely arbitrary and would exclude those occasional cases presenting after a longer interval, they believed that it might improve the specificity and its practical usefulness [134].

In a retrospective multicentre study from France, a diagnosis of cryptococcosis revealing HIV-infection (OR 4.8), presence of fungemia at baseline (OR 6.1), CD4 cell count of less than 7/μL (OR 4.0) and starting HAART within 2 months of diagnosis of cryptococcosis (OR 5.5) were identified in a multivariate model as independent risk factors for development of IRIS [136]. Another retrospective cohort study from USA showed that patients who had started HAART within 30 days after the diagnosis of cryptococcosis were more likely to develop IRIS (RR 1.73, 95% CI 1.03–2.29; $P = .031$) [135]. On the contrary, Bicanic et al. in a prospective observational study conducted in South Africa on 65 antiretroviral naïve patients affected by CM were unable to find any association with fungal burden, baseline CD4 cell count, HIV viral load and time to start of HAART, and the subsequent development of IRIS [149]. They showed that a more rapid and strong immunological response measured at 6 months (220 versus 124 CD4 cells/μL, $P = 0.01$) was the only variable associated with development of IRIS [149]. Finally, in Thailand the investigators found a higher baseline cryptococcal antigen as the only risk factor associated with development of IRIS [150].

Interestingly in a prospective study conducted in a cohort of ART-naïve Ugandans that aimed to identify serum biomarkers predictive of IRIS development, a 4-fold higher baseline concentrations of cryptococcal antigen was observed among patients who developed IRIS in comparison with those who did not develop IRIS [152]. In the same study higher levels of IL-4 and IL-17 and lower levels of TNF-α, granulocyte colony-stimulating factor (G-CSF), granulocyte-macrophage colony-stimulating factor (GM-CSF), and vascular endothelial growth factor (VEGF) were predictive of IRIS with a receiver operating characteristic (ROC) curve of 0.82. The same group showed that a paucity of inflammation in the cerebrospinal fluid at the time of CM is associated with failure to sterilize CSF at 2 weeks and subsequent risk of developing IRIS [153].

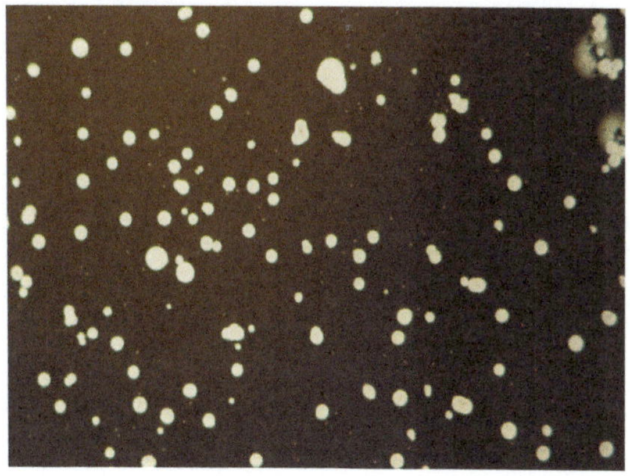

FIGURE 3: India ink preparation of cerebrospinal fluid showing yeast cells some of which budding surrounded by large capsule (Courtesy Dr Giuseppe Giuliani).

Clinical presentation of paradoxical IRIS can range from the more frequent picture of relapsing meningitis with raised intracranial pressure and negative CSF culture [13, 130, 135, 136, 138–140, 145, 149, 150, 154–158] to other less frequent central nervous system diseases (i.e., cerebral cryptococcoma, intramedullary abscess, cerebellitis with mass effect, visual and hearing loss, and radiculitis) [135, 136, 146, 147, 159–163] or alternatively may present with extraneural pictures (Table 3). Lymphadenopathy [128, 135, 136, 145, 147, 151, 158, 164], pulmonary disease, including cavitating,necrotizing and nodular lesions [130, 136, 165], subcutaneous abscess and erosive bone lesions [129, 164, 165] are the extraneural manifestations of paradoxical cryptococcal IRIS. The clinical manifestations of ART-associated cryptococcosis (comprising also unmasking disease) are essentially similar, with a predominance of meningitis [110, 129, 135, 149], lymphadenopathy, and subcutaneous abscesses [166–170].

Cryptococcal IRIS, especially when presenting with CNS manifestation, is a potentially lethal disease [136, 140, 145, 149, 151, 157] with an average fatality of about 20% [141]. Different approaches in the management of this complication have been employed including anti-inflammatory steroidal [136, 145, 155, 156, 160, 164], and nonsteroidal therapy [164, 165], thalidomide [136], anti-TNF monoclonal antibody [171], surgery [130, 136, 147, 151], and antifungal therapy (including increased dosage, change of drug or resumed antifungal therapy) [129, 130, 151, 154, 155, 157, 159].

9. Laboratory Diagnosis

A definitive diagnosis of CM is made by positive CSF culture and/or direct identification of the organism by means of India ink staining (Figure 3). *Cryptococcus neoformans*, however, is able to disseminate and infect most areas of the body (i.e., lung, skin, lymph node, spleen, liver, prostate, eye, bone, bone marrow, heart, thyroid, adrenal gland, muscle) and thus it can

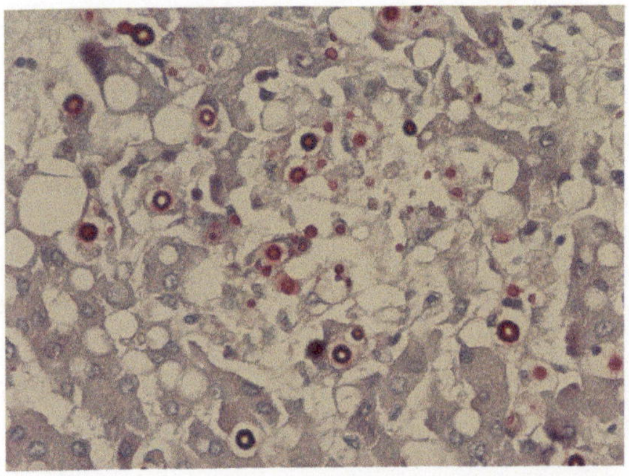

Figure 4: Liver histology showing PAS-positive yeast cells in a case of disseminated cryptococcosis (Courtesy Dr. Carlo Parravicini).

be cultured or shown by histopathology as well from different body specimens (Figure 4). Blood cultures are reported to be positive in 47–70% of HIV-infected patients as compared to 21% of HIV-uninfected patients with CM (Table 1).

A presumptive diagnosis of CM can be made on the basis of a positive cryptococcal antigen (CrAg) using a latex agglutination or an enzyme immunoassay kit. Cryptococcal antigen testing on blood and CSF is a highly reliable and rapid diagnostic technique with excellent sensitivity and specificity [172]. Sensitivity of CSF cryptococcal antigen test is 92% to 96% in patients with culture-proven CM (Table 1). False positive results are associated with rarer infections due to *Trichosporon beigelii*, *Capnocytophaga canimorsus*, and *Stomatococcus mucilaginosus* and, on the contrary, false negative results are observed either with poorly encapsulated organisms and low fungal burden or the prozone phenomenon [173–175].

HIV-positive patients usually have very high serum and CSF CrAg titres than their HIV-negative counterpart as a reflection of the higher yeast burden and, in the pre-HAART era, both were predictive of mycological failure and poor outcome [8, 13]. In one cohort study conducted in Uganda among HIV-infected adults, detectable cryptococcal antigenemia preceded symptoms by a median of 22 days and approximately 11% of people had cryptococcal antigenaemia for more than 100 days [28].

In areas of high prevalence of cryptococcosis, the use of serum CrAg as a screening test is helpful to identify those HIV-infected people with advanced disease at risk of developing cryptococcal meningitis and who might benefit of a preemptive antifungal treatment together with antiretroviral therapy [107–110, 113]. A summary of studies reporting on detection of CrAg is reported in Table 2 [28, 106–116].

Using a cut-off value of >1:8 the CrAg assay was 100% sensitive and 96% specific for predicting incident CM during the first year of HAART [109]. Subsequently, in a prospective observational study conducted in Kampala (Uganda), Meya and coworkers showed that CrAg testing targeting people with severe immunodeficiency (less than 100 CD4+ cell/μL) was a cost-effective measure showing 71% survival at 30-month of those treated with fluconazole together with HAART compared with 100% deaths within 2 months in those treated only with HAART [110].

In 2009, a new lateral flow assay (LFA) characterized by rapidity (5–15 minutes), stability at room temperature, and affordability (1.5 to 2.5 US $) was developed for the detection of cryptococcal antigen on serum, CSF, and urine [198]. All the above mentioned characteristics made it an ideal test to be used at point-of-care (POC) in resource-limited countries. This dipstick assay has been evaluated and validated against EIA positive sera and *Cryptococcus* positive blood culture from HIV-positive patients from Thailand, showing sensitive ranging from 96% to 100%, respectively [199]. In another retrospective study using serum, plasma and urine from patients with HIV-associated cryptococcal meningitis sensitivity was 100% for serum and plasma and 98% for urine [200]. It has been suggested that the ratio of titres measured by latex agglutination (LA) in comparison with LFA is 1:5 [201] but a small study found imperfect agreement (LFA:LA 1.53 with confidence limits from 0.13 to 18.1) [202]. Based on all the above mentioned studies, it has been proposed to integrate CrAg as a screening test into routine HIV care not only in resource-limited settings but also in western countries [200, 202, 203].

Finally two studies showed cross-reactivity between the Platelia *Aspergillus* galactomannan assay and serum from patients with cryptococcal meningitis with positive results ranging from 13.6 to 63.3% [204, 205].

10. Prognosis and Outcome

Left untreated CM is a uniformly fatal disease but even with antifungal treatment the outcome is influenced either by factors associated with the host and the underlying diseases and the fungus [206]. Several studies have confirmed that abnormal mental status [14, 74, 207], high cerebrospinal fungal burden (demonstrated by high cryptococcal antigen titers or colony forming unit) [20, 74, 76, 77, 122, 183, 184, 207], disseminated infection [20], wasting syndrome (low body mass index) [83] symptomatic elevated ICP [121], low CSF leukocyte cell counts [14, 71], lack of flucytosine treatment during induction phase [20], induction treatment with low dose fluconazole [82, 85, 207] are factors associated with poor outcome of AIDS-related CM.

In the Antiretroviral Therapy Cohort Collaboration study (including 15 cohorts with over 31,000 HIV-positive patients without prior AIDS-defining events who started HAART), cryptococcosis ranked third (after non-Hodgkin lymphoma and progressive multifocal leukoencephalopathy), as a cause of death overall and within the first 6 months after the beginning of therapy [208]. However, the introduction of HAART has witnessed a marked increase of survival of patients with cryptococcal meningitis either in resource poor- and in high-income countries [13, 14, 209]. The 14-day survival rates among antiretroviral-naïve persons with CM was 49% in 2001-02 and 80% in 2006 in Kampala, Uganda [14]. However, the 1-year survival rate in Uganda remains 4-fold worse than in France and 2-fold worse than in Thailand even with the availability of HAART [20, 210]. Another

Table 2: Summary of published studies regarding cryptococcal antigenaemia in HIV-positive patients.

Author, year of publication, reference	Country	Type of study/Population	CrAg asymptomatic prevalence	All CrAg positive	Comment
			Africa		
Desmet et al., 1998 [106]	Kinshasa, Zaire	Cohort/450 adults	15/450 (3.3%)	55/450 (12.2%)	29 out of 44 had CSF positive microscopy/culture for *C. neoformans*
French et al., 2002 [28]	Entebbe, Uganda	Cohort/1372 adults	7/77 (9.1%)	77/1372 (6.6%)	CrAg preceded onset of symptoms by a median of 22 days
Tassie et al., 2003 [107]	Mbarara, Uganda	Cohort/197 adults	8/197 (4.1%)	21/197 (10.7%)	13 pts had CM
Liechty et al., 2007 [108]	Kampala, Uganda	Retrospective/395 adults	22/377 (5.8)	44/395 (11.1)	7 pts newly diagnosed with CM, 3 of whom had a positive serum CrAg at baseline; asymptomatic CrAg independent risk factor for death (RR 6.6)
Jarvis et al., 2009 [109]	Cape Town, South Africa	Retrospective/707 adults	25/707 (3.5)*	46/707 (7%)	13 out of 46 (28%) developed new or relapsed CM; CrAg independent risk factor for death (HR 3.1)
Meya et al., 2010 [110]	Kampala, Uganda	Prospective cohort/609 adults	33/592 (5.6%) 26/295 (8.8% incidence) < 100 CD4+/μL 7/298 (2.3%) > 100 CD4+/μL	50/609 (8.2%)	17 had pre-Art diagnosed CM; preemptive treatment cost-effective (NNTac 6.5; NNTad 10)
Mamoojee et al., 2011 [111]	Kumasi, Ghana	Retrospective/92 adults	2/92 (2%)	2/92 (2%)	This study suggested a limited value of CrAg testing in this area
Oyella et al., 2012 [112]	Kampala, Uganda	Cross-sectional/367 adults	45/367 (12.2%)	69/367 (18.8%)	Only 30 pts undergo lumbar puncture; 24 out of 30 had CM
			South-east Asia		
Micol et al., 2007 [113]	Phnom Penh, Cambodia	Prospective cohort/327 adults	10/327 (3.1%)	58/327 (17.7 %)	41 pts had CM
Pongsai et al., 2010 [114]	Bangkok, Thailand	Retrospective/131 adults	8/131 (6.1%)	12/131 (9.2%)	3 out of 12 had CM, 1 pulmonary cryptococcosis
			Europe and USA		
Feldmesser et al., 1996 [115]	USA	Case series/10 adults	7/10 (70%)	10	First study about isolated CrAg
Patel et al., 2013 [116]	London, UK	Retrospective/157 adults	1/157 (0.6%)	7/157 (4.4%)	7 pts diagnosed with CM

CrAg: cryptococcal antigenemia, CM: cryptococcal meningitis, UK: United Kingdom; RR: relative risk; HR: hazard ratio; NNTac: number needed to treat to avoid a case; NNTad: number needed to treat to avoid death.
*Only patients without a history of cryptococcal meningitis were considered.

important point is the still high early mortality associated with CM that is apparently not influenced by HAART: 18% probability of death versus 21% at 3 months, respectively, in the pre-HAART and post-HAART period in France or 15% deaths at 2 weeks and 31% at 10 weeks in four cohorts in Thailand, Uganda, and South Africa [209, 210].

11. Antifungal Treatment

Several clinical trials or cohort studies regarding antifungal therapy for AIDS-associated CM have been performed and published over the last 22 years and are summarized in Table 4 [74, 76, 85, 177–182, 185–197]. However, it is worth noting that much of these studies have been hampered by several drawbacks such as low number of patients enrolled, low dosages of antifungal employed, different end-points, short follow-up. Current management of AIDS-associated CM is largely based on the results of the landmark randomized trial published over a decade ago [76]. It is based on three distinct phases: induction, consolidation, and maintenance therapy. The induction phase is aimed to achieve rapid fungicidal activity to obtain CSF sterility using the combination of amphotericin B deoxycholate (0.7 mg/kg/day) and 5- fluorocytosine (100 mg/kg/day) for two weeks. The combination of amphotericin B deoxycholate (AmB) and fluorocytosine (5-FC) is more rapidly fungicidal than amphotericin B alone and is associated with a trend towards a higher proportion of patients achieving a sterile CSF at 2 weeks and a reduced relapse rate [76]. The consolidation phase is the subsequent 8-week treatment period with either fluconazole (400 mg/day) or itraconazole (400 mg/day) as an alternative for patients with fluconazole intolerance. The maintenance phase or secondary prophylaxis of treatment for CM in HIV-infected subjects is imperative in order to prevent the high relapse rate of this meningitis. Oral fluconazole at a dosage of 200 mg/day has been shown to be superior to weekly intravenous AmB [211], placebo [212], or oral itraconazole [213]. Although the above mentioned treatment is endorsed by IDSA guidelines as the recommended first line treatment of AIDS-associated CM [123], it is far from being completely satisfactory because during the induction phase, it is unable to achieve CSF sterility in all patients and it is associated with a still high acute mortality; moreover, one of its component (i.e., 5-FC) is not available in most developing countries where CM is prevalent. One of the goals that needs to be achieved in the treatment of CM, especially among immunocompromised patients, is that of rapidly and efficiently reduce the huge burden of yeast cells in the CSF. In this regard in an elegant randomized study performed in Thailand, using for the first time the rate of reduction in CSF colony forming units from serial quantitative CSF cultures, Brouwer and coworkers demonstrated that the combination of AmB plus 5-FC had the highest and most rapid fungicidal activity compared to AmB alone, AmB plus fluconazole or all the three drugs together [183]. Since AmB shows concentration-dependent antifungal activity, the same group conducted a randomized controlled trial in 64 HIV-infected antiretroviral naïve patients to compare the standard of care with a higher drug dosage (i.e., 1 mg/kg/day) [185]. Although they showed that the higher dosage had a significantly greater early fungicidal activity compared to the standard dose (−0.56 log cfu/mL versus −0.45 log cfu/mL, $P = .02$), mortality at 2 and 10 weeks was not statistically different in the two arms [185].

However, analyzing combined data of early fungicidal activity collected from different cohorts, Bicanic and coworkers were able to show that the magnitude of this was inversely associated with mortality at 2 and 10 weeks and in a multivariate models (that included altered mental status and fungal burden), it remained independently associated with mortality [207]. As discussed by the Authors it is unknown if this relationship is linear or if exists a threshold value above which no further benefit of early fungicidal activity will be observed.

In consideration of the fact that 5-FC is presently unavailable in several resource-limited areas where, on the contrary, fluconazole might be obtained free of charge through the Pfizer program or as a cheap generic drug, a phase II randomized open label trial was conducted in Thailand and USA comparing three arms (AmB at 0.7 mg/kg versus AmB at the same dosage plus fluconazole 400 mg or 800 mg per day) [188]. Using a composite efficacy end-point (CSF negative culture, stable neurological function, and survival) the arm employing higher dosage of fluconazole showed the better response (53.7 versus 28.3 versus 42.5) at 2 weeks [188]. The 2011 WHO guidelines for the management of cryptococcal disease in HIV-infected subjects strongly recommend treatment with amphotericin-based regimens [214] but in the real life a strategy employing fluconazole monotherapy is generally used. High-dose fluconazole (1200 mg/day) plus 5-FC with or without a short-course (7 days) of AmB has been shown to significantly enhance early fungicidal activity and more rapid fungal clearance form CSF although the studies were not powered for clinical end-points [192, 197].

A very interesting decision analysis study based on the results of cryptococcal trials in resource-limited areas and expected life assumptions, provided some evidence that a short-course (1-week) of AmB (1 mg/kg/d) associated with high-dose fluconazole (1200 mg/d) for 2 weeks is the most cost-effective induction treatment among the 6 regimens evaluated [215].

The French CryptoA/D prospective observational study performed on both HIV-positive or negative patients with a first episode of CM showed that also in the "real life" the best regimen for induction therapy is the combination of AmB and 5-FC [20]. Treatment failure at week 2 was documented in 26% of patients receiving AmB+5-FC in contrast with 56% with any other treatments ($P < 0.001$). Moreover, a 5-FC prescription shorter than 14 days was one of the variables independently associated with treatment failure at 3 months of follow-up confirming the results of the study of van der Horst [20, 76]. Interestingly the Authors documented that only 49% of French clinicians adhered to the recommendations of the IDSA guidelines to use the combination therapy for meningoencephalitis [20]. In a multivariate analysis the use of AmB+5-FC rather than

Table 3: Clinical manifestations of paradoxical and ART-associated cryptococcosis.

Clinical syndrome	References
Paradoxical cryptococcal IRIS	
Meningitis	[13, 130, 135, 136, 138–140, 145, 149, 150, 154–158]
Other CNS-IRIS manifestations	
(i) Intracranial space-occupying lesion/s	[136, 146, 159, 160]
(ii) Meningoradiculitis	[163]
(iii) Hearing loss	[161]
Lymphadenopathy	[135, 136, 145, 147, 151, 158, 164]
Cutaneous and/or soft-tissue lesions	[130, 165, 176]
Pneumonia or pulmonary nodules	[130, 136, 145]
ART-associated cryptococcal IRIS	
Unmasking meningitis	[129, 135]
Lymphadenopathy	[166, 169]
Cutaneous and/or soft-tissue lesions	[168, 170]
Pneumonia	[167]

Table 4: Summary of main clinical studies of antifungal induction phase for AIDS-associated cryptococcal meningitis since 1990.

Author, year of publication, reference	Study design/location	Drugs	Duration of treatment	Number of cases versus comparators	Clinical response (%)	Mycological response (%) or (EFA)^	Overall (clinical + mycological) response (%)	Mortality (%)
Larsen et al., 1990 [177]	RCT/USA	Flu (400 mg) versus AmB (0.7 mg/kg) for 1 week then three-times weekly + 5FC (150 mg/kg)	10 weeks	14 versus 6	63	75	43 versus 100	19 versus 0 ($P = 0.27$)
Saag et al., 1992 [74]	RCT (2 : 1)/USA	Flu (200 mg) versus AmB (0.4 mg/kg)	10 weeks	131 versus 63	60 versus 67	43 versus 46 (10 weeks)	44 versus 40	15 versus 8 (2 weeks) 14 versus 18
De Gans et al., 1992 [178]	RCT (non-blinded)/The Netherlands	Itra (400 mg) versus AmB (0.3 mg/kg) + 5FC (150 mg/kg)	6 weeks	12 versus 10	NR	NR	42 versus 100	0
Coker et al., 1993 [179]	OS/Multicentre (Europe)	LAMB (4 mg/kg/d)	2 weeks	23	74	66.7	NR	0
Menichetti et al., 1996 [180]	Cohort/Italy	Flu (800–1000 mg/d)	3 weeks	14	54.5 (10 weeks)	NR	67.1	18.2
van Der Horst et al., 1997 [76]	RCT/USA	AmB (0.7 mg/kg) + 5FC (100 mg/kg) versus AmB (0.7 mg/kg)	2 weeks	202 versus 179	78 versus 83	60 versus 51 (2 weeks)	NR	Overall 5.5 (2 weeks); 3.9 (10 weeks)
Leenders et al., 1997 [181]	RCT/The Netherlands	L-AmB (4 mg/kg) versus Amb (0.7 mg/kg)	3 weeks	15 versus 13	87 versus 83 (10 weeks)	73 versus 38 (3 weeks)		Overall 10.7
Mayanja-Kizza et al., 1998 [182]	RCT/Uganda	Flu (200 mg/d) + 5FC (150 mg/kg/d) versus Flu (200 mg/d)	8 weeks	30 versus 28	NR	NR	32 versus 12	60 versus 84 (2 weeks); 68 versus 88 (6 months)
Brouwer et al., 2004 [183]	RCT/Thailand	AmB (0.7 mg/kg) + FC (100 mg/kg) versus AmB (0.7 mg/kg) versus AmB (0.7 mg/kg) + Flu (400 mg) + FC (100 mg/kg) versus AmB (0.7 mg/kg) + Flu (400 mg)	2 weeks	15 versus 16 versus 16 versus 16	NR	−0.54 versus −0.31 versus −0.38 versus −0.39^	64 (10 weeks)	Overall 14.6 (2 weeks); 21.9 (10 weeks)
Schaars et al., 2006 [85]	Retrospective chart review/South Africa	Flu (200 mg/d) year 1991–2000 Flu (400 mg/d) 2001		77 versus 128	NR	NR	NR	23.4 versus 26.6
Bicanic et al., 2007 [184]	POT/South Africa	AmB (1 mg/kg) versus Flu 400 mg	10 weeks	49 versus 5	67 versus 25*	−0.48 versus −0.02^	38 versus 0†	Overall mortality 17 (2 weeks); 37 (10 weeks)
Bicanic et al., 2008 [185]	RCT/South Africa	AmB (1 mg/kg) + 5FC (100 mg) versus AmB (0.7 mg/kg) + 5FC (100 mg)	2 weeks	34 versus 30	74 versus 79*	−0.56 versus −0.45^	60†	3 versus 9 (2 weeks); 21 versus 26 (10 weeks). Overall mortality 24 (10 weeks) and no differences between groups

Table 4: Continued.

Author, year of publication, reference	Study design/location	Drugs	Duration of treatment	Number of cases versus comparators	Clinical response (%)	Mycological response (%) or (EFA)^	Overall (clinical + mycological) response (%)	Mortality (%)
Longley et al., 2008 [186]	Cohort/Uganda	Flu (800 mg) versus Flu (1200 mg) then 400 mg	2 weeks + 8 weeks	30 versus 30	NR	−0.07 versus −0.18^	40 versus 52*	37 versus 22 (2 weeks) 60 versus 48 (10 weeks)
Dammert et al., 2008 [187]	Cohort/Perù	AmB (0.7 mg/kg/d)	2-3 weeks	47	NR	25 (2 weeks) 68 (10 weeks)	70 (10 weeks)	13 (2 weeks) 22 (10 weeks)
Pappas et al., 2009 [188]	RCT/USA and Thailand	AmB (0.7 mg/kg) versus AmB (0.7 mg/kg) + Flu (400 mg) versus AmB (0.7 mg/kg) + Flu (800 mg)	2 weeks	46 versus 48 versus 41	42.5 versus 28.3 versus 52.3	NR	71.4 versus 84.2 versus 83.3 (10 weeks)	22 versus 17 versus 18.4 (10 weeks)
Hamill et al., 2010 [189]	RCT/USA and Canada	LamB (3 mg/kg/d) versus LamB (6 mg/kg/d) versus AmB (0.7 mg/kg/d)	2 weeks (11–21 days)	86 versus 94 versus 87	65.8 versus 75.3 versus 65.8 (2 weeks) 70.5 versus 72.9 versus 81.5 (10 weeks)	58.3 versus 48 versus 47.5 (2 weeks) 60 versus 70.7 versus 78.7	67.5 versus 73.7 versus 75.5 (10 weeks)	14 versus 9.6 versus 11.5 (10 weeks) Overall mortality at 10 weeks 11.6%
Lightowler et al., 2010 [190]	Cohort/South Africa	AmB (0.7 mg/kg/d) versus Flu (400 mg/d)	2 weeks	148 versus 28	NR	NR	Fluconazole associated with 5.1 RR of death at 28 days	Overall 28 (2 weeks); 32.3 (10 weeks)
Falci et al., 2010 [191]	Pilot/Brazil	AmB (0.7 mg/kg/d) continuous infusion (24-h) + FC (100 mg/k/d)	2 weeks	12	NR	−0.37^	80	10 (2 weeks); 10 (10 weeks)
Nussbaum et al., 2010 [192]	RCT/Malawi	Flu (1200 mg/d) versus Flu (1200 mg/d) + FC (100 mg/kg/d)	2 weeks	20 versus 21	NR	−0.11 versus −0.28^	NR	10 versus 37 (2 weeks); 43 versus 58 (10 weeks) Overall 48.8
Jadhav et al., 2010 [193]	RCT/India	LamB (1 mg/kg) versus LamB (3 mg/kg)	3 weeks	11 versus 15	NR	NR	36.6 versus 54	Overall 27 (10 weeks)
Loyse et al., 2012 [194]	RCT/South Africa	AmB (0.7–1 mg/kg) + 5FC (100 mg/d) versus AmB (0.7–1 mg/kg/d) + Flu (800 mg/d) versus AmB (0.7–1 mg/kg) + Flu (1200 mg/d) versus AmB (0.7–1 mg/kg) + Vor (600 mg/d)	2 weeks	21 versus 22 versus 24 versus 14	NR	−0.41 versus −0.38 versus −0.41 versus −0.44^	NR	Overall 12 (2 weeks); 29 (10 weeks) (no statistically significant differences among groups)
Muzoora et al., 2012 [195]	Cohort/Uganda	Flu (1200 mg/d) + AmB (1 mg/kg/d)	2 weeks	30	NR	−0.31 (2 weeks)^	NR	23 (2 weeks); 28 (10 weeks)

Table 4: Continued.

Author, year of publication, reference	Study design/location	Drugs	Duration of treatment	Number of cases versus comparators	Clinical response (%)	Mycological response (%) or (EFA)^	Overall (clinical + mycological) response (%)	Mortality (%)
Jarvis et al., 2012 [196]	RCT/South Africa	AmB (1 mg/kg/d) + 5FC (100 mg/kg/d) versus AmB (1 mg/kg/d) + 5FC (100 mg/kg/d) + IFNγ (100 μg) 2 doses versus AmB (1 mg/kg/d) + 5FC (100 mg/kg/d) + IFNγ (100 μg) 6 doses	2 weeks	31 versus 29 versus 30	NR	−0.49 versus 0.64 versus −0.64^	NR	32 versus 33 versus 27 (10 weeks) Overall 14 (2 weeks) 27 (10 weeks)
Jackson et al., 2012 [197]	RCT/Malawi	Flu (1200 mg/d) + AmB (1 mg/kg/d) versus Flu (1200 mg/d) + 5FC (100 mg/kg/d) + AmB (1 mg/kg/d for 7 days)	2 weeks	20 versus 20	NR	−0.38 versus −0.50^	NR	No statistically significant differences at 2 and 10 weeks between the arms

RCT: randomized controlled trial; OS: open label study; NR: not reported; EFA: early fungicidal activity ^expressed as mean log CFU/mL; Flu: fluconazole; amB: amphotericin B deox; Itra: itraconazole; 5FC: 5-fluorocytosine; LAMB: liposomal amphotericin B; IFNγ: interferon-gamma; Vor: voriconazole; *percentage of patients surviving at weeks 10: †proportion of patients surviving after 1 year of followup.

AmB was independently associated with a high CSF CrAg titre whereas the prescription of AmB+5-FC rather than fluconazole was independently associated with high CSF CrAg titre and younger age. One might suppose that older patients are treated with fluconazole because of the better profile of tolerability but this choice exposes patients to a risk of worst outcome as it has been clearly documented.

Although AmB is still recommended as the drug of choice for induction therapy of CM by authoritative guidelines [123, 214], its use is frequently complicated by infusion-related adverse effects and nephrotoxicity that can affect mortality [216]. Results from small studies have indicated that liposomal amphotericin B (L-AMB) may represent a safer alternative to AmB with similar mycological success rates [179, 181]. A multicenter double-blind randomized comparative study performed in USA and Canada using 2 different dosages of L-AMB (3 and 6 mg/kg/day) versus conventional AmB (0.7 mg/kg/day) found similar results for primary efficacy end-point (negative CSF culture at week 2) and in the mortality rate in the 3 groups of patients (13.9%, 9.5%, and 11.5%, respectively, in the 3 and 6 mg of L-AMB and in the conventional AmB) [189]. Patients treated with L-AMB had a significantly lower incidence of infusion-related reactions compared with those treated with AmB ($P < .001$) and less nephrotoxicity with the lower dosage of L-AMB ($P = .004$). Thus the results of this study confirmed that the main advantage using L-AMB instead of AmB in the treatment of AIDS-associated cryptococcosis is a better tolerability without any significant improvement in the outcome. Recently the expert committee panel of the British HIV Association recommended the use of L-AMB (4 mg/kg/d) as preferred amphotericin B preparation for the induction therapy of AIDS-associated CM [217]. On the basis of economic considerations, other UK experts argued strongly against this endorsement [218]. Finally, two new questions, that will be discussed in the next session, emerged as the consequence of the implementation of very efficacious antiretroviral therapy in the HIV setting: (1) the appropriate time of starting ARV (antiretroviral) therapy after the diagnosis of CM; (2) the time and threshold of CD4+ lymphocytes at which maintenance therapy can be safely discontinued.

12. When to Start ARV Therapy and When Discontinue Antifungal Maintenance Therapy

Among HIV-infected patients with advanced disease such as those with a diagnosis of CM, there is general agreement that ARV therapy should be started as soon as possible since its deferral is associated with further HIV-related diseases and increased mortality. However, the risk of severe and potentially fatal IRIS associated with an unsterilized CSF infection is an argument against an early or concomitant (with antifungal therapy) ARV therapy. An open-label randomized strategy study of early (within 2 weeks) versus deferred (after acute therapy for opportunistic infection was completed) ARV therapy among subjects with different opportunistic infections demonstrated that the early strategy was associated with fewer AIDS progression and death [219]. However this study was underpowered with to regard CM and presented a low incidence than expected of IRIS (7%). In sharp contrast with the results of the above mentioned study, another open-label prospective study conducted in Zimbabwe showed a 3-fold greater risk of mortality in the early ARV group (within 72 hours after CM diagnosis) in comparison with the delayed ARV group (after 10 weeks of treatment with fluconazole) [220]. Worth noting the Cryptococcal Optimal ART Timing (COAT) study conducted in Uganda and South Africa under the US National Institute of Health sponsorship was ended prematurely after an interim analysis found a 1.7 times worse survival observed among patients receiving early ARV treatment (http://www.niaid.nih.gov/news/newsreleases/2012/Pages/COAT.aspx).

It has been supposed but not proved that the fungistatic effect of fluconazole used in one study [220] as opposed to the fungicidal action of AmB used in the other study [219] could account for an increased risk of IRIS [221]. On the ground of this uncertainty guidelines offer options to start ARV therapy between 2 and 10 weeks after antifungal therapy [123, 214, 222]. The conditional recommendation of the WHO guidelines that indicates a different time option of deferred ARV initiation according to the drug regimen used in the induction and consolidation treatment seems reasonable [214].

The question regarding when antifungal maintenance therapy can be safely discontinued in patients responding to ARV therapy and at what threshold of CD4+ lymphocytes it should be done has been so far addressed in five case studies [223–227], three observational cohorts [228–230], and in one randomized controlled trial [231]. A total of 227 patients have been evaluated following discontinuation of prophylaxis: they had a median CD4+ cell count ranging from 167 to 297 cells/μL, a median duration of HAART ranging from 6 to 42.5 months and a median follow-up ranging from 9 to 28.4 months after discontinuation [232]. The calculated incidence of relapse was very low and varied from 0 to 1.53 per 100 PY thus providing the basis for the indication of discontinue maintenance therapy after at least 12 months of antifungal therapy with undetectable HIVRNA (>3 months) and a sustained CD4+ cell count > 100 cells/μL [123].

13. Prevention

In the pre-HAART era, a randomized clinical trial comparing fluconazole 200 mg/day with clotrimazole troches for prevention of fungal infections in AIDS patients demonstrated a sevenfold reduction in the risk of cryptococcosis [233]. Subsequently several other studies some of which not designed for cryptococcal prevention demonstrated that weekly administration of fluconazole at different dosages (ranging from 100 mg up to 400 mg) was successful as primary prophylaxis of CM in patients with advanced HIV disease [234–236]. However, all these studies were performed in the pre-HAART era and the policy of primary prophylaxis for CM was not recommended because of the lack of evidence of any survival benefit, the high cost associated and the risk of development of fungal resistance.

In contrast with the above mentioned lack of survival benefit a randomized double-blind placebo-controlled study performed in Thailand showed a reduction of overall mortality (HR 4.3) in patients receiving weekly fluconazole (400 mg) compared to placebo although the study had a low statistical power with wide confidence intervals for the mortality benefit (0.9–19.8) [237]. A case-control study performed in a metropolitan area of United States characterized by a high prevalence of indigent population and with a low prevalence of HAART use (12–23%) showed a protective role of azole use in preventing invasive cryptococcal disease [238].

Modelling of data from a high endemic region for cryptococcosis in resource-limited settings suggested that screening for cryptococcal antigen with preemptive treatment was more cost-effective in patients with CD4+ lymphocytes between 51–100 cells/μL with primary prophylaxis better when CD4+ are below 50 cells/μL [239].

Finally, a large double-blind randomized placebo controlled trial conducted in Africa provided evidence that fluconazole (200 mg) three times weekly was effective as primary prophylaxis against cryptococcal disease both before and during the early ARV therapy [240]. Moreover, although fluconazole therapy did not influence the all-cause mortality, it indeed reduced the mortality due to cryptococcosis. The results of this study make scientific strength to one of the possible strategy to be implemented in high-risk patients living in high-risk setting to protect against development of cryptococcal disease until immune reconstitution occurs.

14. Conclusions

Cryptococcal meningitis remains a major cause of morbidity and mortality among HIV-positive patients especially in resource-poor areas. ART is responsible of a dramatic improvement of outcome but it is associated with the possible onset of IRIS that is potentially fatal. In this regard, the optimal timing of ART beginning after the diagnosis of HIV-associated cryptococcal meningitis is unclear. Screening severe immunocompromised HIV-positive patients with the new lateral flow assay to detect CrAg is highly cost effective.

References

[1] B. J. Park, K. A. Wannemuehler, B. J. Marston, N. Govender, P. G. Pappas, and T. M. Chiller, "Estimation of the current global burden of cryptococcal meningitis among persons living with HIV/AIDS," *AIDS*, vol. 23, no. 4, pp. 525–530, 2009.

[2] E. W. Bratton, N. El Husseini, C. A. Chastan et al., "Comparison and temporal trends of three groups with cryptococcosis: HIV-infected, solid organ transplant, and HIV-negative/non-transplant," *PLoS One*, vol. 7, Article ID e43582, 2012.

[3] F. Sanfelice, "Contributo alla morfologia e biologia dei blastomiceti che si sviluppano nei succhi di alcuni frutti," *Annali di Igiene*, vol. 5, pp. 232–262, 1894.

[4] O. Busse, "Uber parasitare zelleinschlusse und threzuchtung," *Zbl Bakt I Abt*, vol. 16, pp. 175–180, 1894.

[5] A. Buschke, "Ueber eine durch coccidien hervegerufene krankheit des menschen," *Deutsche Medizinische Wochenschrift*, vol. 21, no. 1, pp. 14–15, 1895.

[6] J. A. Barnett, "A history of research on yeasts 14:1 medical yeasts—part 2: *Cryptococcus neoformans*," *Yeast*, vol. 27, no. 11, pp. 875–904, 2010.

[7] S. L. Chuck and M. A. Sande, "Infections with *Cryptococcus neoformans* in the acquired immunodeficiency syndrome," *The New England Journal of Medicine*, vol. 321, no. 12, pp. 794–799, 1989.

[8] F. Dromer, S. Mathoulin, B. Dupont, and A. Laporte, "Epidemiology of cryptococcosis in France: a 9-year survey (1985–1993). French Cryptococcosis Study Group," *Clinical Infectious Diseases*, vol. 23, no. 1, pp. 82–90, 1996.

[9] B. Speed and D. Dunt, "Clinical and host differences between infections with the two varieties of *Cryptococcus neoformans*," *Clinical Infectious Diseases*, vol. 21, no. 1, pp. 28–34, 1995.

[10] S. A. Mirza, M. Phelan, D. Rimland et al., "The changing epidemiology of cryptococcosis: an update from population-based active surveillance in 2 large metropolitan areas, 1992–2000," *Clinical Infectious Diseases*, vol. 36, no. 6, pp. 789–794, 2003.

[11] L. J. R. van Elden, A. M. E. Walenkamp, M. M. Lipovsky et al., "Declining number of patients with cryptococcosis in the Netherlands in the era of highly active antiretroviral therapy," *AIDS*, vol. 14, no. 17, pp. 2787–2788, 2000.

[12] F. Dromer, S. Mathoulin-Pélissier, A. Fontanet, O. Ronin, B. Dupont, and O. Lortholary, "Epidemiology of HIV-associated cryptococcosis in France (1985–2001): comparison of the pre- and post-HAART eras," *AIDS*, vol. 18, no. 3, pp. 555–562, 2004.

[13] S. Antinori, A. L. Ridolfo, M. Fasan et al., "AIDS-associated cryptococcosis: a comparison of epidemiology, clinical features and outcome in the pre- and post-HAART eras. Experience of a single centre in Italy," *HIV Medicine*, vol. 10, no. 1, pp. 6–11, 2009.

[14] A. Kambugu, D. B. Meya, J. Rhein et al., "Outcomes of cryptococcal meningitis in Uganda before and after the availability of highly active antiretroviral therapy," *Clinical Infectious Diseases*, vol. 46, no. 11, pp. 1694–1701, 2008.

[15] J. N. Jarvis, A. Boulle, A. Loyse et al., "High ongoing burden of cryptococcal disease in Africa despite antiretroviral roll out," *AIDS*, vol. 23, no. 9, pp. 1182–1183, 2009.

[16] J. R. Harris, M. D. Lindsley, S. Henchaichon et al., "High prevalence of cryptococcal infection among HIV-infected patients hospitalized with pneumonia in Thailand," *Clinical Infectious Diseases*, vol. 54, no. 5, pp. e43–e50, 2012.

[17] K. J. Kwon-Chung, T. Boekhout, J. W. Fell, and M. Diaz, "Proposal to conserve the name *Cryptococcus gattii* against *C. hondurianus* and *C. bacillisporus* (*Basidiomycota, Hymenomycetes, Tremellomycetidae*)," *Taxon*, vol. 51, no. 4, pp. 804–806, 2002.

[18] K. J. Kwon-Chung and A. Varma, "Do major species concepts support one, two or more species within *Cryptococcus neoformans*?" *FEMS Yeast Research*, vol. 6, no. 4, pp. 574–587, 2006.

[19] X. Lin and J. Heitman, "The biology of the *Cryptococcus neoformans* species complex," *Annual Review of Microbiology*, vol. 60, pp. 69–105, 2006.

[20] F. Dromer, S. Mathouline-Pélissier, O. Launay, O. Lotholary, and The French Cryptococcosis Study Group, "Determinants of disease presentation and outcome during cryptococcosis: the CryptoA/D study," *PLoS Medicine*, vol. 4, no. 2, article e21, 2007.

[21] D. H. Mitchell, T. C. Sorrell, A. M. Allworth et al., "Cryptococcal disease of the CNS in immunocompetent hosts: influence of cryptococcal variety on clinical manifestations and outcome," *Clinical Infectious Diseases*, vol. 20, no. 3, pp. 611–616, 1995.

[22] S. C. Chen, M. A. Slavin, C. H. Heath et al., "Clinical manifestations of *Cryptococcus gattii* infection: determinants of neurological sequelae and death," *Clinical Infectious Diseases*, vol. 55, no. 6, pp. 789–798, 2012.

[23] T. Boekhout, B. Theelen, M. Diaz et al., "Hybrid genotypes in the pathogenic yeast *Cryptococcus neoformans*," *Microbiology*, vol. 147, no. 4, pp. 891–907, 2001.

[24] T. Khawcharoenporn, A. Apisarnthanarak, and L. M. Mundy, "Non-neoformans cryptococcal infections: a systematic review," *Infection*, vol. 35, no. 2, pp. 51–58, 2007.

[25] M. E. Brandt, L. C. Hutwagner, L. A. Klug et al., "Molecular subtype distribution of *Cryptococcus neoformans* in four areas of the United States," *Journal of Clinical Microbiology*, vol. 34, no. 4, pp. 912–917, 1996.

[26] J. N. Steenbergen and A. Casadevall, "Prevalence of *Cryptococcus neoformans* var. *neoformans* (serotype D) and *Cryptococcus neoformans* var. *grubii* (serotype A) isolates in New York City," *Journal of Clinical Microbiology*, vol. 38, no. 5, pp. 1974–1976, 2000.

[27] S. Chen, T. Sorrell, G. Nimmo et al., "Epidemiology and host- and variety-dependent characteristics of infection due to *Cryptococcus neoformans* in Australia and New Zealand," *Clinical Infectious Diseases*, vol. 31, no. 2, pp. 499–508, 2000.

[28] N. French, K. Gray, C. Watera et al., "Cryptococcal infection in a cohort of HIV-1-infected Ugandan adults," *AIDS*, vol. 16, no. 7, pp. 1031–1038, 2002.

[29] M. M. Nishikawa, M. S. Lazera, G. G. Barbosa et al., "Serotyping of 467 *Cryptococcus neoformans* isolates from clinical and environmental sources in Brazil: analysis of host and regional patterns," *Journal of Clinical Microbiology*, vol. 41, no. 1, pp. 73–77, 2003.

[30] W. Meyer, A. Castaneda, S. Jackson, M. Huynh, E. Castaneda, and The IberoAmerican Cryptococcal Study group, "Molecular typing of IberoAmerican *Cryptococcus neoformans* isolates," *Emerging Infectious Diseases*, vol. 9, no. 2, pp. 189–195, 2003.

[31] A. P. Litvintseva, R. Thakur, L. B. Reller, and T. G. Mitchell, "Prevalence of clinical isolates of *Cryptococcus gattii* serotype C among patients with AIDS in sub-Saharan Africa," *Journal of Infectious Diseases*, vol. 192, no. 5, pp. 888–892, 2005.

[32] S. Chaturvedi, M. Dyavaiah, R. A. Larsen, and V. Chaturvedi, "*Cryptococcus gattii* in AIDS patients, southern California," *Emerging Infectious Diseases*, vol. 11, no. 11, pp. 1686–1692, 2005.

[33] M. A. Viviani, M. Cogliati, M. C. Esposto et al., "Molecular analysis of 311 *Cryptococcus neoformans* isolates from a 30-month ECMM survey of cryptococcosis in Europe," *FEMS Yeast Research*, vol. 6, no. 4, pp. 614–619, 2006.

[34] J. Lizarazo, M. Linares, C. de Bedout, A. Rastrepo, C. I. Agudelo, and Castaneda C y Grupo Colombiano para el Studio de la Criptococosis, "Estudio clínico y epidemiológico de la criptococosis en Colombia: resultados de nueve años de la encuesta nacional, 1997–2005," *Biomedica*, vol. 27, no. 1, pp. 94–109, 2007.

[35] M. Capoor, D. Nair, M. Deb, B. Gupta, and P. Aggarwal, "Clinical and mycological profile of cryptococcosis in a tertiary care hospital," *Indian Journal of Medical Microbiology*, vol. 25, no. 4, pp. 401–404, 2007.

[36] J. Chen, A. Varma, M. R. Diaz, A. P. Litvintseva, K. K. Wollenberg, and K. J. Kwon-Chung, "*Cryptococcus neoformans* strains and infection in apparently immunocompetent patients, China," *Emerging Infectious Diseases*, vol. 14, no. 5, pp. 755–762, 2008.

[37] M. R. Capoor, P. Mandal, M. Deb, P. Aggarwal, and U. Banerjee, "Current scenario of cryptococcosis and antifungal susceptibility pattern in India: a cause for reappraisal," *Mycoses*, vol. 51, no. 3, pp. 258–265, 2008.

[38] K. J. Kwon-Chung and J. E. Bennett, "Epidemiologic differences between the two varieties of *Cryptococcus neoformans*," *American Journal of Epidemiology*, vol. 120, no. 1, pp. 123–130, 1984.

[39] D. H. Ellis, "*Cryptococcus neoformans* var. *gattii* in Australia," *Journal of Clinical Microbiology*, vol. 25, no. 2, pp. 430–431, 1987.

[40] D. H. Ellis and T. J. Pfeiffer, "Natural habitat of *Cryptococcus neoformans* var. *gattii*," *Journal of Clinical Microbiology*, vol. 28, no. 7, pp. 1642–1644, 1990.

[41] S. E. Kidd, F. Hagen, R. L. Tscharke et al., "A rare genotype of *Cryptococcus gattii* caused the cryptococcosis outbreak on Vancouver Island (British Columbia, Canada)," *Proceedings of the National Academy of Sciences of the United States of America*, vol. 101, no. 49, pp. 17258–17263, 2004.

[42] E. Galanis and L. MacDougall, "Epidemiology of *Cryptococcus gattii*, British Columbia, Canada, 1999–2007," *Emerging Infectious Diseases*, vol. 16, no. 2, pp. 251–257, 2010.

[43] E. J. Byrnes III, R. J. Bildfell, S. A. Frank, T. G. Mitchell, K. A. Marr, and J. Heitman, "Molecular evidence that the range of the Vancouver island outbreak of *Cryptococcus gattii* infection has expanded into the Pacific Northwest in the United States," *Journal of Infectious Diseases*, vol. 199, no. 7, pp. 1081–1086, 2009.

[44] A. Chowdhary, H. S. Randahawa, T. Boekhout, F. Hagen, C. H. Klaassen, and J. F. Meis, "Temperate climate niche for *Cryptococcus gattii* in Northern Europe," *Emerging Infectious Diseases*, vol. 18, no. 1, pp. 172–174, 2012.

[45] K. Okamoto, S. Hatakeyama, S. Itoyama et al., "*Cryptococcus gattii* genotype VGIIa infection in man, Japan, 2007," *Emerging Infectious Diseases*, vol. 16, no. 7, pp. 1155–1157, 2010.

[46] S. E. Kidd, Y. Chow, S. Mak et al., "Characterization of environmental sources of the human and animal pathogen *Cryptococcus gattii* in British Columbia, Canada, and the Pacific Northwest of the United States," *Applied and Environmental Microbiology*, vol. 73, no. 5, pp. 1433–1443, 2007.

[47] D. J. Springer and V. Chaturvedi, "Projecting global occurrence of *Cryptococcus gattii*," *Emerging Infectious Diseases*, vol. 16, no. 1, pp. 14–20, 2010.

[48] M. A. Viviani, S. Antinori, M. Cogliati et al., "European Confederation of Medical Mycology (ECMM) prospective survey of cryptococcosis: report from Italy," *Medical Mycology*, vol. 40, no. 5, pp. 507–517, 2002.

[49] F. R. Knight, D. W. Mackenzie, B. G. Evans, K. Porter, N. J. Barrett, and G. C. White, "Increasing incidence of cryptococcosis in the United Kingdom," *Journal of Infection*, vol. 27, no. 2, pp. 185–191, 1993.

[50] R. A. Hajjeh, M. E. Brandt, and R. W. Pinner, "Emergence of cryptococcal disease: epidemiologic perspectives 100 years after its discovery," *Epidemiologic Reviews*, vol. 17, no. 2, pp. 303–320, 1995.

[51] L. Kaufman and S. Blumer, "Cryptococcosis: the awakening giant," in *Proceedings of the 4th International Conference on the Mycoses*, pp. 176–182, Washington, DC, USA, 1978.

[52] C. D. Holtzer, M. A. Jacobson, W. K. Hadley et al., "Decline in the rate of specific opportunistic infections at San Francisco General Hospital, 1994–1997," *AIDS*, vol. 12, no. 14, pp. 1931–1933, 1998.

[53] J. F. Molez, "The historical question of acquired immunodeficiency syndrome in the 1960s in the Congo River basin area in relation to cryptococcal meningitis," *American Journal of Tropical Medicine and Hygiene*, vol. 58, no. 3, pp. 273–276, 1998.

[54] M. Scarborough, S. B. Gordon, C. J. M. Whitty et al., "Corticosteroids for bacterial meningitis in adults in sub-Saharan Africa," *The New England Journal of Medicine*, vol. 357, no. 24, pp. 2441–2450, 2007.

[55] R. S. Heyderman, I. T. Gangaidzo, J. G. Hakim et al., "Cryptococcal meningitis in human immunodeficiency virus-infected patients in Harare, Zimbabwe," *Clinical Infectious Diseases*, vol. 26, no. 2, pp. 284–289, 1998.

[56] J. G. Hakim, I. T. Gangaidzo, R. S. Heyderman et al., "Impact of HIV infection on meningitis in Harare, Zimbabwe: a prospective study of 406 predominantly adult patients," *AIDS*, vol. 14, no. 10, pp. 1401–1407, 2000.

[57] C. Békondi, C. Bernede, N. Passone et al., "Primary and opportunistic pathogens associated with meningitis in adults in Bangui, Central African Republic, in relation to human immunodeficiency virus serostatus," *International Journal of Infectious Diseases*, vol. 10, no. 5, pp. 387–395, 2006.

[58] J. N. Jarvis, A. Boulle, A. Loyse et al., "High ongoing burden of cryptococcal disease in Africa despite antiretroviral roll out," *AIDS*, vol. 23, no. 9, pp. 1182–1183, 2009.

[59] S. Bamba, O. Lortholary, A. Sawadogo, A. Millogo, R. T. Guiguemdé, and S. Bretagne, "Decreasing incidence of cryptococcal meningitis in West Africa in the era of highly active antiretroviral therapy," *AIDS*, vol. 26, no. 8, pp. 1039–1041, 2012.

[60] S. Sukroongreung, K. Kitiniyom, C. Nilakul, and S. Tantimavanich, "Pathogenicity of basidiospores of *Filobasidiella neoformans* var. *neoformans*," *Medical Mycology*, vol. 36, no. 6, pp. 419–424, 1998.

[61] A. Idnurm, Y. S. Bahn, K. Nielsen, X. Lin, J. A. Fraser, and J. Heitman, "Deciphering the model pathogenic fungus *Cryptococcus neoformans*," *Nature Reviews Microbiology*, vol. 3, no. 10, pp. 753–764, 2005.

[62] S. H. M. Chen, M. F. Stins, S. H. Huang et al., "*Cryptococcus neoformans* induces alterations in the cytoskeleton of human brain microvascular endothelial cells," *Journal of Medical Microbiology*, vol. 52, no. 11, pp. 961–970, 2003.

[63] Y. C. Chang, M. F. Stins, M. J. McCaffery et al., "Cryptococcal yeast cells invade the central nervous system via transcellular penetration of the blood-brain barrier," *Infection and Immunity*, vol. 72, pp. 4985–4995, 2004.

[64] M. Alvarez and A. Casadevall, "Phagosome extrusion and host-cell survival after *Cryptococcus neoformans* phagocytosis by macrophages," *Current Biology*, vol. 16, no. 21, pp. 2161–2165, 2006.

[65] C. Charlier, K. Nielsen, S. Daou, M. Brigitte, F. Chretien, and F. Dromer, "Evidence of a role for monocytes in dissemination and brain invasion by *Cryptococcus neoformans*," *Infection and Immunity*, vol. 77, no. 1, pp. 120–127, 2009.

[66] F. Visnegarwala, E. A. Graviss, C. E. Lacke et al., "Acute respiratory failure associated with cryptococcosis in patients with AIDS: analysis of predictive factors," *Clinical Infectious Diseases*, vol. 27, no. 5, pp. 1231–1237, 1998.

[67] J. A. Driver, C. A. Saunders, B. Heinze-Lacey, and A. M. Sugar, "Cryptococcal pneumonia in AIDS: is cryptococcal meningitis preceded by clinically recognizable pneumonia?" *Journal of Acquired Immune Deficiency Syndromes and Human Retrovirology*, vol. 9, no. 2, pp. 168–171, 1995.

[68] S. Deok-Jong Yoo, W. Worodria, J. L. Davis et al., "The prevalence and clinical course of HIV-associated pulmonary cryptococcosis in Uganda," *Journal of Acquired Immune Deficiency Syndromes*, vol. 54, no. 3, pp. 269–274, 2010.

[69] M. L. Wong, P. Back, G. Candy, G. Nelson, and J. Murray, "Cryptococcal pneumonia in African miners at autopsy," *International Journal of Tuberculosis and Lung Disease*, vol. 11, no. 5, pp. 528–533, 2007.

[70] J. R. Harris, M. D. Lindsley, S. Henchaichton et al., "High prevalence of cryptococcal infection among HIV-infected patients hospitalized with pneumonia in Thailand," *Clinical Infectious Diseases*, vol. 54, pp. e43–e50, 2012.

[71] K. Angstwurm, W. Sokolowska-Koehler, C. Stadelmann, E. Schielke, and J. R. Weber, "Fulminant cryptococcal meningitis as presenting feature in a patient with AIDS," *European Journal of Neurology*, vol. 11, no. 5, pp. 353–354, 2004.

[72] A. Zuger, E. Louie, R. S. Holzman, M. S. Simberkoff, and J. J. Rahal, "Cryptococcal disease in patients with the acquired immunodeficiency syndrome. Diagnostic features and outcome of treatment," *Annals of Internal Medicine*, vol. 104, no. 2, pp. 234–240, 1986.

[73] R. A. Clark, D. Greer, W. Atkinson, G. T. Valainis, and N. Hyslop, "Spectrum of *Cryptococcus neoformans* infection in 68 patients infected with human immunodeficiency virus," *Reviews of Infectious Diseases*, vol. 12, no. 5, pp. 768–777, 1990.

[74] M. S. Saag, W. G. Powderly, G. A. Cloud et al., "Comparison of amphotericin B with fluconazole in the treatment of acute AIDS-associated cryptococcal meningitis," *The New England Journal of Medicine*, vol. 326, no. 2, pp. 83–89, 1992.

[75] C. Darras-Joly, S. Chevret, M. Wolff et al., "*Cryptococcus neoformans* infection in France: epidemiologic features of and early prognostic parameters for 76 patients who were infected with human immunodeficiency virus," *Clinical Infectious Diseases*, vol. 23, no. 2, pp. 369–376, 1996.

[76] C. M. van Der Horst, M. S. Saag, G. A. Cloud et al., "Treatment of cryptococcal meningitis associated with the acquired immunodeficiency syndrome," *The New England Journal of Medicine*, vol. 337, pp. 15–21, 1997.

[77] S. Antinori, L. Galimberti, C. Magni et al., "*Cryptococcus neoformans* infection in a cohort of Italian AIDS patients: natural history, early prognostic parameters, and autopsy findings," *European Journal of Clinical Microbiology and Infectious Diseases*, vol. 20, no. 10, pp. 711–717, 2001.

[78] U. Jongwutiwes, S. Sungkanuparph, and S. Kiertiburanakul, "Comparison of clinical features and survival between cryptococcosis in human immunodeficiency virus (HIV)-positive and HIV-negative patients," *Japanese Journal of Infectious Diseases*, vol. 61, no. 2, pp. 111–115, 2008.

[79] M. Hong Nguyen, S. Husain, C. J. Clancy et al., "Outcomes of central nervous system cryptococcosis vary with host immune function: results from a multi-center, prospective study," *Journal of Infection*, vol. 61, no. 5, pp. 419–426, 2010.

[80] M. Y. S. Moosa and Y. M. Coovadia, "Cryptococcal meningitis in Durban, South Africa: a comparison of clinical features, laboratory findings, and outcome for human immunodeficiency virus (HIV)-positive and HIV-negative patients," *Clinical Infectious Diseases*, vol. 24, no. 2, pp. 131–134, 1997.

[81] J. Bogaerts, D. Rouvroy, H. Taelman et al., "AIDS-associated cryptococcal meningitis in Rwanda (1983–1992): epidemiologic and diagnostic features," *Journal of Infection*, vol. 39, no. 1, pp. 32–37, 1999.

[82] P. Mwaba, J. Mwansa, C. Chintu et al., "Clinical presentation, natural history, and cumulative death rates of 230 adults with primary cryptococcal meningitis in Zambian AIDS patients treated under local conditions," *Postgraduate Medical Journal*, vol. 77, no. 914, pp. 769–773, 2001.

[83] K. M. McCarthy, J. Morgan, K. A. Wannemuehler et al., "Population-based surveillance for cryptococcosis in an antiretroviral-naive South African province with a high HIV seroprevalence," *AIDS*, vol. 20, no. 17, pp. 2199–2206, 2006.

[84] J. D. Trachtenberg, A. D. Kambugu, M. McKellar et al., "The medical management of central nervous system infections in Uganda and the potential impact of an algorithm-based approach to improve outcomes," *International Journal of Infectious Diseases*, vol. 11, no. 6, pp. 524–530, 2007.

[85] C. F. Schaars, G. A. Meintjes, C. Morroni, F. A. Post, and G. Maartens, "Outcome of AIDS-associated cryptococcal meningitis initially treated with 200 mg/day or 400 mg/day of fluconazole," *BMC Infectious Diseases*, vol. 6, article 118, 2006.

[86] R. Rozenbaum and A. J. R. Goncalves, "Clinical epidemiological study of 171 cases of cryptococcosis," *Clinical Infectious Diseases*, vol. 18, no. 3, pp. 369–380, 1994.

[87] C. H. Lu, W. N. Chang, H. W. Chang, and Y. C. Chuang, "The prognostic factors of cryptococcal meningitis in HIV-negative patients," *Journal of Hospital Infection*, vol. 42, no. 4, pp. 313–320, 1999.

[88] C. C. Shih, Y. C. Chen, S. C. Chang, K. T. Luh, and W. C. Hsieh, "Cryptococcal meningitis in non-HIV-infected patients," *QJM*, vol. 93, no. 4, pp. 245–251, 2000.

[89] P. G. Pappas, J. R. Perfect, G. A. Cloud et al., "Cryptococcosis in human immunodeficiency virus-negative patients in the era of effective azole therapy," *Clinical Infectious Diseases*, vol. 33, no. 5, pp. 690–699, 2001.

[90] S. Kiertiburanakul, S. Wirojtananugoon, R. Pracharktam, and S. Sungkanuparph, "Cryptococcosis in human immunodeficiency virus-negative patients," *International Journal of Infectious Diseases*, vol. 10, no. 1, pp. 72–78, 2006.

[91] D. W. Denning, R. W. Armstrong, M. Fishman, and D. A. Stevens, "Endophthalmitis in a patient with disseminated cryptococcosis and AIDS who was treated with itraconazole," *Reviews of Infectious Diseases*, vol. 13, no. 6, pp. 1126–1130, 1991.

[92] J. R. C. Crump, S. G. Elner, V. M. Elner, and C. A. Kauffman, "Cryptococcal endophthalmitis: case report and review," *Clinical Infectious Diseases*, vol. 14, no. 5, pp. 1069–1073, 1992.

[93] R. R. Battu, J. Biswas, N. Jayakumar, H. N. Madhavan, N. Kumarsamy, and S. Solomon, "Papilloedema with peripapillary retinal haemorrhages in an acquired immunodeficiency syndrome (AIDS) patient with cryptococcal meningitis," *Indian Journal of Ophthalmology*, vol. 48, no. 1, pp. 47–49, 2000.

[94] J. Duggan and H. M. Walls, "Ocular complications of cryptococcal meningitis in patients with HIV: report of two cases and review of the literature," *Journal of the International Association of Physicians in AIDS Care*, vol. 11, pp. 283–288, 2012.

[95] S. R. D. Johnston, E. L. Corbett, O. Foster, S. Ash, and J. Cohen, "Raised intracranial pressure and visual complications in AIDS patients with cryptococcal meningitis," *Journal of Infection*, vol. 24, no. 2, pp. 185–189, 1992.

[96] A. M. Tortorano, M. A. Viviani, A. L. Rigoni, M. Cogliati, A. Roverselli, and A. Pagano, "Prevalence of serotype D in *Cryptococcus neoformans* isolates from HIV positive and HIV negative patients in Italy," *Mycoses*, vol. 40, no. 7-8, pp. 297–302, 1997.

[97] F. Dromer, S. Mathoulin, B. Dupont, L. Letenneur, and O. Ronin, "Individual and environmental factors associated with infection due to *Cryptococcus neoformans* serotype D. French Cryptococcosis Study Group," *Clinical Infectious Diseases*, vol. 23, no. 1, pp. 91–96, 1996.

[98] L. R. Martinez, J. Garcia-Rivera, and A. Casadevall, "*Cryptococcus neoformans* var. *neoformans* (serotype D) strains are more susceptible to heat than *C. neoformans* var. *grubii* (serotype A) strains," *Journal of Clinical Microbiology*, vol. 39, no. 9, pp. 3365–3367, 2001.

[99] C. E. Gonzalez, D. Shetty, L. L. Lewis, B. U. Mueller, P. A. Pizzo, and T. J. Walsh, "Cryptococcosis in human immunodeficiency virus-infected children," *Pediatric Infectious Disease Journal*, vol. 15, no. 9, pp. 796–800, 1996.

[100] J. Abadi, S. Nachman, A. B. Kressel, and L. A. Pirofski, "Cryptococcosis in children with AIDS," *Clinical Infectious Diseases*, vol. 28, no. 2, pp. 309–313, 1999.

[101] T. Gumbo, G. Kadzirange, J. Mielke, I. T. Gangaidzo, and J. G. Hakim, "*Cryptococcus neoformans* meningoencephalitis in African children with acquired immunodeficiency syndrome," *Pediatric Infectious Disease Journal*, vol. 21, no. 1, pp. 54–56, 2002.

[102] S. Likasitwattanakul, B. Poneprasert, and V. Sirisanthana, "Cryptococcosis in HIV-infected children," *Southeast Asian Journal of Tropical Medicine and Public Health*, vol. 35, no. 4, pp. 935–939, 2004.

[103] S. T. Meiring, V. C. Quan, C. Cohen et al., "A comparison of paediatric- and adult-onset cryptococcosis detected through population-based surveillance in South Africa, 2005–2007," *AIDS*, vol. 26, pp. 2307–2314, 2012.

[104] N. S. Joshi, B. T. Fisher, P. A. Prasad, and T. E. Zaoutis, "Epidemiology of cryptococcal infection in hospitalized children," *Pediatric Infectious Disease Journal*, vol. 29, no. 12, pp. e91–e95, 2010.

[105] C. B. Severo, M. O. Xavier, A. F. Gazzoni, and L. C. Severo, "Cryptococcosis in children," *Paediatric Respiratory Reviews*, vol. 10, no. 4, pp. 166–171, 2009.

[106] P. Desmet, K. D. Kayembe, and C. de Vroey, "The value of cryptococcal serum antigen screening among HIV-positive/AIDS patients in Kinshasa, Zaire," *AIDS*, vol. 3, no. 2, pp. 77–78, 1989.

[107] J. M. Tassie, L. Pepper, C. Fogg et al., "Systematic screening of cryptococcal antigenemia in HIV-positive adults in Uganda," *Journal of Acquired Immune Deficiency Syndromes*, vol. 33, no. 3, pp. 411–412, 2003.

[108] C. A. Liechty, P. Solberg, W. Were et al., "Asymptomatic serum cryptococcal antigenemia and early mortality during antiretroviral therapy in rural Uganda," *Tropical Medicine and International Health*, vol. 12, no. 8, pp. 929–935, 2007.

[109] J. N. Jarvis, S. D. Lawn, M. Vogt, N. Bangani, R. Wood, and T. S. Harrison, "Screening for cryptococcal antigenemia in patients accessing an antiretroviral treatment program in South Africa," *Clinical Infectious Diseases*, vol. 48, no. 7, pp. 856–862, 2009.

[110] D. B. Meya, Y. C. Manabe, B. Castelnuovo et al., "Cost-effectiveness of serum cryptococcal antigen screening to prevent deaths among HIV-infected persons with a $CD4^+$ cell count ≤ 100 cells/μL who start HIV therapy in resource-limited settings," *Clinical Infectious Diseases*, vol. 51, no. 4, pp. 448–455, 2010.

[111] Y. Mamoojee, S. Shakoor, R. L. Gorton et al., "Short Communication: low seroprevalence of cryptococcal antigenaemia in

patients with advanced HIV infection enrolling in an antiretroviral programme in Ghana," *Tropical Medicine and International Health*, vol. 16, no. 1, pp. 53–56, 2011.

[112] J. Oyella, D. Meya, F. Bajunirwe, and M. R. Kamya, "Prevalence and factors associated with cryptococcal antigenemia among severely immunosuppressed HIV-infected adults in Uganda: a cross-sectional study," *Journal of the International AIDS Society*, vol. 15, article 15, 2012.

[113] R. Micol, O. Lortholary, B. Sar et al., "Prevalence, determinants of positivity, and clinical utility of cryptococcal antigenemia in Cambodian HIV-infected patients," *Journal of Acquired Immune Deficiency Syndromes*, vol. 45, no. 5, pp. 555–559, 2007.

[114] P. Pongsai, K. Atamasirikul, and S. Sungkanuparph, "The role of serum cryptococcal antigen screening for the early diagnosis of cryptococcosis in HIV-infected patients with different ranges of CD4 cell counts," *Journal of Infection*, vol. 60, no. 6, pp. 474–477, 2010.

[115] M. Feldmesser, C. Harris, S. Reichberg, S. Khan, and A. Casadevall, "Serum cryptococcal antigen in patients with AIDS," *Clinical Infectious Diseases*, vol. 23, no. 4, pp. 827–830, 1996.

[116] S. Patel, G. Y. Shin, I. Wijewardana et al., "The prevalence of cryptococcal antigenemia in newly diagnosed HIV patients in a Southwest London cohort," *The Journal of Infection*, vol. 66, no. 1, pp. 75–79, 2013.

[117] R. J. Leggiadro, M. W. Kline, and W. T. Hughes, "Extrapulmonary cryptococcosis in children with acquired immunodeficiency syndrome," *Pediatric Infectious Disease Journal*, vol. 10, no. 9, pp. 658–662, 1991.

[118] S. C. Lee, D. W. Dickson, and A. Casadevall, "Pathology of cryptococcal meningoencephalitis: analysis of 27 patients with pathogenetic implications," *Human Pathology*, vol. 27, no. 8, pp. 839–847, 1996.

[119] D. W. Denning, R. W. Armstrong, B. H. Lewis, and D. A. Stevens, "Elevated cerebrospinal fluid pressures in patients with cryptococcal meningitis and acquired immunodeficiency syndrome," *American Journal of Medicine*, vol. 91, no. 3, pp. 267–272, 1991.

[120] J. R. Graybill, J. Sobel, M. Saag et al., "Diagnosis and management of increased intracranial pressure in patients with AIDS and cryptococcal meningitis," *Clinical Infectious Diseases*, vol. 30, no. 1, pp. 47–54, 2000.

[121] T. Bicanic, A. E. Brouwer, G. Meintjes et al., "Relationship of cerebrospinal fluid pressure, fungal burden and outcome in patients with cryptococcal meningitis undergoing serial lumbar punctures," *AIDS*, vol. 23, no. 6, pp. 701–706, 2009.

[122] A. Loyse, H. Wainwright, J. N. Jarvis et al., "Histopathology of the arachnoid granulations and brain in HIV-associated cryptococcal meningitis: correlation with cerebrospinal fluid pressure," *AIDS*, vol. 24, no. 3, pp. 405–410, 2010.

[123] J. R. Perfect, W. E. Dismukes, F. Dromer et al., "Clinical practice guidelines for the management of cryptococcal disease: 2010 update by the Infectious Diseases Society of America," *Clinical Infectious Diseases*, vol. 50, no. 3, pp. 291–322, 2010.

[124] S. Antinori, A. L. Ridolfo, E. Gianelli, M. Piazza, C. Gervasoni, and A. d'Arminio Monforte, "The role of lumbar puncture in the management of elevated intracranial pressure in patients with AIDS-associated cryptococcal meningitis," *Clinical Infectious Diseases*, vol. 31, no. 5, pp. 1309–1310, 2000.

[125] R. D. Fessler, J. Sobel, L. Guyot et al., "Management of elevated intracranial pressure in patients with cryptococcal meningitis," *Journal of Acquired Immune Deficiency Syndromes and Human Retrovirology*, vol. 17, no. 2, pp. 137–142, 1998.

[126] K. F. Macsween, T. Bicanic, A. E. Brouwer, H. Marsh, D. C. Macallan, and T. S. Harrison, "Lumbar drainage for control of raised cerebrospinal fluid pressure in cryptococcal meningitis: case report and review," *Journal of Infection*, vol. 51, no. 4, pp. e221–e224, 2005.

[127] W. Manosuthi, S. Sungkanuparph, S. Chottanapund et al., "Temporary external lumbar drainage for reducing elevated intracranial pressure in HIV-infected patients with cryptococcal meningitis," *International Journal of STD and AIDS*, vol. 19, no. 4, pp. 268–271, 2008.

[128] M. C. Bach, P. W. Tally, and E. W. Godofsky, "Use of cerebrospinal fluid shunts in patients having acquired immunodeficiency syndrome with cryptococcal meningitis and uncontrollable intracranial hypertension," *Neurosurgery*, vol. 41, no. 6, pp. 1280–1283, 1997.

[129] M. L. Woods II, R. MacGinley, D. P. Eisen, and A. M. Allworth, "HIV combination therapy: partial immune restitution unmasking latent cryptococcal infection," *AIDS*, vol. 12, no. 12, pp. 1491–1494, 1998.

[130] E. R. Jenny-Avital and M. Abadi, "Immune reconstitution cryptococcosis after initiation of successful highly active antiretroviral therapy," *Clinical Infectious Diseases*, vol. 35, no. 12, pp. e128–133, 2002.

[131] N. Singh, O. Lortholary, B. D. Alexander et al., "An immune reconstitution syndrome-like illness associated with *Cryptococcus neoformans* infection in organ transplant recipients," *Clinical Infectious Diseases*, vol. 40, no. 12, pp. 1756–1761, 2005.

[132] P. R. Ingram, R. Howman, M. F. Leahy, and J. R. Dyer, "Cryptococcal immune reconstitution inflammatory syndrome following alemtuzumab therapy," *Clinical Infectious Diseases*, vol. 44, no. 12, pp. e115–e117, 2007.

[133] J. Cadena, G. R. Thompson III, T. T. Ho, E. Medina, D. W. Hughes, and T. F. Patterson, "Immune reconstitution inflammatory syndrome after cessation of the tumor necrosis factor α blocker adalimumab in cryptococcal pneumonia," *Diagnostic Microbiology and Infectious Disease*, vol. 64, no. 3, pp. 327–330, 2009.

[134] L. J. Haddow, R. Colebunders, G. Meintjes et al., "Cryptococcal immune reconstitution inflammatory syndrome in HIV-1-infected individuals: proposed clinical case definitions," *The Lancet Infectious Diseases*, vol. 10, no. 11, pp. 791–802, 2010.

[135] S. A. Shelburne, J. Darcourt, A. C. White Jr. et al., "The role of immune reconstitution inflammatory syndrome in AIDS-related *Cryptococcus neoformans* disease in the era of highly active antiretroviral therapy," *Clinical Infectious Diseases*, vol. 40, no. 7, pp. 1049–1052, 2005.

[136] O. Lortholary, A. Fontanet, N. Mémain, A. Martin, K. Sitbon, and F. Dromer, "Incidence and risk factors of immune reconstitution inflammatory syndrome complicating HIV-associated cryptococcosis in France," *AIDS*, vol. 19, no. 10, pp. 1043–1049, 2005.

[137] L. J. Haddow, M. Y. Moosa, A. Mosam, P. Moodley, R. Parboosing, and P. J. Easterbrook, "Incidence, clinical spectrum, risk factors and impact of HIV-associated immune reconstitution inflammatory syndrome in South Africa," *PLoS One*, vol. 7, Article ID e40623, 2012.

[138] D. M. Murdoch, W. D. F. Venter, C. Feldman, and A. Van Rie, "Incidence and risk factors for the immune reconstitution inflammatory syndrome in HIV patients in South Africa: a prospective study," *AIDS*, vol. 22, no. 5, pp. 601–610, 2008.

[139] C. Michelet, C. Arvieux, C. François et al., "Opportunistic infections occurring during highly active antiretroviral treatment," *AIDS*, vol. 12, no. 14, pp. 1815–1822, 1998.

[140] S. D. Lawn, L. G. Bekker, L. Myer, C. Orrell, and R. Wood, "Cryptococcocal immune reconstitution disease: a major cause of early mortality in a South African antiretroviral programme," *AIDS*, vol. 19, no. 17, pp. 2050–2052, 2005.

[141] M. Müller, S. Wandel, R. Colebunders, S. Attia, H. Furrer, and M. Egger, "Immune reconstitution inflammatory syndrome in patients starting antiretroviral therapy for HIV infection: a systematic review and meta-analysis," *The Lancet Infectious Diseases*, vol. 10, no. 4, pp. 251–261, 2010.

[142] S. D. Lawn and R. Wood, "Immune reconstitution inflammatory syndrome," *The Lancet Infectious Diseases*, vol. 10, no. 12, pp. 833–834, 2010.

[143] F. J. Mateen and A. Nath, "Central nervous system-immune reconstitution inflammatory syndrome in resource-limited settings. Current burden and future needs," *AIDS*, vol. 26, pp. 1851–1855, 2012.

[144] D. L. Wiesner and D. R. Boulware, "*Cryptococcus*-Related Immune Reconstitution Inflammatory Syndrome (IRIS): pathogenesis and its Clinical Implications," *Current Fungal Infection Reports*, vol. 5, no. 4, pp. 252–261, 2011.

[145] S. A. Shelburne III, R. J. Hamill, M. C. Rodriguez-Barradas et al., "Immune reconstitution inflammatory syndrome: emergence of a unique syndrome during highly active antiretroviral therapy," *Medicine*, vol. 81, no. 3, pp. 213–227, 2002.

[146] G. Breton, D. Seilhean, P. Chérin, S. Herson, and O. Benveniste, "Paradoxical intracranial cryptococcoma in a human immunodeficiency virus-infected man being treated with combination antiretroviral therapy," *American Journal of Medicine*, vol. 113, no. 2, pp. 155–157, 2002.

[147] J. Rambeloarisoa, D. Batisse, J. B. Thiebaut et al., "Intramedullary abscess resulting from disseminated cryptococcosis despite immune restoration in a patient with AIDS," *Journal of Infection*, vol. 44, no. 3, pp. 185–188, 2002.

[148] S. Sungkanuparph, U. Jongwutiwes, and S. Kiertiburanakul, "Timing of cryptococcal immune reconstitution inflammatory syndrome after antiretroviral therapy in patients with AIDS and cryptococcal meningitis," *Journal of Acquired Immune Deficiency Syndromes*, vol. 45, no. 5, pp. 595–596, 2007.

[149] T. Bicanic, G. Meintjes, K. Rebe et al., "Immune reconstitution inflammatory syndrome in HIV-associated cryptococcal meningitis: a prospective study," *Journal of Acquired Immune Deficiency Syndromes*, vol. 51, no. 2, pp. 130–134, 2009.

[150] S. Sungkanuparph, S. G. Filler, P. Chetchotisakd et al., "Cryptococcal immune reconstitution inflammatory syndrome after antiretroviral therapy in AIDS patients with cryptococcal meningitis: a prospective multicenter study," *Clinical Infectious Diseases*, vol. 49, no. 6, pp. 931–934, 2009.

[151] D. J. Skiest, L. J. Hester, and R. D. Hardy, "Cryptococcal immune reconstitution inflammatory syndrome: report of four cases in three patients and review of the literature," *Journal of Infection*, vol. 51, no. 5, pp. e289–e297, 2005.

[152] D. R. Boulware, D. B. Meya, T. L. Bergemann et al., "Clinical features and serum biomarkers in HIV immune reconstitution inflammatory syndrome after cryptococcal meningitis: a prospective cohort study," *PLoS Medicine*, vol. 7, no. 12, Article ID e1000384, 2010.

[153] D. R. Boulware, S. C. Bonham, D. B. Meya et al., "Paucity of initial cerebrospinal fluid inflammation in cryptococcal meningitis is associated with subsequent immune reconstitution inflammatory syndrome," *Journal of Infectious Diseases*, vol. 202, no. 6, pp. 962–970, 2010.

[154] S. K. Cinti, W. S. Armstrong, and C. A. Kauffman, "Case report. Recurrence of increased intracranial pressure with antiretroviral therapy in an AIDS patient with cryptococcal meningitis," *Mycoses*, vol. 44, no. 11-12, pp. 497–501, 2001.

[155] M. D. King, C. A. Perlino, J. Cinnamon, and J. A. Jernigan, "Paradoxical recurrent meningitis following therapy of cryptococcal meningitis: an immune reconstitution syndrome after initiation of highly active antiretroviral therapy," *International Journal of STD and AIDS*, vol. 13, no. 10, pp. 724–726, 2002.

[156] J. R. Boelaert, K. H. Goddeeris, L. J. Vanopdenbosch, and J. W. Casselman, "Relapsing meningitis caused by persistent cryptococcal antigens and immune reconstitution after the initiation of highly active antiretroviral therapy," *AIDS*, vol. 18, no. 8, pp. 1223–1224, 2004.

[157] J. York, I. Bodi, I. Reeves, P. Riordan-Eva, and P. J. Easterbrook, "Raised intracranial pressure complicating cryptococcal meningitis: immune reconstitution inflammatory syndrome or recurrent cryptococcal disease?" *Journal of Infection*, vol. 51, no. 2, pp. 165–171, 2005.

[158] E. R. da Cunha Colombo, D. J. Mora, and M. L. Silva-Vergara, "Immune reconstitution inflammatory syndrome (IRIS) associated with *Cryptococcus neoformans* infection in AIDS patients," *Mycoses*, vol. 54, no. 4, pp. e178–e182, 2011.

[159] A. M. Cattelan, M. Trevenzoli, L. Sasset, M. Lanzafame, U. Marchioro, and F. Meneghetti, "Multiple cerebral cryptococcomas associated with immune reconstitution in HIV-1 infection," *AIDS*, vol. 18, no. 2, pp. 349–351, 2004.

[160] A. Venkataramana, C. A. Pardo, J. C. McArthur et al., "Immune reconstitution inflammatory syndrome in the CNS of HIV-infected patients," *Neurology*, vol. 67, no. 3, pp. 383–388, 2006.

[161] N. Khanna, R. Nüesch, C. Buitrago-Tellez, M. Battegay, and H. H. Hirsch, "Hearing loss after discontinuing secondary prophylaxis for cryptococcal meningitis: relapse or immune reconstitution?" *Infection*, vol. 34, no. 3, pp. 163–168, 2006.

[162] R. N. Khurana, M. Javaheri, and N. Rao, "Ophthalmic manifestations of immune reconstitution inflammatory syndrome associated with *Cryptococcus neoformans*," *Ocular Immunology and Inflammation*, vol. 16, no. 4, pp. 185–190, 2008.

[163] A. Brunel, A. Makinson, N. Menjot de Champfleur et al., "HIV-related immune reconstitution cryptococcal meningoradiculitis: corticosteroid response," *Neurology*, vol. 73, no. 20, pp. 1705–1707, 2009.

[164] P. Blanche, B. Gombert, C. Ginsburg et al., "HIV combination therapy: immune restitution causing cryptococcal lymphadenitis dramatically improved by anti-inflammatory therapy," *Scandinavian Journal of Infectious Diseases*, vol. 30, no. 6, pp. 615–616, 1998.

[165] R. Manfredi, F. Pieri, S. Pileri, and F. Chiodo, "The changing face of AIDS-related opportunism: cryptococcosis in the highly active antiretroviral therapy (HAART) era. Case reports and literature review," *Mycopathologia*, vol. 148, no. 2, pp. 73–78, 1999.

[166] M. Trevenzoli, A. M. Cattelan, F. Rea et al., "Mediastinitis due to cryptococcal infection: a new clinical entity in the HAART era," *Journal of Infection*, vol. 45, no. 3, pp. 173–179, 2002.

[167] U. Legendre, M. Battegay, I. Nuttli, P. Dalquen, and R. Nüesch, "Simultaneous occurrence of 2 HIV-related immunereconstitution diseases after initiation of highly active antiretroviral

therapy," *Scandinavian Journal of Infectious Diseases*, vol. 33, no. 5, pp. 388–389, 2001.

[168] R. Lehloenya and G. Meintjes, "Dermatologic manifestations of the immune reconstitution inflammatory syndrome," *Dermatologic Clinics*, vol. 24, no. 4, pp. 549–570, 2006.

[169] M. Tahir, S. K. Sharma, S. Sinha, and C. J. Das, "Immune reconstitution inflammatory syndrome in a patient with cryptococcal lymphadenitis as the first presentation of acquired immunodeficiency syndrome," *Journal of Postgraduate Medicine*, vol. 53, no. 4, pp. 250–252, 2007.

[170] L. J. Haddow, F. Sahid, and M. Y. S. Moosa, "Cryptococcal breast abscess in an HIV-positive patient: arguments for reviewing the definition of immune reconstitution inflammatory syndrome," *Journal of Infection*, vol. 57, no. 1, pp. 82–84, 2008.

[171] A. M. Sitapati, C. L. Kao, E. R. Cachay, H. Masoumi, R. S. Wallis, and W. C. Mathews, "Treatment of HIV-related inflammatory cerebral cryptococcoma with adalimumab," *Clinical Infectious Diseases*, vol. 50, no. 2, pp. e7–e10, 2010.

[172] S. Antinori, A. Radice, L. Galimberti, C. Magni, M. Fasan, and C. Parravicini, "The role of cryptococcal antigen assay in diagnosis and monitoring of cryptococcal meningitis," *Journal of Clinical Microbiology*, vol. 43, no. 11, pp. 5828–5829, 2005.

[173] E. J. McManus and J. M. Jones, "Detection of a *Trichosporon beigelii* antigen cross-reactive with *Cryptococcus neoformans* capsular polysaccharide in serum from a patient with disseminated Trichosporon infection," *Journal of Clinical Microbiology*, vol. 21, no. 5, pp. 681–685, 1985.

[174] A. M. Stamm and S. S. Polt, "False-negative cryptococcal antigen test," *Journal of the American Medical Association*, vol. 244, no. 12, p. 1359, 1980.

[175] B. P. Currie, L. F. Freundlich, M. A. Soto, and A. Casadevall, "False-negative cerebrospinal fluid cryptococcal latex agglutination tests for patients with culture-positive cryptococcal meningitis," *Journal of Clinical Microbiology*, vol. 31, no. 9, pp. 2519–2522, 1993.

[176] R. Burton, N. Gogela, K. Rebe, M. McNally, and G. Meintjes, "Cryptococcal immune reconstitution inflammatory syndrome presenting with erosive bone lesions, arthritis and subcutaneous abscesses," *AIDS*, vol. 23, no. 17, pp. 2371–2373, 2009.

[177] R. A. Larsen, M. A. E. Leal, and L. S. Chan, "Fluconazole compared with amphotericin B plus flucytosine for cryptococcal meningitis in AIDS. A randomized trial," *Annals of Internal Medicine*, vol. 113, no. 3, pp. 183–187, 1990.

[178] J. de Gans, P. Portegies, G. Tiessens et al., "Itraconazole compared with amphotericin B plus flucytosine in AIDS patients with cryptococcal meningitis," *AIDS*, vol. 6, no. 2, pp. 185–190, 1992.

[179] R. J. Coker, M. Viviani, B. G. Gazzard et al., "Treatment of cryptococcosis with liposomal amphotericin B (AmBisome) in 23 patients with AIDS," *AIDS*, vol. 7, no. 6, pp. 829–835, 1993.

[180] F. Menichetti, M. Fiorio, A. Tosti et al., "High-dose fluconazole therapy for cryptococcal meningitis in patients with AIDS," *Clinical Infectious Diseases*, vol. 22, no. 5, pp. 838–840, 1996.

[181] A. C. A. P. Leenders, P. Reiss, P. Portegies et al., "Liposomal amphotericin B (AmBisome) compared with amphotericin and both followed by oral fluconazole in the treatment of AIDS-associated cryptococcal meningitis," *AIDS*, vol. 11, no. 12, pp. 1463–1471, 1997.

[182] H. Mayanja-Kizza, K. Oishi, S. Mitarai et al., "Combination therapy with fluconazole and flucytosine for cryptococcal meningitis in ugandan patients with AIDS," *Clinical Infectious Diseases*, vol. 26, no. 6, pp. 1362–1367, 1998.

[183] A. E. Brouwer, A. Rajanuwong, W. Chierakul et al., "Combination antifungal therapies for HIV-associated cryptococcal meningitis: a randomised trial," *Lancet*, vol. 363, no. 9423, pp. 1764–1767, 2004.

[184] T. Bicanic, G. Meintjes, R. Wood et al., "Fungal burden, early fungicidal activity, and outcome in cryptococcal meningitis in antiretroviral-naïve or antiretroviral-experienced patients treated with amphotericin B or fluconazole," *Clinical Infectious Diseases*, vol. 45, no. 1, pp. 76–80, 2007.

[185] T. Bicanic, R. Wood, G. Meintjes et al., "High-dose amphotericin B with flucytosine for the treatment of cryptococcal meningitis in HIV-infected patients: a randomized trial," *Clinical Infectious Diseases*, vol. 47, no. 1, pp. 123–130, 2008.

[186] N. Longley, C. Muzoora, K. Taseera et al., "Dose response effect of high-dose fluconazole for HIV-associated cryptococcal meningitis in southwestern Uganda," *Clinical Infectious Diseases*, vol. 47, no. 12, pp. 1556–1561, 2008.

[187] P. Dammert, B. Bustamante, E. Ticona et al., "Treatment of cryptococcal meningitis in Peruvian AIDS patients using amphotericin B and fluconazole," *Journal of Infection*, vol. 57, no. 3, pp. 260–265, 2008.

[188] P. G. Pappas, P. Chetchotisakd, R. A. Larsen et al., "A phase II randomized trial of amphotericin B alone or combined with fluconazole in the treatment of HIV-associated cryptococcal meningitis," *Clinical Infectious Diseases*, vol. 48, no. 12, pp. 1775–1783, 2009.

[189] R. J. Hamill, J. D. Sobel, W. El-Sadr et al., "Comparison of 2 doses of liposomal amphotericin B and conventional amphotericin B deoxycholate for treatment of AIDS-associated acute cryptococcal meningitis: a randomized, double-blind clinical trial of efficacy and safety," *Clinical Infectious Diseases*, vol. 51, no. 2, pp. 225–232, 2010.

[190] J. V. J. Lightowler, G. S. Cooke, P. Mutevedzi, R. J. Lessells, M. L. Newell, and M. Dedicoat, "Treatment of cryptococcal meningitis in KwaZulu-Natal, South Africa," *PLoS One*, vol. 5, no. 1, Article ID e8630, 2010.

[191] D. R. Falci, L. W. Lunardi, C. G. Ramos, M. B. Bay, V. R. Aquino, and L. Z. Goldani, "Continuous infusion of amphotericin B deoxycholate in the treatment of cryptococcal meningoencephalitis: analysis of safety and fungicidal activity," *Clinical Infectious Diseases*, vol. 50, no. 5, pp. e26–e29, 2010.

[192] J. C. Nussbaum, A. Jackson, D. Namarika et al., "Combination flucytosine and high-dose fluconazole compared with fluconazole monotherapy for the treatment of cryptococcal meningitis: a randomized trial in Malawi," *Clinical Infectious Diseases*, vol. 50, no. 3, pp. 338–344, 2010.

[193] M. P. Jadhav, A. Bamba, V. M. Shinde et al., "Liposomal amphotericin B (Fungisome) for the treatment of cryptococcal meningitis in HIV/AIDS patients in India: a multicentric, randomized controlled trial," *Journal of Postgraduate Medicine*, vol. 56, no. 2, pp. 71–75, 2010.

[194] A. Loyse, D. Wilson, G. Meintjes et al., "Comparison of the early fungicidal activity of high-dose fluconazole, voriconazole, and flucytosine as second line drugs given in combination with amphotericin B for the treatment of HIV-associated cryptococcal meningitis," *Clinical Infectious Diseases*, vol. 54, no. 1, pp. 121–128, 2012.

[195] C. R. Muzoora, T. Kabanda, G. Ortu et al., "Short course amphotericin B with high dose fluconazole for HIV-associated cryptococcal meningitis," *Journal of Infection*, vol. 64, no. 1, pp. 76–81, 2012.

[196] J. N. Jarvis, G. Meintjes, K. Rebe et al., "Adjunctive interferon-γ immunotherapy for the treatment of HIV-associated cryptococcal meningitis: a randomized controlled trial," *AIDS*, vol. 26, pp. 1105–1113, 2012.

[197] A. T. Jackson, J. C. Nussbaum, J. Phulusa et al., "A phase II randomized controlled trial adding oral flucytosine to high-dose fluconazole, with short-course amphotericin B, for cryptococcal meningitis," *AIDS*, vol. 26, no. 11, pp. 1363–1370, 2012.

[198] M. D. Lindsley, N. Mekha, H. C. Baggett et al., "Evaluation of a newly developed lateral flow immunoassay for the diagnosis of cryptococcosis," *Clinical Infectious Diseases*, vol. 53, no. 4, pp. 321–325, 2011.

[199] J. N. Jarvis, A. Percival, S. Bauman et al., "Evaluation of a novel point-of-care cryptococcal antigen test on serum, plasma and urine from patients with HIV-associated cryptococcal meningitis," *Clinical Infectious Diseases*, vol. 53, pp. 1019–1023, 2011.

[200] R. Rajasingham, D. B. Meya, and D. R. Boulware, "Integrating cryptococcal antigen screening and pre-emptive treatment into routine HIV care," *Journal of Acquired Immune Deficiency Syndromes*, vol. 59, pp. e85–e91, 2012.

[201] B. J. McMullan, C. Halliday, T. C. Sorrell et al., "Clinical utility of the cryptococcal antigen lateral flow assay in a diagnostic mycology laboratory," *PLoS One*, vol. 7, Article ID e49541, 2012.

[202] J. N. Jarvis, N. Govender, T. Chiller et al., "Cryptococcal antigen screening and preemptive therapy in patients initiating antiretroviral therapy in resource-limited settings. A proposed algorithm for clinical implementation," *Journal of the International Association of Physicians in AIDS Care*, vol. 11, pp. 374–379, 2012.

[203] R. Rajasingham and D. R. Boulware, "Reconsidering cryptococcal antigen screening in the U.S. among persons with CD4<100 cells/mcL," *Clinical Infectious Diseases*, vol. 55, pp. 1742–1744, 2012.

[204] Y. T. Huang, C. C. Hung, C. H. Liao, H. Y. Sun, S. C. Chang, and Y. C. Chen, "Detection of circulating galactomannan in serum samples for diagnosis of *Penicillium marneffei* infection and cryptococcosis among patients infected with human immunodeficiency virus," *Journal of Clinical Microbiology*, vol. 45, no. 9, pp. 2858–2862, 2007.

[205] M. O. Xavier, A. C. Pasqualotto, I. C. E. Cardoso, and L. C. Severo, "Cross-reactivity of *Paracoccidioides brasiliensis*, *Histoplasma capsulatum*, and *Cryptococcus* species in the commercial platelia *Aspergillus* enzyme immunoassay," *Clinical and Vaccine Immunology*, vol. 16, no. 1, pp. 132–133, 2009.

[206] J. R. Perfect, "The triple threat of cryptococcosis: it's the body site, the strain, and/or the host," *mBio*, vol. 3, no. 4, pp. e00165–e00112, 2012.

[207] T. A. Bicanic, C. Muzoora, A. E. Brouwer et al., "Independent association between rate of clearance of infection and clinical outcome of HIV-associated cryptococcal meningitis: analysis of a combined cohort of 262 patients," *Clinical Infectious Diseases*, vol. 49, no. 5, pp. 702–709, 2009.

[208] Antiretroviral Therapy Cohort Collaboration, "Variable impact on mortality of AIDS-defining events diagnosed during combination antiretroviral therapy: not all AIDS-defining conditions are created equal," *Clinical Infectious Diseases*, vol. 48, no. 8, pp. 1138–1151, 2009.

[209] O. Lortholary, G. Poizat, V. Zeller et al., "Long-term outcome of AIDS-associated cryptococcosis in the era of combination antiretroviral therapy," *AIDS*, vol. 20, pp. 2183–2191, 2006.

[210] U. Jongwutiwes, S. Kiertiburanakul, and S. Sungkanuparph, "Impact of antiretroviral therapy on the relapse of cryptococcosis and survival of HIV-infected patients with cryptococcal infection," *Current HIV Research*, vol. 5, no. 3, pp. 355–360, 2007.

[211] W. G. Powderly, M. S. Saag, G. A. Cloud et al., "A controlled trial of fluconazole or amphotericin B to prevent relapse of cryptococcal meningitis in patients with the acquired immunodeficiency syndrome," *The New England Journal of Medicine*, vol. 326, no. 12, pp. 793–798, 1992.

[212] S. A. Bozzette, R. A. Larsen, J. Chiu et al., "A placebo-controlled trial of maintenance therapy with fluconazole after treatment of cryptococcal meningitis in the acquired immunodeficiency syndrome," *The New England Journal of Medicine*, vol. 324, no. 9, pp. 580–584, 1991.

[213] M. S. Saag, G. A. Cloud, J. R. Graybill et al., "A comparison of itraconazole versus fluconazole as maintenance therapy for AIDS-associated cryptococcal meningitis," *Clinical Infectious Diseases*, vol. 28, no. 2, pp. 291–296, 1999.

[214] WHO, *Rapid Advice. Diagnosis, Prevention and Management of Cryptococcal Disease in HIV-Infected Adults, Adolescents and Children*, WHO Press, Geneva, Switzerland, 2011, http://whqlibidoc.who.int/publications/2011/9789241502979_eng.pdf.

[215] R. Rajasingham, M. A. Rolfes, K. E. Birkenkamp, D. B. Meya, and D. R. Boulware, "Cryptococcal meningitis treatment strategies in resource-limited settings. A cost-effectiveness analysis," *PLoS Medicine*, vol. 9, Article ID e1001316, 2012.

[216] D. W. Bates, L. Su, D. T. Yu et al., "Mortality and costs of acute renal failure associated with amphotericin B therapy," *Clinical Infectious Diseases*, vol. 32, no. 5, pp. 686–693, 2001.

[217] M. Nelson, H. Manji, and E. Wilkins, "Central nervous system opportunistic infections. British HIV association and British Infection Association guidelines for the treatment of opportunistic infection in HIV-seropositive individuals," *HIV Medicine*, vol. 12, supplement 2, pp. 8–24, 2011.

[218] T. Bicanic, D. Ogden, I. Whitney, A. Loyse, and J. Jarvis, "British HIV association opportunistic infection guidelines: in defence of amphotericin B deoxycholate," *HIV Medicine*, vol. 13, pp. 636–637, 2012.

[219] A. R. Zolopa, J. Andersen, W. Powderly et al., "Early antiretroviral therapy reduces AIDS progression/death in individuals with acute opportunistic infections: a multicenter randomized strategy trial," *PLoS One*, vol. 4, no. 5, Article ID e5575, 2009.

[220] A. T. Makadzange, C. E. Ndhlovu, K. Takarinda et al., "Early versus delayed initiation of antiretroviral therapy for concurrent HIV infection and cryptococcal meningitis in sub-saharan Africa," *Clinical Infectious Diseases*, vol. 50, no. 11, pp. 1532–1538, 2010.

[221] P. M. Grant, L. Komarow, J. Andersen et al., "Risk factor analyses for immune reconstitution inflammatory syndrome in a randomized study of early vs. deferred ART during an opportunistic infection," *PloS One*, vol. 5, no. 7, Article ID e11416, 2010.

[222] K. McCarthy and G. Meintjes, "Guidelines for the prevention, diagnosis and management of cryptococcal meningitis and disseminated cryptococcosis in HIV-infected patients," *Southern African Journal of HIV Medicine*, vol. 28, no. 3, pp. 25–35, 2007.

[223] E. Martínez, M. A. García-Viejo, M. A. Marcos et al., "Discontinuation of secondary prophylaxis for cryptococcal meningitis in HIV-infected patients responding to highly active antiretroviral therapy," *AIDS*, vol. 14, no. 16, pp. 2615–2617, 2000.

[224] F. Rollot, P. Bossi, R. Tubiana et al., "Discontinuation of secondary prophylaxis against cryptococcosis in patients with

AIDS receiving highly active antiretroviral therapy," *AIDS*, vol. 15, no. 11, pp. 1448–1449, 2001.

[225] N. C. Nwokolo, M. Fisher, B. G. Gazzard, and M. R. Nelson, "Cessation of secondary prophylaxis in patients with cryptococcosis," *AIDS*, vol. 15, no. 11, pp. 1438–1439, 2001.

[226] J. A. Aberg, R. W. Price, D. M. Heeren, and B. Bredt, "A pilot study of the discontinuation of antifungal therapy for disseminated cryptococcal disease in patients with acquired immunodeficiency syndrome, following immunologic response to antiretroviral therapy," *Journal of Infectious Diseases*, vol. 185, no. 8, pp. 1179–1182, 2002.

[227] W. H. Sheng, C. C. Hung, M. Y. Chen, S. M. Hsieh, and S. C. Chang, "Successful discontinuation of fluconazole as secondary prophylaxis for cryptococcosis in AIDS patients responding to highly active antiretroviral therapy," *International Journal of STD and AIDS*, vol. 13, no. 10, pp. 702–705, 2002.

[228] O. Kirk, P. Reiss, C. Uberti-Foppa et al., "Safe interruption of maintenance therapy against previous infection with four common HIV-associated opportunistic pathogens during potent antiretroviral therapy," *Annals of Internal Medicine*, vol. 137, no. 4, pp. 239–250, 2002.

[229] C. Mussini, P. Pezzotti, J. M. Miró et al., "Discontinuation of maintenance therapy for cryptococcal meningitis in patients with AIDS treated with highly active antiretroviral therapy: an international observational study," *Clinical Infectious Diseases*, vol. 38, no. 4, pp. 565–571, 2004.

[230] H. Y. Sun, M. Y. Chen, C. F. Hsiao, S. M. Hsieh, C. C. Hung, and S. C. Chang, "Endemic fungal infections caused by *Cryptococcus neoformans* and *Penicillium marneffei* in patients infected with human immunodeficiency virus and treated with highly active anti-retroviral therapy," *Clinical Microbiology and Infection*, vol. 12, no. 4, pp. 381–388, 2006.

[231] A. Vibhagool, S. Sungkanuparph, P. Mootsikapun et al., "Discontinuation of secondary prophylaxis for cryptococcal meningitis in human immunodeficiency virus-infected patients treated with highly active antiretroviral therapy: a prospective, multicenter, randomized study," *Clinical Infectious Diseases*, vol. 36, no. 10, pp. 1329–1331, 2003.

[232] S. Antinori, "Molluscum or a mimic? Add *Penicillium marneffei!*," *American Journal of Medicine*, vol. 120, no. 11, pp. e19–e20, 2007.

[233] W. G. Powderly, D. M. Finkelstein, J. Feinberg et al., "A randomized trial comparing fluconazole with clotrimazole troches for the prevention of fungal infections in patients with advanced human immunodeficiency virus infection," *The New England Journal of Medicine*, vol. 332, no. 11, pp. 700–705, 1995.

[234] V. J. Quagliarello, C. Viscoli, and R. I. Horwitz, "Primary prevention of cryptococcal meningitis by fluconazole in HIV-infected patients," *Lancet*, vol. 345, no. 8949, pp. 548–552, 1995.

[235] J. A. Newton, S. A. Tasker, W. D. Bone et al., "Weekly fluconazole for the suppression of recurrent thrush in HIV-seropositive patients: impact on the incidence of disseminated cryptococcal infection," *AIDS*, vol. 9, no. 11, pp. 1286–1287, 1995.

[236] D. V. Havlir, M. P. Dube, J. A. McCutchan et al., "Prophylaxis with weekly versus daily fluconazole for fungal infections in patients with AIDS," *Clinical Infectious Diseases*, vol. 27, no. 6, pp. 1369–1375, 1998.

[237] P. Chetchotisakd, S. Sungkanuparph, B. Thinkhamrop, P. Mootsikapun, and P. Boonyaprawit, "A multicentre, randomized, double-blind, placebo-controlled trial of primary cryptococcal meningitis prophylaxis in HIV-infected patients with severe immune deficiency," *HIV Medicine*, vol. 5, no. 3, pp. 140–143, 2004.

[238] P. T. Cantey, D. S. Stephens, and D. Rimland, "Prevention of cryptococcosis in HIV-infected patients with limited access to highly active antiretroviral therapy: evidence for primary azole prophylaxis," *HIV Medicine*, vol. 6, no. 4, pp. 253–259, 2005.

[239] R. Micol, A. Tajahmady, O. Lortholary et al., "Cost-effectiveness of primary prophylaxis of AIDS associated cryptococcosis in Cambodia," *PLoS One*, vol. 5, no. 11, Article ID e13856, 2010.

[240] R. Parkes-Ratanshi, K. Wakeham, J. Levin et al., "Primary prophylaxis of cryptococcal disease with fluconazole in HIV-positive Ugandan adults: a double-blind, randomised placebo-controlled trial," *Lancet Infectious Diseases*, vol. 11, pp. 933–941, 2011.

Rapid Point-of-Care Testing for Detection of HIV and Clinical Monitoring

D. R. Arora,[1] Megha Maheshwari,[1,2] and B. Arora[3]

[1] *Department of Microbiology, SGT Medical College, Budhera, Gurgaon, Haryana 123505, India*
[2] *Shri Guru Gobind Singh Tricentenary Medical College, Village Budhera, Gurgaon, Haryana 123505, India*
[3] *Department of Pathology, SGT Medical College, Budhera, Gurgaon, Haryana 123505, India*

Correspondence should be addressed to Megha Maheshwari; megha0gera51@gmail.com

Academic Editors: D. Aunis, L. Gray, C. Petrovas, J. Poudrier, and A. B. Williams

Reversing and arresting the epidemic of HIV are a challenge for any country. Early diagnosis and rapid initiation of treatment remain a key strategy in the control of HIV. Technological advances in the form of low-cost rapid point-of-care tests have completely transformed the diagnosis and management of HIV, especially in resource limited settings, where health infrastructure is poor and timely access to medical care is a challenge. Point-of-care devices have proven to be easy to transport, operate, and maintain, and also lower-skilled staff is equally able to perform these tests as compared to trained laboratory technicians. Point-of-care tests allow rapid detection of HIV allowing for rapid initiation of therapy, monitoring of antiretroviral therapy and drug toxicity, and detection of opportunistic infections and associated illnesses.

1. Introduction

Testing and treatment are key elements in the effort to control HIV, and testing services are rightly considered as the gateway to the treatment facilities. Data suggest that HIV-infected individuals who are aware of their status are more likely to adopt risk reduction behaviour than those who are not as discussed by Higgins et al. [1]. With a diagnosis of AIDS, consideration may be given to the initiation of antiretroviral treatment, which reduces viral load and infectivity as discussed by Rotheram-Borus et al. [2]. From a public health perspective, it is advisable to recommend testing to those at risk for HIV and to make testing easily accessible. The idea is to detect every HIV positive whether it belongs to high risk group, a pregnant woman, or a patient of tuberculosis or reproductive tract infection approaching the health system for health needs and refer him/her to the nearest antiretroviral therapy (ART) centre. Providing quality laboratory services for HIV testing to all those who need it is a challenging task.

2. Point-of-Care Tests for HIV

Point-of-care (POC) testing of HIV refers to the practice undertaken by health care professionals of providing pretest counseling, posttest counseling, and a preliminary HIV antibody result at the time of testing outside of a designated laboratory. The standard methods of HIV testing (enzyme linked immunosorbent assay (ELISA) or western blot with confirmatory testing using p24 antigen detection or viral nucleic acid detection) can take several days for result availability as discussed by Arora et al. [3]. A significant proportion of individuals who agree to undergo HIV serologic testing do not return to the HIV testing site to receive their test results as discussed elsewhere [4–6]. POC testing of HIV attempts to address delay in detection of HIV status by providing preliminary antibody results. POC tests can be most useful in resource limited settings (RLS) or outreach settings where there is lack of well-trained laboratory technicians, poor physical infrastructure, extremes of climate, and lack of uninterrupted power supply, all of which impact the use of laboratory technologies.

Rapid HIV test kits are designed to test for HIV antibodies. These deliver results within about 20 minutes of a specimen being taken; so, results are available within a single consultation. Rapid test devices (RTDs) are typically capillary flow tests for use on whole blood (e.g., fingerprick), plasma, urine, or oral fluid as discussed elsewhere [7–10]. They detect

HIV antibodies against HIV 1 and 2 antigens produced by oligopeptide synthesis or recombinant DNA technology. Quick turnaround time, ease of sampling, performance and reading results, no requirement of cold chain, and specialized equipment make these tests highly suitable in RLS. Since, oral fluid/saliva testing is more convenient, noninvasive and safe for laboratory workers, it can serve as an alternative for screening as well as surveillance purposes as discussed by Garg et al. [11]. Oral fluid sampling for HIV could particularly benefit the uptake among children and injectable drug users who may have collapsed blood vessels. However, not all RTDs are usable at the point-of-care (e.g., they require serum separation but still give results in a few minutes). Any HIV POC test approved for use is required to have sensitivity and specificity equivalent to HIV screening test kits (ELISA) approved for laboratory use as discussed by Shott et al. [12]. Currently, seven FDA approved HIV RTDs are available in the market [13].

The field has also advanced with the development of over-the-counter (OTC) self-testing options for HIV and multiplexed platforms that allow for simultaneous detection of infections associated with HIV, such as hepatitis B and C and syphilis. Researchers believed that home testing could be valuable "in empowering individuals to manage their HIV risks; in helping couples to learn their partners' HIV status before the initiation of sexual relations; and in addressing the three principal barriers to wider HIV-test acceptance: stigma, convenience, and privacy" as described by Walensky and Paltiel [14]. FDA approved the OraQuick In-Home HIV Test, the first over-the-counter home use rapid HIV test kit to detect the presence of antibodies to HIV-1 and HIV-2 [15].

Fourth generation HIV RTDs that detect both antigen and antibodies (ARCHITECT HIV Ag/Ab Combo Assay, Alere Determine HIV 1/2 Ag/Ab Combo assay) are being developed. They allow for early detection of HIV infection, prior to the emergence of HIV antibodies, therefore reducing the window period of antibody detection [16]. These tests, however, need validation and extensive performance evaluation in diverse field settings.

3. When to Use the HIV POC Test Kits

POC testing of HIV is not designed for screening the general population; it is to be used to screen patients at high risk for HIV. The rapid turnaround time associated with its use can guide urgent decision making. This makes it suitable for use in targeted clinical scenarios where the immediate administration of antiretroviral drugs is recommended to reduce the risk of transmission or in cases where the patient's management may be altered by the availability of a reactive test result.

3.1. Obstetric Settings. Testing pregnant women for HIV at the time of labor and delivery is the last opportunity for prevention of mother-to-child HIV transmission (PMTCT) measures, particularly in settings where women do not receive adequate antenatal care. However, HIV testing and counseling of pregnant women in labor is a challenge, especially in resource-constrained settings. In India, many rural women present for delivery without any prior antenatal care. Those who do get antenatal care are not always tested for HIV, because of deficiencies in the provision of HIV testing and counseling services as discussed elsewhere [17, 18]. POC testing should be provided to women with risk factors for HIV infection, but no recorded HIV status presenting in established labour as access to immediate HIV results improves the judicious use of antiretroviral prophylaxis as discussed by Cohen et al. [19].

3.2. Blood and Body Fluid Exposure/Health Care Worker Occupational Exposure. Knowledge of the source of the individual's HIV status during an evaluation of blood and body fluid exposure can help to determine more precisely those situations where HIV prophylaxis might be useful. HIV POC testing of source individuals offers an opportunity to eliminate anxiety and the unnecessary use of postexposure prophylaxis in the exposed person.

3.3. Acutely Ill Patients. In some clinical situations, it may be critical to have a rapid HIV diagnosis so that immediate and appropriate therapy or further diagnostic work-up can be provided, for example, a patient with risk factors for HIV who presents with pneumonia for which differential diagnosis would include *Pneumocystis jirovecii* pneumonia or patients undergoing hemodialysis.

3.4. An Individual at High Risk for HIV Acquisition. Consenting patients who are at high risk for HIV (needle stick source, from endemic area, injectable drug users, sexual partner with AIDS or positive HIV, history of unprotected sexual intercourse, multiple sex partners, sex partner of high risk person(s), sex worker, and homosexual men) and who have not had an HIV test in the previous 3 months, or who are unaware of their HIV status as discussed by D. R. Arora and B. Arora [20].

3.5. Patients Attending Sexually Transmitted Diseases (STD) Clinics. POC testing is acceptable, feasible, and leads to timely entry of people with HIV positive tests into the health care facility as discussed by Kendrick et al. [21]. Also among the STD clinic attendees presenting with genital ulcer, HIV reactivity (4%) was found to be statistically significant as discussed by Arora et al. [22].

4. Challenges in POC Testing

4.1. Counseling. POC HIV testing requires pre- and posttest counseling to be modified from the usual HIV counseling that accompanies standard HIV testing. However, certain clinical situations may make detailed pretest counseling difficult, for example, rapid testing for pregnant women in labour. In these situations, informed consent for testing is a minimum requirement. Informed consent is a process of communication that enables a person to make a reasonable and informed decision. Pretest counseling is critical in preparing patients for the implications of the test, and in cases of reactive test results, ensuring that they return for confirmatory test results. Posttest counseling provides information on risk behaviour, potential links to community resources, and rationale for behaviour changes needed to reduce risk. In the case of a nonreactive test result, the counseling session provides the opportunity for an exchange of information on the individual's perceived risks and cofactors and on harm reduction and prevention. Patients with risk activities in the last 3 months may not have detectable antibodies at the time of the test. These patients should be counseled as to the need for repeated HIV testing and on the need to protect their partners when engaging in high risk activities. With reactive test results, the implications are just as great in terms of reduction in risk of transmission, provision of health care information, and referral to ART centres.

4.2. Quality Assurance. In contrast to the situation in standard HIV testing, the health care workers in the POC setting assume responsibility for specimen collection, testing, and counseling of the patient. Adequate resources, appropriate training, and the implementation of quality assurance practices will be critical in ensuring the proper administration of the test and the correct interpretation of the test result.

4.3. Regulatory Approval. Rapid HIV test kits must be licensed for use in the country.

4.4. Performance Characteristics of Rapid Test Devices. RTDs are generally satisfactory for the detection of uncomplicated HIV infection (or its absence) but are less sensitive than lab-based ELISAs and automated systems for detecting early infections (seroconversion). Also specificity of RTDs is lower than conventional ELISAs although it can be improved by immediate repeat of all RTD positives as discussed by Kagulire et al. [23]. Since these may not be reliable in the "window" period and appropriate repeat testing should be advised, no currently available RTDs incorporate HIV p24 antigen detection in contrast to the commonly used conventional combination ELISA laboratory tests which are more sensitive in early HIV infection.

4.5. Ethical Implications. Ease of testing might lead to people being tested without their voluntary, specific, and informed consent. This is a particular risk where patients are anaesthetised (e.g., occupational exposure) or unable to communicate (e.g., woman in labour) or otherwise lack capacity to make decisions.

4.6. Staff Training. Appropriate training on the use of kits, reading of results, detection of errors, quality assurance, counseling, and regular assessment of staff who will be performing POC testing is required for providing point-of-care testing as discussed by Kabra and Kanugo [24].

4.7. Patients with a (Preliminary) Positive Test. A small number of people who are not HIV infected will produce a positive (reactive) result when tested with an HIV antibody test kit, including the rapid test. Because of this, all reactive test results must be confirmed using a laboratory-based confirmatory test. The importance for confirmatory testing at an approved HIV testing laboratory needs to be emphasized to rule out the possibility of a false-positive result in the rapid HIV test and to confirm a true positive result.

5. Cost-Benefit Evaluation of HIV POC Testing

Costs and adverse events associated with the use of HIV POC tests (labour, training, test kit, and cost of antiretroviral medication in response to false reactive result) will be compared to the cost and adverse events associated with untreated HIV infection resulting in transmission to the newborn (among women with no prenatal testing), use of antiretroviral medications when not required (in cases of occupational exposure), and increased morbidity and mortality associated with delay in HIV status detection of an acutely ill patient. The cost-effectiveness of routine HIV screening in health care settings, even in relatively low-prevalence populations, is similar to that of commonly accepted interventions, and such programs should be expanded as discussed by Sanders et al. [25].

6. Clinical Monitoring of Patients

Access to antiretroviral therapy (ART) has increased dramatically over the past decade in low- and middle-income countries. However, successful management of HIV requires patients receiving ART to be monitored routinely to assess treatment efficacy and detect treatment failure due to drug resistance. The standard of care to monitor ART is quantitative viral load testing based on plasma HIV RNA concentration as discussed by Volberding and Deeks [26]. Although CD4 count has also been used to monitor ART, recent studies suggest that it may not detect early treatment failure adequately as discussed by Moore et al. [27]. POC test for CD4 count could help clinicians in resource limited settings to decide when to start antiretroviral treatment, and a POC test for viral load would be of great value in identifying treatment failure and the need for second-line treatment. POC devices for CD4 immunologic monitoring and viral load assay are currently being evaluated as discussed elsewhere [28–30]. If validated, these devices could rapidly and accurately identify CD4 counts with minimal operator training, infrastructural setup, and with less cost than standard laboratory-based equipment such as flow cytometers for CD4 count or RT-PCR for viral load assay. PIMA analyzer (Alere, Inc., Waltham, MA, USA) is a WHO prequalified simple, effective point-of-care CD4 count test. It gives a CD4 count in 20 minutes from a finger stick or venous sample. Recent evaluations in Zimbabwe and Mozambique have shown good performance in comparison to flow cytometry as discussed elsewhere [27, 28]. VISITECT CD4 is a disposable, semiquantitative point-of-care rapid test for the determination of CD4 counts in whole blood. VISITECT CD4 can guide treatment decisions at the point-of-care, without the need for extensive training or sophisticated equipment. The test is a convenient solution for use in laboratories and remote clinics worldwide and provides a visual "TREAT" or "NO TREAT" result within 40 minutes [31].

Antiretroviral drugs, especially stavudine (nucleoside reverse transcriptase inhibitors), are associated with severe side effects such as lactic acidosis, pancreatitis, and hepatitis as discussed by Arora et al. [32]. POC tests for toxicity monitoring (e.g., lactate, renal function tests, and liver function tests) are also being evaluated as discussed elsewhere [33, 34] and will help in monitoring drug toxicity in patients. Tuberculosis is one of the most common opportunistic infection in developing countries as discussed by Arora et al. [35]. Therefore, there will also be a need for rapid POC detection of opportunistic infections.

7. Conclusion

Decentralization of laboratory services is required to detect the maximum possible number of HIV-positive patients and to put them on antiretroviral therapy. Accurate HIV rapid test devices are available but are not yet widely used. They may improve patient care especially in outreach settings for hard to reach groups and in obstetric management. The particular public health interest in the use of point-of-care testing for HIV is its ability to contribute to health goals which include preventing new HIV infections, reducing the number of HIV individuals who are unaware of their status, and promoting linkage of HIV-positive individuals to care. The ethical framework surrounding informed consent for a rapid test is the same as for a standard blood test, but the dissemination of testing and potential lack of experience of staff administering tests and handling the results requires careful consideration.

References

[1] D. L. Higgins, C. Galavott, K. R. O'Reilly et al., "Evidence for the effects of HIV antibody counseling and testing on risk behaviours," *Journal of American Medical Association*, vol. 266, no. 17, pp. 2419–2429, 1991.

[2] M. J. Rotheram-Borus, P. A. Newman, and M. A. Etzel, "Effective detection of HIV," *Journal of Acquired Immune Deficiency Sydromes*, vol. 25, no. 2, pp. S105–S114, 2000.

[3] D. R. Arora, V. Gupta, S. Gupta, and B. Arora, "Laboratory diagnosis of acquired immunodeficiency syndrome (AIDS)—a review," *Indian Journal of Sexually Transmitted Diseases*, vol. 21, pp. 59–68, 2000.

[4] R. O. Valdiserri, M. Moore, A. R. Gerber, C. H. Campbell, B. A. Dillon Jr., and G. R. West, "A study of clients returning for counseling after HIV testing: implications for improving rates of return," *Public Health Reports*, vol. 108, no. 1, pp. 12–18, 1993.

[5] Centers for Disease Control and Prevention, "Update: HIV counseling and testing using rapid tests—United States, 1995," *Morbidity Mortality Weekly Report*, vol. 47, pp. 211–215.

[6] G. Tao, B. M. Branson, W. J. Kassler, and R. A. Cohen, "Rates of receiving HIV test results: data from the U.S. National Health Interview Survey for 1994 and 1995," *Journal of Acquired Immune Deficiency Syndromes and Human Retrovirology*, vol. 22, no. 4, pp. 395–400, 1999.

[7] S. C. Kagulire, P. D. Stamper, P. Opendi et al., "Performance of two commercial immunochromatographic assays for rapid detection of antibodies specific to human immunodeficiency virus types 1 and 2 in serum and urine samples in a rural community-based research setting (Rakai, Uganda)," *Clinical and Vaccine Immunology*, vol. 14, no. 6, pp. 738–740, 2007.

[8] B. Taye, Y. Woldeamanuel, and E. Kebede, "Diagnostic detection of human immunodeficincy virus type-1 antibodies in urine, Jimma Hospital, south west Ethiopa," *Ethiopian Medical Journal*, vol. 44, no. 4, pp. 363–368, 2006.

[9] S. J. S. Pascoe, L. F. Langhaug, J. Mudzori, E. Burke, R. Hayes, and F. M. Cowan, "Field evaluation of diagnostic accuracy of an oral fluid rapid test for HIV, tested at point-of-service sites in rural Zimbabwe," *AIDS Patient Care and STDs*, vol. 23, no. 7, pp. 571–576, 2009.

[10] R. L. Hamers, I. H. de Beer, H. Kaura, M. van Vugt, L. Caparos, and T. F. Rinke de Wit, "Diagnostic accuracy of 2 oral fluid-based tests for HIV surveillance in Namibia," *Journal of Acquired Immune Deficiency Syndromes*, vol. 48, no. 1, pp. 116–118, 2008.

[11] N. Garg, V. Gautam, P. Sgill, B. Arora, and D. R. Arora, "Comparison of salivary and serum antibody detection in HIV-1 infection by ELISA and rapid methods in India," *Tropical Doctor*, vol. 36, no. 2, pp. 108–109, 2006.

[12] J. P. Shott, R. M. Galiwango, and S. J. Reynolds, "A quality management approach to implementing point-of-care technologies for HIV diagnosis and monitoring in sub-Saharan Africa," *Journal of Tropical Medicine*, vol. 2012, Article ID 651927, 8 pages, 2012.

[13] 2013, http://www.fda.gov/forconsumers/byaudience/forpatientadvocates/hivandaidsactivities/ucm117922.htm.

[14] R. P. Walensky and A. D. Paltiel, "Rapid HIV testing at home: does it solve a problem or create one?" *Annals of Internal Medicine*, vol. 145, no. 6, pp. 459–462, 2006.

[15] 2013, http://www.fda.gov/forconsumers/consumerupdates/ucm310545.htm.

[16] http://alerehiv.com/hiv-screening/alere-determine-hiv-12-agab-combo/.

[17] N. P. Pai, R. Barick, J. P. Tulsky et al., "Impact of round-the-clock, rapid oral fluid HIV testing of women in labor in rural India," *PLoS Medicine*, vol. 5, no. 5, article e92, 2008.

[18] F. A. Bello, O. O. Ogunbode, O. A. Adesina, O. Olayemi, O. M. Awonuga, and I. F. Adewole, "Acceptability of counselling and testing for HIV infection in women in labour at the University College Hospital, Ibadan, Nigeria," *African Health Sciences*, vol. 11, no. 1, pp. 30–35, 2011.

[19] M. H. Cohen, B. Branson, Y. Olszewski et al., "Effective Point—of—care Rapid HIV testing at labour and delivery," in *Proceedings of the 9th Conference on Retroviruses and Opportunistic Infections at Program and Abstracts*, Foundation for Retrovirology and Human health, Boston, Mass, USA, 2003.

[20] D. R. Arora and B. Arora, "Retroviridae," in *Textbook of Microbiology*, pp. 586–604, CBS Publishers, New Delhi, India, 4th edition, 2012.

[21] S. R. Kendrick, K. A. Kroc, D. Withum, R. J. Rydman, B. M. Branson, and R. A. Weinstein, "Outcomes of offering rapid point-of-care HIV testing in a sexually transmitted disease clinic," *Journal of Acquired Immune Deficiency Syndromes*, vol. 38, no. 2, pp. 142–146, 2005.

[22] D. R. Arora, V. Gautam, P. S. Gill, B. Arora, and V. Gupta, "Haryana state in India, still a low HIV prevalence state," *Sexually Transmitted Infections*, vol. 80, no. 4, pp. 325–326, 2004.

[23] S. C. Kagulire, P. Opendi, P. D. Stamper et al., "Field evaluation of five rapid diagnostic tests for screening of HIV-1 infections

in rural Rakai, Uganda," *International Journal of STD and AIDS*, vol. 22, no. 6, pp. 308–309, 2011.

[24] S. Kabra and R. Kanugo, "Monitoring quality of HIV testing at point of care facilities in India," *Indian Journal of Medical Microbiology*, vol. 30, no. 2, pp. 129–130, 2012.

[25] G. D. Sanders, A. M. Bayoumi, V. Sundaram et al., "Cost-effectiveness of screening for HIV in the era of highly active antiretroviral therapy," *New England Journal of Medicine*, vol. 352, no. 6, pp. 570–585, 2005.

[26] P. A. Volberding and S. G. Deeks, "Antiretroviral therapy and management of HIV infection," *The Lancet*, vol. 376, no. 9734, pp. 49–62, 2010.

[27] D. Moore, A. Awor, R. Downing et al., "CD4(+) T cell count monitoring does not accurately identify HIV-infected adults with virologic failure receiving antiretroviral therapy," *Journal of Acquired Immne Deficiency Syndrome*, vol. 49, pp. 477–484, 2008.

[28] S. Mtapuri-Zinyowera, M. Chideme, D. Mangwanya et al., "Evaluation of the PIMA point-of-care CD4 analyzer in VCT clinics in Zimbabwe," *Journal of Acquired Immune Deficiency Syndromes*, vol. 55, no. 1, pp. 1–7, 2010.

[29] I. V. Jani, N. E. Sitoe, P. L. Chongo et al., "Accurate CD4 T-cell enumeration and antiretroviral drug toxicity monitoring in primary healthcare clinics using point-of-care testing," *AIDS*, vol. 25, no. 6, pp. 807–812, 2011.

[30] B. A. Rohrman, V. Leautaud, E. Molyneux, and R. R. Richards-Kortum, "A lateral flow assay for quantitative detection of amplified HIV-1 RNA," *PLoS ONE*, vol. 7, no. 9, article e45611, 2012.

[31] 2013, http://www.omegadiagnostics.com/CD4.

[32] D. R. Arora, V. Gautam, P. S. Gill, and N. Mishra, "Recent advances in antiretroviral therapy in HIV infection," *Journal of the Indian Medical Association*, vol. 108, no. 1, pp. 29–34, 2010.

[33] C. C. Moore, S. T. Jacob, R. Pinkerton et al., "Point-of-care lactate testing predicts mortality of severe sepsis in a predominantly HIV type 1-infected patient population in Uganda," *Clinical Infectious Diseases*, vol. 46, no. 2, pp. 215–222, 2008.

[34] J. Yu, L. Ge, J. Huang, S. Wang, and S. Ge, "Microfluidic paper-based chemiluminescence biosensor for simultaneous determination of glucose and uric acid," *LAb on a Chip*, vol. 11, pp. 1286–1291, 2011.

[35] D. R. Arora, V. Gautam, S. Sethi, and B. Arora, "A 16-year study of HIV seroprevalence and HIV-related diseases in a teaching tertiary care hospital in India," *International Journal of STD and AIDS*, vol. 15, no. 3, pp. 178–182, 2004.

Prevalence of Intestinal Parasitic Infection among HIV Positive Persons Who Are Naive and on Antiretroviral Treatment in Hiwot Fana Specialized University Hospital, Eastern Ethiopia

Zelalem Teklemariam,[1] Degu Abate,[1] Habtamu Mitiku,[1] and Yadeta Dessie[2]

[1] *Department of Medical Laboratory Sciences, College of Health and Medical Sciences, Haramaya University, P.O. Box 235, Harar, Ethiopia*
[2] *Department of Public Health, College of Health and Medical Sciences, Haramaya University, P.O. Box 235, Harar, Ethiopia*

Correspondence should be addressed to Zelalem Teklemariam; zelalemtmariam@yahoo.com

Academic Editors: D. Aunis, H. C. Mwandumba, C. Petrovas, and J. Poudrier

Background. Intestinal parasitic infection affects the health and quality of life of people living with HIV. This study was aimed to determine the prevalence of intestinal parasites among HIV positive individuals who are naive and who are on antiretroviral treatment (ART) in Hiwot Fana Specialized University Hospital, Eastern Ethiopia. *Methods.* A comparative cross-sectional study was conducted on 371 (112 ART-naive group and 259 on ART) HIV positive individuals. Stool specimens were collected and examined by direct wet mount, formol ether concentration technique, and modified ziehl-Neelsen methods. *Results.* The overall prevalence of intestinal parasitic infections was 33.7%; it was significantly higher among the study participants who were ART-naive group (45.5%) (AOR: 2.60(1.56,4.34)) and diarrheic (53.3%) (AOR: 2.30(1.34,3.96)) and with CD_4 count <200 cells/μL (46%) (AOR: 2.07(1.06,4.04)). The most commonly identified parasites were *Entamoeba histolytica/E. dispar* (13.5%), *Giardia lamblia* (8.1%), *Strongyloides stercoralis* (4.0%), and *Cryptosporidium* species (2.2%). *Conclusion.* HIV positive individuals with diarrhea and low CD_4 count and ART naive groups were more infected with intestinal parasites than their counterparts. Early stool examination and treatment of intestinal parasites for HIV/AIDS patients is essential.

1. Introduction

Globally about 3.5 billion people are infected with intestinal parasite. Out of whom, 450 million are suffering from its illness [1, 2]. The prevalence of intestinal parasitic infection is high in Sub-Saharan Africa, where the majority of HIV/AIDS cases are from [2, 3]. Parasites are common infections among HIV/AIDS patients [4–7]. Diarrhea causing opportunistic parasites like *Cryptosporidium parvum* and *Isospora belli* is common among HIV positive persons with CD_4 count less than 200 cells/μL [4, 5].

Antiretroviral treatment (ART) increases the length and quality of life and productivity of patients by improving survival and decreasing the incidence of opportunistic infections in people with HIV through reduction of the viral load and increasing the level of CD_4 cells [8]. Nevertheless, in Ethiopia, few studies have tried to investigate the extent of intestinal parasitic infections in relation to ART experiences and CD4 count [4, 5].

Therefore, we investigated the prevalence of intestinal parasites among HIV positive persons who were naive and who were on ART in Hiwot Fana Specialized University Hospital, Eastern Ethiopia.

2. Material and Methods

2.1. Study Setting. The study was conducted in Hiwot Fana Specialized University Hospital, Harar, Ethiopia. It is a teaching hospital of Haramaya University. The hospital is found in Harari National Regional State which is one of the Federal Democratic Republic of Ethiopia regional states located 515 km from Addis Ababa. In Harar, there are six hospitals and eight health centers. The health service coverage of the region was estimated to be above 100%. A comparative cross-sectional study was conducted among Naive and on ART HIV positive persons in Hiwot Fana Specialized University Hospital from March to April, 2011.

2.2. Study Participant. The study population was all the HIV positive individuals who were on ART and pre ART care in the ART unit of the hospital during the study period. Individuals who were on parasitic treatments during the data collection period were excluded. The prevalence of intestinal parasites among ART-naive group HIV positive individuals was taken as 50% and to detect a difference of 15% between the two groups with the assumption of 95% confidence level (CL), power of 80% (0.84) and ratio 2 : 1 of those on ART and ART-naive group. Double proportion formula was applied to calculate the sample size which was 274 on ART and 137 ART-naive group. A 5% nonresponse rate was added and the final calculated sample size was 431. Study participants were selected by simple random sampling techniques.

2.3. Data Collection and Laboratory Investigation Procedures

2.3.1. Stool Collection and Examination. Small pieces of labeled clean plastic sheets and wooden applicator sticks were distributed and the participants were instructed to bring sizable stool specimen of their own. With the provision of specimen, each participant was interviewed for sociodemographic variables. Each stool specimen was initially assessed for consistency. Then, it was examined by direct wet mount method using normal saline (0.85% NaCl solution) at Hiwot Fana Specialized University Hospital Laboratory in order to prevent the loss of motile stage of parasites. Lugol's iodine was used to detect the cyst of intestinal parasites. The remaining sample was preserved with 10% formalin and transported to the laboratory of Medical Laboratory Sciences Department Haramaya University. In the laboratory, it was examined by formol ether concentration technique and modified Zeihl-Neelsen method (for detection of opportunistic parasites—*Cryptosporidium* species, *Cyclospora cayetanensis,* and *Isospora belli*) [9]. The most recent CD_4 T-cells counts of the participants were obtained from their ART fellow-up record in the hospital.

2.4. Data Processing and Analysis. Data were entered into Epideta Version 3.1 and transported to SPSS Version 16 software for analysis. The prevalence of intestinal parasites was determined in relation to different variables Pearson's chi square test was used to assess statistical significance difference between proportions. Bivariate and multivariate analyses were performed to assess crude and adjusted ratio. A statistical test result was reported as significant when its P value was less than 0.05.

2.5. Ethical Consideration. Ethical clearance was obtained from Haramaya University Colleges of Health and Medical Sciences Institutional Research and Ethical Review Committee. All the participants were explained about the purpose and their right to participate or not to participate in this study. Those who gave their written consent participated in this study. Moreover, all personal information of the participants was kept confidential. Those participants who were found positive for intestinal parasitic infection were treated free of charge using the standard drugs by nurses in ART unit. ART follow-up record was also retrieved by nurses working in ART unit.

3. Results

3.1. Sociodemographic Characteristics of Study Participants. A total of 259 on ART and 112 ART-naive group HIV positive clients participated in the study, and the response rate was 86.7%. The mean age of the participants was 33.6 (SD ±10.04) and many of the ART-naive group (68.5%) and on ART (70%) participants were female. The majority of the study subjects were in the age group of 25–34, married, daily laborers, and urban dwellers (Table 1).

3.2. The Distribution of Parasite Species. The overall prevalence of intestinal parasites among the study participants was 33.7% (125/371). It was significantly higher in the ART-naive group (45.5% (51/112)) compared to those on ART (28.6% (74/259)) (P = 0.002). Some were infected with nonopportunistic (31.8%) and very few with opportunistic (3.5%) parasites.

Eleven parasite species were detected: *Entamoeba histolytica/Entamoeba dispar* (13.4% on ART-naive group and 13.5% on ART group ($P > 0.05$)) and *Giardia lamblia* (7.1% on ART-naive group and 8.5% on ART group) were the common ones. Opportunistic parasites like Crypotospriudum (7.1%) and *Isospora belli* (4.5%) were found only in ART-naive group group.

Some of the ART-naive group (26.8%) and few of the on ART (17.4%) subjects were diarrheic ($P < 0.05$); most of them were infected with *G. lamblia* ($P > 0.05$), Crypotospriudum species, *I. belli, and S. Stercolaris.* The overall prevalence of intestinal parasites was significantly higher among diarrheic (53.3% (40/75)) as compared to nondiarrheic (28.7% (85/296)) study participants ($P < 0.05$) (Table 2).

About 31% (31/100), 17.3% (34/196), and 13.3% (10/75) of the study participants with CD_4 count less than 200 cells/μL, 200–499 cells/μL and greater than or equal to 500 cells/μL, respectively, were diarrheic. The prevalence of diarrhea is significant in participants with CD_4 count less than 200 cells/μL ($P = 0.005$).

In the bivariate analysis, age, sex, occupation, residence, education, and marital status of the participants did not show significant association with prevalence of intestinal parasites. Participants with CD_4 count less than 200 cells/μL (COR: 1.93; CI: 1.03, 3.61), diarrheic (COR: 2.84; CI: 1.69, 4.77), and ART-naive group (COR: 2.09; CI: 1.32, 3.31) had higher risk of intestinal parasites. The participants with CD_4 count < 200 cells/μL were 2.07 times more likely to be infected with intestinal parasites than those with CD_4 count ≥500 cells/μL. The diarrheic participants and the ART-naive group ones were 2.30 and 2.60 times more likely to be infected with intestinal parasites (Table 3).

TABLE 1: Sociodemographic characteristics of naïve ART and on ART HIV positive study participants at Hiwot Fana Specialized University Hospital, Harar, Eastern Ethiopia, 2011.

Variables	Naïve ART *N* (%)	On ART *N* (%)	Total *N* (%)
Age (in year)			
15–24	35 (31.5%)	40 (15.6%)	75 (20.4)
25–34	51 (45.9%)	121 (47.3%)	172 (46.9)
≥35	25 (22.5%)	95 (37.1%)	120 (32.7)
Sex			
Male	35 (31.5)	76 (29.3)	111 (30)
Female	76 (68.5)	183 (70.7)	259 (70)
Educational status			
Illiterate	27 (24.1)	56 (21.6)	83 (22.4)
Read and write	3 (2.7)	7 (2.7)	10 (2.7)
Elementary school	49 (43.8)	94 (36.3)	143 (38.5)
High school and above	33 (29.5)	102 (39.4)	135 (36.4)
Marital status			
Single	30 (27.5)	56 (21.6)	86 (23.4)
Married	55 (50.5)	112 (43.2)	167 (45.4)
Divorced	14 (12.8)	55 (21.2)	69 (18.8)
Widowed	10 (9.2)	36 (13.9)	46 (12.5)
Occupation			
Government employee	14 (12.8)	56 (21.8)	70 (19.1)
Nongovernmental organization	5 (4.6)	13 (5.1)	18 (4.9)
Farmer	2 (1.8)	11 (4.3)	13 (3.6)
Merchants	23 (21.1)	47 (18.3)	70 (19.1)
Daily laborer	27 (24.8)	66 (25.7)	93 (25.4)
House wife	19 (17.4)	26 (10.1)	45 (12.3)
Students	1 (0.9)	3 (1.2)	4 (1.1)
Other	12 (11.0)	16 (6.2)	28 (7.7)
No job	6 (5.5)	19 (7.4)	25 (6.8)
Residence			
Rural	23 (21.3)	65 (25.3)	88 (24.1)
Urban	85 (78.7)	192 (74.2)	277 (75.9)

TABLE 2: Intestinal parasite species identified with ART and diarrheic status of HIV positive study participants at Hiwot Fana Specialized University Hospital, Harar, Eastern Ethiopia, 2011.

Parasite species	Naïve ART ($N = 112$) Number of pos. (%)	On ART ($N = 259$) Number of pos. (%)	Total ($N = 371$) Number of pos. (%)	*P* value	Diarrheic ($n = 75$) Number of pos. (%)	Nondiarrheic ($n = 296$) Number of pos. (%)	*P* value
Entamoeba histolytica/E. dispar	15 (13.4)	35 (13.5)	50 (13.5)	0.975	10 (13.3)	40 (13.5)	0.967
Giardia lamblia	8 (7.1)	22 (8.5)	30 (8.1)	0.661	9 (12)	21 (7.1)	0.164
Strongyloides stercoralis	6 (5.4)	9 (3.5)	15 (4.0)	—	9 (12)	6 (2)	—
Crypotospriudum species	8 (7.1)	0 (0)	8 (2.2)		7 (9.3)	1 (0.3)	—
Hookworm	3 (2.7)	4 (1.5)	7 (1.9)	—	0 (0)	7 (2.4)	—
Isospora belli	5 (4.5)	0 (0)	5 (1.3)	—	5 (6.7)	0 (0)	—
Hymenolepis nana	1 (0.9)	4 (1.5)	5 (1.3)	—	0 (0)	5 (1.7)	—
Taenia saginata	0 (0)	3 (1.2)	3 (0.8)	—	0	3 (1.0)	—
Ascaris lumbricoides	2 (1.8)	1 (0.4)	3 (0.8)	—	1 (1.3)	2 (0.7)	—
Schistosoma mansoni	2 (1.8)	1 (0.4)	3 (0.8)	—	1 (1.3)	2 (0.7)	
Enterobius vermicularis	2 (1.8)	0 (0)	2 (0.5)	—	0 (0)	2 (0.7)	—

TABLE 3: Associating intestinal parasite with CD4 count and diarrheic and ART status among HIV positive study participants at Hiwot Fana Specialized University Hospital, Eastern Ethiopia, 2011.

Variables	No examined (% pos.)	Crude odds ratio (95% confidence interval)	*P* value	Adjusted odds ratio (95% confidence interval)	*P* value
CD_4 count (cells/μL)					
≥500	75 (30.7)	1		1	
200–499	196 (28.6)	0.90 (0.51, 1.62)	0.734	0.78 (0.42, 1.42)	0.409
<200	100 (46)	1.93 (1.03, 3.61)	0.041	2.07 (1.06, 4.04)	0.034
Diarrheic status					
Nondiarrheic	296 (28.7)	1		1	
Diarrheic	75 (53.3)	2.84 (1.69, 4.77)	0.000	2.30 (1.34, 3.96)	0.003
ART status					
On ART	259 (28.6)	1		1	
Naïve ART	112 (45.5)	2.09 (1.32, 3.31)	0.002	2.60 (1.56, 4.34)	0.000

4. Discussions

Intestinal parasitic infections are the major causes of morbidity and mortality in HIV positive patients [4–7, 10]. In this study, about 33.7% of the participants were infected with intestinal parasites. The result is almost similar to the ones reported from Afar, Ethiopia [5], Cameroon [11], and Saudi Arabia [12], but lower than those from Jimma [13], Hawassa [4], Bahir Dar [14], Dire Dawa and Afar [5] of Ethiopia, India [15], Kenya [16], and Jakarta [17]. But it is higher than a finding in Senegal [18]. The difference in the prevalence might be due to differences in geographical location, sensitivity of diagnostic techniques, study participants' immunity status, environmental hygiene, socioeconomic status, access to safe water supply, or other.

Several species of protozoa and other intestinal parasites have been associated with acute and chronic diarrhea and even weight loss in HIV/AIDS patients [19, 20]. In this study, *Entamoeba histolytica/E. dispar* and *Giardia lamblia* were the commonest nonopportunistic protozoa. The overall prevalence of *Entamoeba histolytica/E. dispar* was 13.5%. The finding is similar with 13% report in Ethiopia [5]. But it is higher than a report in Ethiopia (4.2%) [14], Saudi Arabia (5.2%) [12], and Jakarta (0.3%) [17]. It is lower than the one in Kenya (58.3%) [16] and Ethiopia (23.8%) [13]. The overall prevalence of *Gardia lamblia* was 8.1%. It is slightly lower than 10.6% in Ethiopia [13]. However, it is higher than report of 1.1% in Ethiopia [14], 0.6% in Senegal, and 1.9% in Jakarta [17]. It is also lower than report of 16.6% in Kenya [16] and 16% in Ethiopia [5].

Opportunistic protozoa like Crypotospriudum species and *Isospora belli* were also identified in this study. The prevalence of Crypotospriudum species was 2.2% and this is lower than the findings from other studies which are found in the range of 4.9% to 15.8% [5, 12–15, 17]. While *Isospora belli* was found at 1.3%. This is lower than other studies which are found in the range of 3.9% to 11.7% [5, 13–15]. The lower prevalence of both parasites in this study might be due to that our study participants are in the ART care who were taking ART and/or treatment for opportunistic infection. The other reason might be due to difference in immunity, diarrheic status, environmental and personal hygiene of the study participants.

Other nonopportunistic intestinal helimiths were identified at the rate of ranging from 0.5% to 4.0%. The highest prevalent helminth was *Strongyloides stercoralis*. This is similar to study carried out in Ethiopia [13], but it is slightly lower than another study in Ethiopia [14] and Saudi Arabia [12]. The effect of *Strongyloides Stercolaris* in HIV infected patients, which is disseminated strongloidiasis, was reported in another study [21].

In this study, we tried to compare the prevalence of intestinal parasites with the diarrheic status, CD_4 count, and ART experience of HIV positive persons. The prevalence of intestinal parasites was significantly higher among diarrheic as compared to nondiarrheic groups. Similar reports are found in other studies [12, 15, 16]. The most common diarrheal causing parasites were *E. histolytica, Gardia lamblia*, Crypotospriudum species, *Isospora belli,* and *Strongyloides stercoralis*. Similarly, there are reports which showed that diarrhea can be caused by opportunistic and nonopportunistic parasites [5, 15, 22].

The association between opportunistic parasitic infection and HIV is widely reported [4, 15, 23]. However, in this study, most of the parasites identified were nonopportunistic. The relationship between nonopportunistic parasite and HIV was not well established. Even though the defense against them might be damaged by HIV, the exposure to this parasites are likely to occur independent of HIV infection but heavier parasitic load might accumulate as well as experience of delayed clearance of parasite in individual with concurrent HIV induced immunosupperssion [23, 24].

The prevalence of intestinal parasites was highly significant among those study participants with CD_4 count <200 cells/μL in this study. This is consistent with other studies [4, 5, 15]. The correlation of CD_4 count with opportunistic parasites could not be assessed because of small number of individuals infected with Crypotospriudum species and *Isospora belli*. However, the association of these two parasites with HIV positive persons, who have CD_4 count <200 cells/μL, is reported in other studies [4, 5, 15, 23]

The prevalence of intestinal parasites was significantly higher when ART-naive group compared to those on ART study participants. Opportunistic parasites, which are Crypotospriudum species and *Isospora belli*, were found only in ART-naive group group. This is similar to study conducted in Ethiopia [5]. ART increases the immunity status HIV positive persons and decreases the incidence of opportunistic infections [8].

The study was not without limitations. The detection method for *Microsoporidia* was not employed and sensitive diagnostic techniques for *Strongyloides stercoralis* and *Enetrobius vermicularis* were not used. Therefore, the prevalence intestinal parasites in our study participant may have been underestimated. HIV negative control groups were not included in this study which was the other limitation.

5. Conclusions

The prevalence of intestinal parasite was high. Opportunistic and nonopportunistic parasites were identified with a different rate. The prevalence of intestinal parasites was higher among those HIV infected individuals with diarrhea, low CD_4 count, and ART-naive group groups. Those results posit the need for considering early detection and treatment of intestinal parasites in HIV infected individuals in order to reduce their morbidity. This seeks great attention by those clinical service providers who are working in the ART unit. Adherence counseling of ART, health information dissemination on environmental, and personal hygiene should also be given to HIV/AIDS patients. In addition further large scale study by using different diagnostic techniques, HIV negative control and assessing predisposing factors of intestinal parasites is recommended.

Acknowledgments

The authors acknowledge Haramaya University for funding this research. They also would like to thank all their study participants, data collectors, and supervisors. Hiwot Fana Specialized University Hospital administration is also strongly acknowledged.

References

[1] World Health Organization (WHO), *Control of Tropical Diseases*, WHO, Geneva, Switzerland, 1998.

[2] WHO, "Prevention of schistosomiasis and soil transmitted helminthiasis: report of WHO Expert Committee," WHO Technical Report Series 912, WHO, Geneva, Switzerland, 2002.

[3] UNAIDS/WHO, *AIDS Epidemic Update*, World Health Organization, Geneva, Switzerland, 2006.

[4] S. Assefa, B. Erko, G. Medhin, Z. Assefa, and T. Shimelis, "Intestinal parasitic infections in relation to HIV/AIDS status, diarrhea and CD_4 T-cell count," *BMC Infectious Diseases*, vol. 9, article 155, 2009.

[5] H. Adamu and B. Petros, "Intestinal protozoan infections among HIV positive persons with and without Antiretroviral Treatment (ART) in selected ART centers in Adama, Afar and Dire-Dawa, Ethiopia," *The Ethiopian Journal Health Development*, vol. 23, no. 2, pp. 133–140, 2009.

[6] A. E. Ibrahim, E. I. Ikeh, A. O. Malu, E. N. Okeke, and J. G. Damen, "Intestinal parasitosis in HIV infected adult with chronic diarrhea at Jos University teaching hospital, Nigeria," *Internet Journal of Parasitic Diseases*, vol. 2, no. 1, 2007.

[7] S. Kumas and S. Anthania, "Intestinal parasitic infection in HIV infected patients with diarrhea in clinic," *Indian Journal of Medical Microbiology*, vol. 20, no. 2, pp. 88–91, 2002.

[8] R. S. Hogg, B. Yip, C. Kully et al., "Improved survival among HIV-infected patients after initiation of triple-drug antiretroviral regimens," *Canadian Medical Association Journal*, vol. 160, no. 5, pp. 659–665, 1999.

[9] M. Cheesbrough, *District Laboratory Practice in Tropical Countries Part 1*, Cambridge University Press, New York, NY, USA, Second edition, 2009.

[10] S. Gupta, S. Narang, V. Nunavath, and S. Singh, "Chronic diarrhoea in HIV patients: prevalence of coccidian parasites," *Indian Journal of Medical Microbiology*, vol. 26, no. 2, pp. 172–175, 2008.

[11] C. Sarfati, A. Bourgeois, J. Menotti et al., "Prevalence of intestinal parasites including microsporidia in human immunodeficiency virus-infected adults in Cameroon: a cross-sectional study," *The American Journal of Tropical Medicine and Hygiene*, vol. 74, no. 1, pp. 162–164, 2006.

[12] W. A. I. Al-Megrin, "Intestinal parasites infection among immunocompromised patients in Riyadh, Saudi Arabia," *Pakistan Journal of Biological Sciences*, vol. 13, no. 8, pp. 390–394, 2010.

[13] Z. T. Mariam, G. Abebe, and A. Mulu, "Opportunistic and other intestinal parasitic infections in AIDS patients, HIV seropositive healthy carriers and HIV seronegative individuals in Southwest Ethiopia," *East African journal of public health*, vol. 5, no. 3, pp. 169–173, 2008.

[14] A. Alemu, Y. Shiferaw, G. Getnet, A. Yalew, and Z. Addis, "Opportunistic and other intestinal parasites among HIV/AIDS patients attending Gambi higher clinic in Bahir Dar city, North West Ethiopia," *Asian Pacific Journal of Tropical Medicine*, vol. 4, no. 8, pp. 661–665, 2011.

[15] R. Naik, H. Ravichandraprakash, P. M. Ukey, V. Vijayanath, G. Shreeharsha, and V. K. Chandak, "Opportunistic intestinal parasitic infections in HIV/AIDS patients presenting with diarrhea and their correlation with CD4+ T-lymphocyte counts," *International Journal of Pharmacy and Biological Sciences*, vol. 2, no. 4, pp. 293–299, 2012.

[16] C. K. Kipyegen, R. S. Shivairo, and R. O. Odhiambo, "Prevalence of intestinal parasites among HIV patients in Baringo, Kenya," *Pan African Medical Journal*, vol. 13, article 37, 2012.

[17] A. Kurniawan, T. Karyadi, S. W. Dwintasari et al., "Intestinal parasitic infections in HIV/AIDS patients presenting with diarrhoea in Jakarta, Indonesia," *Transactions of the Royal Society of Tropical Medicine and Hygiene*, vol. 103, no. 9, pp. 892–898, 2009.

[18] B. Faye, R. C. Tine, J. L. Ndiaye et al., "Impact of intestinal parasites on intensity of HIV infection in senegal," *Journal of Antivirals and Antiretrovirals*, vol. 2, no. 1, pp. 11–12, 2010.

[19] G. Feitosa, A. C. Bandeira, D. P. Sampaio, R. Badaró, and C. Brites, "High prevalence of giardiasis and stronglyloidiasis

among HIV-infected patients in Bahia, Brazil," *The Brazilian Journal of Infectious Diseases*, vol. 5, no. 6, pp. 339–344, 2001.

[20] K. Modjarrad, I. Zulu, D. T. Redden, L. Njobvu, D. O. Freedman, and S. H. Vermund, "Prevalence and predictors of intestinal helminth infections among human immunodeficiency virus type 1-infected adults in an urban African setting," *The American Journal of Tropical Medicine and Hygiene*, vol. 73, no. 4, pp. 777–782, 2005.

[21] R. Ramanathan and T. B. Nutman, "Strongyloides stercoralis infection in the immunocompromised host," *Current Infectious Disease Reports*, vol. 10, no. 2, pp. 105–110, 2008.

[22] W. V. Kit, "Intestinal parasitic infections in Thai HIV- infected patients with different immunity status," *BMC Gastroenterology*, vol. 1, article 3, 2001.

[23] M. Awole, S. Gebre-Selassie, T. Kassa, and G. Kibru, "Prevalence of intestinal parasites in South-Western Ethiopia," *The Ethiopian Journal of Health Development*, vol. 17, no. 1, pp. 71–78, 2003.

[24] T. Evering and L. M. Weiss, "The immunology of parasite infections in immunocompromised hosts," *Parasite Immunology*, vol. 28, no. 11, pp. 549–565, 2006.

11

Innate Immune Evasion Strategies by Human Immunodeficiency Virus Type 1

Debjani Guha and Velpandi Ayyavoo

Department of Infectious Diseases and Microbiology, Graduate School of Public Health, University of Pittsburgh, 130 Desoto Street, Pittsburgh, PA 15261, USA

Correspondence should be addressed to Velpandi Ayyavoo; velpandi@pitt.edu

Academic Editors: B. Joos, H. C. Mwandumba, and C. Petrovas

Host immune components play both beneficial and pathogenic roles in human immunodeficiency virus type 1 (HIV-1) infection. During the initial stage of viral infection, a complex network of innate immune factors are activated. For instance, the immune cells express a number of inflammatory proteins including cytokines, chemokines, and antiviral restriction factors. These factors, specifically, interferons (IFNs) play a crucial role in antiviral defense system by modulating the downstream signaling events, by inducing maturation of dendritic cells (DCs), and by activation of macrophages, natural killer (NK) cells, and B and T cells. However, HIV-1 has evolved to utilize a number of strategies to overcome the antiviral effects of the host innate immune system. This review discusses the pathways and strategies utilized by HIV-1 to establish latent and persistent infection by defeating host's innate defense system.

1. Introduction

During the early phase of infection, hosts mount innate immune response that comprises defense mechanisms to protect the hosts from invading pathogens in an antigen independent manner. This immune response is the first and a rapid response launched against a variety of microorganisms. The innate immune system can distinguish between self and foreign proteins and responds accordingly. This nonspecific immune response is activated primarily by the structural motifs of invading pathogens. The major cell types that play key roles in innate immune response against invading pathogens include macrophages, dendritic cells, neutrophils, natural killer cells, mast cells, eosinophils, and basophils. Most of the innate effector cells produce inflammatory factors that function as chemical messengers. Among these molecules, IFNs are the most effective in elucidating antiviral immune responses [1]. Additionally, cytokines and chemokines also play important roles as chemoattractants controlling leukocytes trafficking. Innate immune response operates through the steps of recognition of the pathogen, signal transduction, and subsequent gene expression to produce the innate immune effector molecules.

The first step is to recognize a pathogen as a foreign object and differentiate it from self-components. When pathogens breach physical barriers such as the skin or oral mucosa, they are recognized by pattern recognition receptors (PRRs) expressed either in the cytoplasm or on cell membranes. PRRs sense and interact with the structurally conserved motifs of proteins and nucleic acids unique to invading pathogens known as pathogen-associated molecular patterns (PAMPs) [2]. The most widely studied PRRs, the toll-like receptors (TLRs), present either on the cell surface or in the endoplasmic compartments, are involved in recognizing microbial PAMPs. For example, TLR2 and TLR4 respond to specific viral glycoproteins; TLR9, TLR3/7, and TLR8 are involved in sensing viral nucleic acids as well as the unmethylated CpG sequence in viral DNA molecules [3]. In addition to TLRs, viral PAMPs are also detected by other PRRs including RIG-like receptors (RLRs), RIG-I, MDA5, C-type lectin receptor (CLR), and DC-SIGN. RIG-I and MDA5 recognize 5′ phosphorylated short and long dsRNA, respectively, whereas, DC-SIGN binds to viral envelop glycoproteins. Cytosolic receptors such as AIM2 and DAI are also identified as respondents of dsDNA [4]. The interaction of viral ligands with host receptors activates the downstream signaling events that in turn switch on specific transcription factors regulating the expression of genes responsible for innate and adaptive immunity interchange. For example, when TLRs bind to viral PAMPs, the intracellular part of TLR binds to MyD88 and activates mitogen activated protein kinase (MAPK) that leads to the activation of NF-κB. Activation of NF-κB promotes regulation of inflammatory cytokine genes and activates interferon regulatory factor (IRF) [5, 6]. IRF induces type I IFNs that function as antiviral and inflammatory agents [7]. Furthermore, IFN is also involved in maturation of DC and regulates the function of macrophages, NK cells, and T and B cells [8]. However, the efficacy of host response depends on a rapid and specific recognition response to invading pathogens. Upon infection, immune cells are activated to modulate their molecular networks to eliminate the pathogen.

2. Strategies of HIV-1 to Evade Innate Immune Response

To overcome these immune effector functions, viruses including retroviruses are evolved to counteract and subvert through various mechanisms [9, 10]. Retroviruses are a diverse family of enveloped RNA viruses that have the ability to evade immune defense system and establish long-term persistence in the infected hosts. HIV-1, one of the retroviruses, utilizes varying strategies compared to other viruses as the PAMPs exposed by the virus are not easily recognized by the PRRs, and hence the virus can escape from proinflammatory and antiviral responses [11]. One possible mechanism by which HIV-1 manages to avoid immune encounter of the host is that HIV-1 can modify its PAMPs by altering or hiding its nucleic acids in the viral capsid in order to mimic the cellular proteins [12]. The ability of genetic variability of HIV-1 is one of the major immune evasion strategies for the virus. The HIV-1 RNA genome can be mutated randomly which helps the virus to evade immune recognition by the host. Error prone viral reverse transcriptase lacking the proofreading activity is responsible for the high mutation rate in HIV-1 [13]. By avoiding the immune recognition, HIV-1 crosses various checkpoints in innate as well as adaptive immune defense machineries of the host. This review emphasizes on some of the mechanisms utilized by HIV-1 to escape host's innate antiviral responses.

3. Evasion of HIV-1 through Mucosal Barriers during Early Infection

HIV-1 enters primarily through the mucosal surfaces of genital or rectal tissues during sexual transmission. Mucosa presents the first line of physical defense against invading pathogens. HIV-1 evades this initial barrier by successfully crossing the mucosa to reach the susceptible host cells and establish the infection. One of the proposed mechanisms is that the virus crosses the mucosal barrier by transcytosis or by capturing dendrites of intraepithelial DCs [14]. Additionally, HIV-1 also utilizes the intercellular spaces to move through the epithelium and achieve contact with the underlying mucosal Langerhans cells and CD4$^+$ T cells [14]. Exposure of HIV-1 or the viral protein gp120 disrupts tight junction proteins and the monolayer integrity of mucosal epithelium by the upregulating inflammatory cytokines that leads to the increased permeability of the virus particles [15]. These studies suggest that HIV-1 may induce defects at the mucosal epithelial barrier, which could activate mucosal T cells and increase the production of inflammatory cytokines [16–18]. A recent study demonstrated the association of $\gamma\delta$ T cells as a major component of mucosal immune system with the early HIV-1 induced events [19]. Breakdown of mucosal barrier is considered as the most crucial event causing HIV-1-associated immune activation.

Following mucosal breaching, HIV-1 establishes acute infection in immune cells present within the mucosa. It has been suggested that the productive HIV-1 infection starts from a single infectious virus particle [20, 21], and the resting CD4$^+$ T cells are the first targets [21–23]. These infected cells disseminate with the help of proinflammatory cytokines such as IL-1, IL-8, IL-6, and GM-CSF to the lymphoid tissues throughout the body including the gut-associated lymphoid tissue (GALT) containing high numbers of CD4$^+$ T cells where the virus replicates at a very high rate. A group of freshly infected CD4$^+$ T cells is generated, thus inducing rapid spread of HIV-1. This results in a peak of viremia or a viral set point followed by induction of CD8$^+$ T lymphocytes, and dramatic loss of CD4$^+$ T cells. Finally the viral load is controlled and maintained at a steady level throughout the chronic phase of HIV-1 infection. Hence, evading the physical barrier posed by the mucosal tissues marks the success of the initial stages of viral infection and spread.

4. Complement System

After penetrating the initial mucosal barrier, complement system confers a major host defense mechanism contributing the restriction in viral replication by triggering the recruitment of inflammatory cells and also by rupturing plasma membranes of undesired cells. Complement system functions as inhibitor as well as beneficiary for HIV-1 infection and pathogenesis. Complement pathways lyse HIV-1 particles and the infected cells to neutralize IgG and IgM-bound viruses. However, HIV-1 overcomes the complement mediated inhibition of viral spread or pathogenesis by activating the classical pathway of complement system by binding C1q with envelope protein gp41 [24]. HIV-1 downregulates expression of host complement receptors that impair monocyte chemotactic responses to inflammatory stimuli (exposure of gp120 decreases C5a expression) [25]. Deposition of C3 and C5a facilitates HIV-1 interaction with complement receptor CR3 and CR4 containing cells including monocytes/macrophages and DCs. HIV-1 gp41 interacts with CR3 and this interaction enhances both viral entry and viral spread in the cells [26]. HIV-1 also binds to CR1 on erythrocytes and CR2 on B cells and exploits these cells to generate C3d-opsonized infectious HIV-1 reservoirs and to spread infection to the uninfected organs [27–29]. In addition to increasing viral infectivity, HIV-1 gp41 and other viral proteins also stimulate the synthesis of C3 in neurons and astrocytes [30]. This increased production of complements is another means of contributing HIV-1-induced neuropathogenesis. Also, gp41 and gp120 recruit factor H, which is responsible for protecting self-cells from complement mediated lysis to multiple binding sites [31, 32]; thus, in turn, it causes decreased complement dependent lysis of infected cells and virus *in vitro* [33]. Another complement regulatory factor CD59 present on HIV-1 envelope prevents complement mediated neutralization of antibody bound viruses [34]. Together, these studies indicate that HIV-1 has evolved to override the complement system induced innate antiviral response to increase viral spread.

5. HIV-1 Induced Changes in Cytokine and Chemokine Profiles

Cytokines and chemokines have the most influential role in HIV-1 pathogenesis, and the virus exploits the network throughout its life cycle. HIV-1 infection results in the activation of immune cells, altered functions of macrophages, NK cells, and DCs, and the activation of B cells [35–41]. Overactivation of immune cells leads to increased production of pro-inflammatory anti-inflammatory cytokines and chemokines including IFNs, tumor necrosis factor (TNF)-α, interleukin-(IL)-1, -2, -4, -8, -6, -10, -15, interferon gamma-induced protein (IP)-10, and monocyte chemotactic protein (MCP)-1 [42, 43]. These cytokines/chemokines either enhance or inhibit HIV-1 replication. With disease progression—a shift from stimulatory Th1 (IL-2, IFN) to inhibitory Th2 (IL-4, IL-10, IL-1, IL-6, IL-8, and TNF), cytokine production takes place [44]. Attachment of HIV-1 envelope protein, gp120, triggers production of CC chemokines CCL2, CCL3, CCL4, and CCL5 that are chemoattractants for DCs, macrophages, and lymphocytes. The expression of these CC chemokines is regulated by cytokines including IL-6, TNF-α, IL-1β, and IL-10, which are also regulated by HIV-1 infection [45]. HIV-1 utilizes different mechanisms to override host cytokine/chemokine networks; for example, HIV-1 transactivator of transcription (Tat) protein mimics β-chemokines and functions as chemoattractant of monocytes/macrophages that leads to increased activation and infection [46]. A previous study has shown which HIV-1 negative regulatory factor (Nef) increases the production and the stimulatory function of proinflammatory cytokines such as IL-1β, IL-12, IL-15, and TNF-α and chemokines such as macrophage inflammatory protein (MIP)-1α, -1β and IL-8 when it interacts with immature DCs [47, 48]. HIV-1 accessory protein viral protein R (Vpr) also alters the level of proinflammatory cytokines [48]. Hence, HIV-1 either by mimicking or by modulating certain cytokines exploits the cytokine network for its replication and survival.

6. Interferons and Signaling Events

Among the cytokines, IFNs play the major role in virus infection and confer the first defense. Type I IFNs (include IFN-α, -β, -ε, -κ, and -ω), the innate cytokines produced by innate immune stimuli, have multiple properties including induction of immune activation, enhanced antigen presentation, and antiviral activity [49]. IFNs are mainly produced by IFN regulatory factors (IRFs) especially IRF3 and IRF7 [50]. They bind to IFN receptor IFNAR1/IFNAR2 at the cell surface and form STAT1/STAT2 dimer, which translocates into the nucleus and triggers downstream signaling pathways that result in activation of interferon-stimulated genes (ISGs). Cellular factors, ISGs, generated from type I and type II IFN, induce signaling events that inhibit HIV-1 replication [51, 52]. Recognition of PAMPs stimulates activation of IFN-induced signaling pathways triggering activation of transcriptions factors including NF-κB, activator protein (AP)-1 and IRF3, which in turn leads to production of proinflammatory cytokines and chemokines and antiviral type I IFN. The innate immune response largely depends on virus-induced signaling pathways to induce IFN response. A recent study indicated the role of tripartite motif containing 22 (TRIM22) induced by IFN-β as an inhibitor of HIV-1 replication [53].

Since IFN has the most potent role in preventing viral replication and eliminating infection, HIV-1 blocks and/or minimizes the IFN production as well as the downstream signaling pathways to prevent immune responses. However, the mechanism(s) by which HIV-1 can manage to escape IFN induced anti-HIV-1 activity is not fully understood. It was documented that HIV-1 gp120 blocks cytokines including IFN and the cytolytic activity of NK cells by interfering with TLR9 activation in pDCs [54]. In a SIV model of central nervous system, it has been shown that SIV infected astrocytes produce monocyte chemotactic protein (MCP)-1 or CCL2 that binds to the CCR2 receptors on macrophages resulting in suppression of specific ISGs such as TRAIL [55]. In macrophages, HIV-1 exploits another cellular factor, suppressor of cytokine signaling (SOCS) 3 to facilitate its replication. SOCS3 inhibits IFN-β signaling in macrophages, and hence it prevents antiviral gene expression that helps HIV-1 replication [56]. Studies also indicated that cellular $3'$ repair exonuclease 1 (TREX1) helps the virus to hide from immune activation [57]. The exonuclease activity of TREX1 degrades excess ssDNA of HIV-1 and thus prevents activation of IFN by this excess HIV-1 DNA. Mutation or dysfunction of TREX1 results in accumulation of HIV-1 DNA and triggers DNA sensors. This activates STING, TBK1, and IRF3 transcription factors. Activated IRF3 translocates into nucleus and enhances IFN response by activating the respective promoters in different cell types [57–59].

The release of IFNs leads to the induction of ISG through JAK/STAT pathways. ISGs induce antiviral response. One of the first ISG linked to antiviral response is the IFN-induced protein kinase R (PKR). It plays an important role, when it binds to dsRNA of viral replication product, forms a dimer by autophosphorylation, and blocks viral replication by inhibiting translation of alpha subunit of elongation initiation factor 2 (eIF2α) in infected cells. HIV-1 infection does not activate PKR. Virus replicates in cells where a high level of TAR binding protein (TRBP) is present. TRBP functions as a strong inhibitor of PKR and eIF2α [60, 61]. TRBP also binds to and serves as a cofactor of Dicer, which is required for biosynthesis of microRNA (miRNA) or RNA interference (RNAi) [62], inhibitors of viral replication. HIV-1 overrides the PKR mediated innate response via two different mechanisms. First, HIV-1 Tat RNA binds to TRBP and inhibits PKR activation; also TRBP becomes unavailable for Dicer binding [63]. Thus HIV-1 exploits TRBP as a link between IFN and RNAi mediated antiviral response. Second, HIV-1 Tat also functions as a substrate homologue of eIF2α and competes for PKR mediated phosphorylation. PKR phosphorylates HIV-1 Tat, and the phosphorylation of Tat is necessary for HIV-1 LTR transactivation [64]. This prevents phosphorylation of eIF2α and enhances viral replication [65]. Another protein adenosine deaminase acting on RNA (ADAR1) is also reported to inhibit PKR activation [60]. Together, these reports support that HIV-1 proteins play a major role in combating IFN responses, thus blocking innate antiviral activity.

7. Plasmacytoid Dendritic Cells (pDCs) Function as Major Source of IFN

After HIV-1 entry into the system, the immediate IFN response is primarily from pDCs. pDCs play the central role in innate immune response against viral pathogens through the secretion of enormous amount of IFN. It expresses TLR7 and TLR9 in addition to CD4, CCR5, and CXCR4 receptors. TLR7 and TLR9 on pDCs bind to ssRNA and unmethylated CpG DNA motif, respectively, and signal through MyD88 that in turn leads to the activation of IRF7 for IFN production. Compared to other blood cells, these cells produce several times more type I IFNs that function as immunostimulatory cytokine to drive mDC maturation [66]. HIV-1 inhibits the innate immune response of pDCs by reducing pDC cell counts in peripheral blood. HIV-1 infected individuals are reported to have lower levels of pDCs compared to uninfected individuals [39]. HIV-1 gp120 exposure suppresses pDC activation and production of proinflammatory cytokines mediated through TLR9 [54]. Other studies have demonstrated that HIV-1 blocks pDC function by suppressing TLR7 and TLR8 [67] and also by inhibiting IFN-α [68]. However, before undergoing HIV-1-induced cell death, pDCs upregulate CCR7 production, accumulate in lymph node, and produce high level of IFN [69]. High plasma level of IFN has been observed during acute HIV-1 infection and also during the late stage of the HIV-1 disease. It has also been reported that IFN enhances disease progression to AIDS [70]. HIV-1 induced production of IFN by pDCs leads to the expression of TNF-related apoptosis inducing ligand (TRAIL) [71], which is involved in triggering apoptosis of uninfected $CD4^+$ T cells [72]. Through TLR7, TRAIL turns pDCs into IFN-producing killer pDCs (IKpDCs) that produce high level of TNF-α [73]. It has also been shown that in addition to IFNs activation of pDCs, HIV-1 also stimulates production of inflammatory cytokines/chemokines including TNF-α, IL-6, CXCL10, CCL4, and CCL5 [74, 75].

8. Functional Dysregulation of Natural Killer (NK) Cells by HIV-1

The immunomodulatory and cytotoxic activities of NK cells are impaired in HIV-1 infected individuals, diminishing the innate and detrimentally affecting the adaptive immune response [76–79]. Analysis of frequency, phenotypes, and function of peripheral blood CD3-CD56+NK subsets in HIV-1+ individuals revealed significantly reduced numbers of total NK cells and a striking shift in NK cell subsets. More specifically, $CD56^{dim}$ populations of HIV-1 infected subjects were markedly diminished (and exhibited functional abnormalities) when compared to IFN-γ producing $CD56^{bright}$ NK cell fractions from the same individuals [79]. HIV-1 infection is characterized by a dramatic increase in inhibitory receptors and loss of activating receptors, particularly, NKp30 on NK cells, resulting in loss of NK cell activity and defective crosstalk with DC [80, 81]. Involvement of HIV-1 in the impairment of NK cell function *in vivo* has also been bolstered indicating an association between NK cell ligand HLA-B Bw4-801 and its receptor; the killer immunoglobulin-like receptor (KIR) 3DS1; expression of HLA/KIR subtypes can be linked to efficient NK cell mediated inhibition of HIV-1 replication and killing of infected targets [82, 83].

The observed NK cell dysregulation is attributed to HIV-1 viral proteins [84, 85]. HIV-1 Nef functions as a potential regulator of NK cell cytotoxicity due to its involvement in MHC class I downregulation on $CD4^+$ cells [86]. The selective downregulation by Nef of HLA A and HLA B but not HLA C or HLA E molecules in infected target cells inhibits NK cell cytotoxicity which confers an additional evasion strategy targeting the antiviral activities of NK cells [87–89]. HIV-1 Tat inhibits LFA-I-mediated Ca^{2+} influx through the binding of L-type Ca^{2+} channel and thereby impairs NK cell cytotoxicity [90, 91]. A linear motif of HIV-1 gp41 induces expression of NKp44L on $CD4^+$ T cells and results in their depletion by selective lysis by $NK44^+$ NK cells [37]. Azzoni et al. showed that virally suppressed children had normal levels of circulating pDCs, mDC, and total NK cells, yet they had sustained depletion of mature NK cell subsets along with diminished IFN-α production by pDC, which is required to enhance NK cell cytolytic responses [92]. HIV-1 treated target cells exhibit selective upregulation of NKG2D receptor on NK cells, and this upregulation is contact dependent and reversible [93]. Expression of these molecules is directly correlated with efficient killing of infected targets as well as controlling viremia, suggesting that innate immune cells play a critical role in immune control.

9. Antiviral Host Restriction Factors

In addition to other innate antiviral factors and innate immune cells, host restriction factors have also been shown to restrict HIV-1 infection in multiple ways. For instance, apolipoprotein B editing catalytic polypeptide (APOBEC3)

Table 1: Role of HIV-1 viral proteins in innate immune evasion.

HIV-1 accessory proteins	Function in innate immune evasion
gp41	(i) Activates classical pathway of complement system (ii) Enhances viral entry and spread through interaction with complement receptor CR3 (iii) Stimulates synthesis of C3 in neurons and astrocytes (iv) Recruits factor H responsible for protecting from complement dependent lysis (v) Induces expression of NKp44L on CD^{4+} T cells and results in their depletion
gp120	(i) Recruits factor H (ii) Induces production of inflammatory cytokines and the CC chemokines (iii) Suppresses pDC activation and produces IFN and other cytokines (iv) Inhibits cytolytic activity of NK cells by interfering with TLR9
Tat	(i) Substrate homologue for eIF2α and competes for PKR mediated phosphorylation (ii) Mimics β-chemokines and functions as chemoattractant for monocytes and macrophages (iii) Inhibits LFA-I mediated Ca^{2+} influx and impairs NK cell cytotoxicity (iv) Interacts with Dicer and inhibits its activity, suppresses miRNA synthesis
Nef	(i) Increases expression of proinflammatory cytokines (ii) Downregulates HLA-A, HLA-B on target cells and inhibits NK cell cytotoxicity (iii) Helps in budding of HIV-1 (iv) Produces viral miRNA in HIV-1 persistently infected cells
Vpr	(i) Alters the levels of proinflammatory cytokines (ii) Upregulates NKG2D receptor on NK cells
Vpu	(i) Causes detachment of viral particle from cell membrane through interaction with tetherin
Vif	(i) Inhibits the packaging of APOBEC3G in virus producer cells causes proteosomal degradation of APOBEC3G

is a member of cytidine deaminase family that has specific anti-HIV-1 property. APOBEC3G incorporates into HIV-1 through interacting with Gag and restricts HIV-1 infection [94, 95]. It mutates cytidine to uridine in negative sense single stranded DNA by deamination resulting in guanosine to adenosine hypermutation in positive sense viral cDNA and thereby makes it vulnerable to nuclease degradation [96, 97]. Current studies show that APOBEC3G functions in deaminase independent manner [98]. However, HIV-1 viral infectivity factor (Vif) protein inhibits the packaging of APOBEC3G in virus producer cells by functioning as an adaptor molecule that links a cullin-5-based E3 ubiquitin ligase complex with APOBEC3G leading to polyubiquitination and targeting APOBEC3G and APOBEC3F to proteosomal degradation [99–101].

Another restriction factor implicated in early steps of HIV-1 replication is tripartite motif-containing 5 (TRIM5). TRIM5 functions as E3 ubiquitin ligase and recognizes the motifs in viral capsid in the cytoplasm of an infected cell. TRIM5 prevents reverse transcription and transports viral genome to the nucleus [102]. Although the exact mechanism of TRIM5 inhibition is unknown, it has been suggested that TRIM5 promotes innate immune signaling, which is enhanced by interaction with viral capsid lattice [103]. TRIM5 binds to the viral capsid and activates the protein's ubiquitin ligase activity resulting in the synthesis of ubiquitin chains. These chains stimulate TAK1 (also known as MAP3 K7) phosphorylation followed by expression of NF-κB-dependent genes. In primates, TRIM5 expression regulates expression of genes by AP-1 and NF-κB activation [103, 104].

Tetherin is another intrinsic restriction factor involved in innate antiviral response. Tetherin/BST2, a glycosylated type II transmembrane protein, prevents budding of newly formed virus particles from plasma membrane of HIV-1 infected cells. Tetherin restricts HIV-1 transmission from one cell to another [105]. Its expression is upregulated by type I IFN. HIV-1 viral protein unique (Vpu) induces detachment of virus particles from cell membrane [106, 107]. Vpu interacts directly or indirectly with tetherin and reduces its expression at the surface. Viruses that are defective in Vpu expression remain tethered to the cell surface [11]. These tethered virus particles are subjected to endocytosis and degraded in lysosomes [12]. Recent studies indicated that the Vpu-like activity has been reported for other viral proteins including Env and Nef [13, 108, 109].

10. Other Regulatory Factors

Studies have shown that HIV-1 infection as well as innate immune response to viral infection could be controlled by host miRNAs [110]. miRNAs are short ~20–22 nucleotide long small noncoding RNA molecules expressed in most organisms [111]. These miRNAs control gene expression by binding to the 3′ UTR region of the target mRNAs. They can regulate the expression of both cellular and viral genes. For example, miR-26a, -34a, 145, and let-7b have been reported to regulate IFN-β in human and macaque cells [112]. Distinct differences in miRNA profiles have been reported in PBMCs infected with HIV-1 compared to control [113]. HIV-1 replication involves downregulation of specific cellular miRNAs (e.g., miR-29), which plays a significant role in controlling HIV-1 life cycle. Hsa-miR-29 binds to the conserved sequence of Nef 3′-LTR, transports HIV-1 mRNA to P-bodies and inhibits translation of viral mRNA [114]. Other miRNAs including miR-150, 223, 198, and 382 have been shown to be downregulated in HIV-1 infected macrophages and are known as anti-HIV-1 miRNAs, as they exert negative effect on the viral replication [115]. Treatment of macrophages with IFN-α and -β increases the expression of these miRNAs confirming their role in HIV-1 replication [56]. Alternatively, HIV-1 has also evolved viral miRNA to counterattack the host machineries. HIV-1 Tat interacts with Dicer, inhibits its activity, and suppresses the miRNA synthesis [116]. HIV-1 also blocks RNA silencing pathways by TRBP [62, 63]. Some viral miRNAs such as TAR miRNA, Nef miRNA (miR-N367), and miR-H1 are expressed, and regulate viral as well as host gene expression to facilitate virus replication and establishment of latency [117].

11. Conclusion

The interaction between host and HIV-1 is complex. The host system utilizes its machinery to defend HIV-1 infection, whereas the virus uses the host's tools as means of its own propagation. Starting at the transmission site (mucosal barrier) to immune activation site (lymph node), HIV-1 utilizes very unique strategies such as modification of its PAMPs, rapid mutation in its RNA to escape immune recognition, downregulation of complement receptors, increased secretion of inflammatory factors, and downregulation of NK cell function to overcome the innate immune response. The role of HIV-1 viral proteins to overcome host innate immunity is specified in Table 1. Current research focuses on understanding how HIV-1 overrides the innate immune system at multiple levels. The understanding of how HIV-1 prevails the host innate immune defense will increase our knowledge that could improve developing therapeutic approach to resist HIV-1 infection and spreading.

References

[1] V. Chieux, D. Hober, W. Chehadeh, and P. Wattré, "Anti-viral proteins: from interferon α to its receptor," *Annales de Biologie Clinique*, vol. 57, no. 3, pp. 283–290, 1999.

[2] G. Hajishengallis, H. Sojar, R. J. Genco, and E. DeNardin, "Intracellular signaling and cytokine induction upon interactions of Porphyromonas gingivalis fimbriae with pattern-recognition receptors," *Immunological Investigations*, vol. 33, no. 2, pp. 157–172, 2004.

[3] V. Racaniello, "Innate immune defenses," 2009, http://www.virology.ws/2009/06/03/innate-immune-defenses/.

[4] A. Takaoka, Z. Wang, M. K. Choi et al., "DAI (DLM-1/ZBP1) is a cytosolic DNA sensor and an activator of innate immune response," *Nature*, vol. 448, no. 7152, pp. 501–505, 2007.

[5] S. Akira, "TLR signaling," *Current Topics in Microbiology and Immunology*, vol. 311, pp. 1–16, 2006.

[6] T. Kawai and S. Akira, "Signaling to NF-κB by Toll-like receptors," *Trends in Molecular Medicine*, vol. 13, no. 11, pp. 460–469, 2007.

[7] M. Yoneyama, W. Suhara, Y. Fukuhara, M. Fukuda, E. Nishida, and T. Fujita, "Direct triggering of the type I interferon system by virus infection: activation of a transcription factor complex containing IRF-3 and CBP/p300," *EMBO Journal*, vol. 17, no. 4, pp. 1087–1095, 1998.

[8] P. M. Pitha, "Innate antiviral response: role in HIV-I infection," *Viruses*, vol. 3, no. 7, pp. 1179–1203, 2011.

[9] W. de Vries, J. Haasnoot, J. van der Velden et al., "Increased virus replication in mammalian cells by blocking intracellular innate defense responses," *Gene Therapy*, vol. 15, no. 7, pp. 545–552, 2008.

[10] R. A. Lever and A. M. L. Lever, "Intracellular defenses against HIV, viral evasion and novel therapeutic approaches," *Journal of the Formosan Medical Association*, vol. 110, no. 6, pp. 350–362, 2011.

[11] M. H. Malim and M. Emerman, "HIV-1 accessory proteins-ensuring viral survival in a hostile environment," *Cell Host and Microbe*, vol. 3, no. 6, pp. 388–398, 2008.

[12] T. Goto, S. J. Kennel, M. Abe et al., "A novel membrane antigen selectively expressed on terminally differentiated human B cells," *Blood*, vol. 84, no. 6, pp. 1922–1930, 1994.

[13] R. Serra-Moreno, B. Jia, M. Breed, X. Alvarez, and D. T. Evans, "Compensatory changes in the cytoplasmic tail of gp41 confer resistance to tetherin/BST-2 in a pathogenic Nef-deleted SIV," *Cell Host and Microbe*, vol. 9, no. 1, pp. 46–57, 2011.

[14] A. J. McMichael, P. Borrow, G. D. Tomaras, N. Goonetilleke, and B. F. Haynes, "The immune response during acute HIV-1 infection: clues for vaccine development," *Nature Reviews Immunology*, vol. 10, no. 1, pp. 11–23, 2010.

[15] A. Nazli, O. Chan, W. N. Dobson-Belaire et al., "Exposure to HIV-1 directly impairs mucosal epithelial barrier integrity allowing microbial translocation," *PLoS Pathogens*, vol. 6, no. 4, Article ID e1000852, 2010.

[16] J. M. Brenchley and D. C. Douek, "The mucosal barrier and immune activation in HIV pathogenesis," *Current Opinion in HIV and AIDS*, vol. 3, no. 3, pp. 356–361, 2008.

[17] B. Kanwar, D. Favre, and J. M. McCune, "Th17 and regulatory T cells: implications for AIDS pathogenesis," *Current Opinion in HIV and AIDS*, vol. 5, no. 2, pp. 151–157, 2010.

[18] D. Horejsh, T. J. Ruckwardt, and C. D. Pauza, "CXCR4-dependent HIV-1 infection of differentiated epithelial cells," *Virus Research*, vol. 90, no. 1-2, pp. 275–286, 2002.

[19] C. Agrati, G. D'Offizi, M.-L. Gougeon et al., "Innate gamma/delta T-cells during HIV infection: terra relatively incognita in novel vaccination strategies?" *AIDS Reviews*, vol. 13, no. 1, pp. 3–12, 2011.

[20] C. A. Derdeyn, J. M. Decker, F. Bibollet-Ruche et al., "Envelope-constrained neutralization-sensitive HIV-1 after heterosexual transmission," *Science*, vol. 303, no. 5666, pp. 2019–2022, 2004.

[21] B. F. Keele, E. E. Giorgi, J. F. Salazar-Gonzalez et al., "Identification and characterization of transmitted and early founder virus envelopes in primary HIV-1 infection," *Proceedings of the National Academy of Sciences of the United States of America*, vol. 105, no. 21, pp. 7552–7557, 2008.

[22] M.-R. Abrahams, J. A. Anderson, E. E. Giorgi et al., "Quantitating the multiplicity of infection with human immunodeficiency virus type 1 subtype C reveals a non-poisson distribution of transmitted variants," *Journal of Virology*, vol. 83, no. 8, pp. 3556–3567, 2009.

[23] J. F. Salazar-Gonzalez, M. G. Salazar, B. F. Keele et al., "Genetic identity, biological phenotype, and evolutionary pathways of transmitted/founder viruses in acute and early HIV-1 infection,"

Journal of Experimental Medicine, vol. 206, no. 6, pp. 1273–1289, 2009.

[24] P. Marschang, C. F. Ebenbichler, and M. P. Dierich, "HIV and complement: role of the complement system in HIV infection," *International Archives of Allergy and Immunology*, vol. 103, no. 2, pp. 113–117, 1994.

[25] C. Speth and M. P. Dierich, "Modulation of cell surface protein expression by infection with HIV-1," *Leukemia*, vol. 13, supplement 1, pp. S99–S105, 1999.

[26] H. Stoiber, I. Frank, M. Spruth et al., "Inhibition of HIV-1 infection in vitro by monoclonal antibodies to the complement receptor type 3 (CR3): an accessory role for CR3 during virus entry?" *Molecular Immunology*, vol. 34, no. 12-13, pp. 855–863, 1997.

[27] E. Horakova, O. Gasser, S. Sadallah et al., "Complement mediates the binding of HIV to erythrocytes," *Journal of Immunology*, vol. 173, no. 6, pp. 4236–4241, 2004.

[28] Z. Bánki, D. Wilflingseder, C. G. Ammann et al., "Factor I-mediated processing of complement fragments on HIV immune complexes targets HIV to CR2-expressing B cells and facilitates B cell-mediated transmission of opsonized HIV to T cells," *Journal of Immunology*, vol. 177, no. 5, pp. 3469–3476, 2006.

[29] S. Döpper, D. Wilflingseder, W. M. Prodinger et al., "Mechanism(s) promoting HIV-1 infection of primary unstimulated T lymphocytes in autologous B cell/T cell co-cultures," *European Journal of Immunology*, vol. 33, no. 8, pp. 2098–2107, 2003.

[30] C. Speth, T. Schabetsberger, I. Mohsenipour et al., "Mechanism of human immunodeficiency virus-induced complement expression in astrocytes and neurons," *Journal of Virology*, vol. 76, no. 7, pp. 3179–3188, 2002.

[31] C. Pinter, A. G. Siccardi, L. Lopalco, R. Longhi, and A. Clivio, "HIV glycoprotein 41 and complement factor H interact with each other and share functional as well as antigenic homology," *AIDS Research and Human Retroviruses*, vol. 11, no. 8, pp. 971–980, 1995.

[32] H. Stoiber, C. Ebenbichler, R. Schneider, J. Janatova, and M. P. Dierich, "Interaction of several complement proteins with gp120 and gp41, the two envelope glycoproteins of HIV-1," *AIDS*, vol. 9, no. 1, pp. 19–26, 1995.

[33] H. Stoiber, C. Pintér, A. G. Siccardi, A. Clivio, and M. P. Dierich, "Efficient destruction of human immunodeficiency virus in human serum by inhibiting the protective action of complement factor H and decay accelerating factor (DAF, CD55)," *Journal of Experimental Medicine*, vol. 183, no. 1, pp. 307–310, 1996.

[34] J. Schmitz, J. P. Zimmer, B. Kluxen et al., "Antibody-dependent complement-mediated cytotoxicity in sera from patients with HIV-1 infection is controlled by CD55 and CD59," *Journal of Clinical Investigation*, vol. 96, no. 3, pp. 1520–1526, 1995.

[35] D. C. Douek, L. J. Picker, and R. A. Koup, "T cell dynamics in HIV-1 infection," *Annual Review of Immunology*, vol. 21, pp. 265–304, 2003.

[36] S. M. Wahl, T. Greenwell-Wild, and N. Vázquez, "HIV accomplices and adversaries in macrophage infection," *Journal of Leukocyte Biology*, vol. 80, no. 5, pp. 973–983, 2006.

[37] V. Vieillard, J. L. Strominger, and P. Debré, "NK cytotoxicity against $CD4^+$ T cells during HIV-1 infection: a gp41 peptide induces the expression of an NKp44 ligand," *Proceedings of the National Academy of Sciences of the United States of America*, vol. 102, no. 31, pp. 10981–10986, 2005.

[38] B. He, X. Qiao, P. J. Klasse et al., "HIV-1 envelope triggers polyclonal Ig class switch recombination through a CD40-independent mechanism involving BAFF and C-type lectin receptors," *Journal of Immunology*, vol. 176, no. 7, pp. 3931–3941, 2006.

[39] M. Müller-Trutwin and A. Hosmalin, "Role for plasmacytoid dendritic cells in anti-HIV innate immunity," *Immunology and Cell Biology*, vol. 83, no. 5, pp. 578–585, 2005.

[40] M. Van Der Vlist, A. M. G. Van Der Aar, S. I. Gringhuis, and T. B. H. Geijtenbeek, "Innate signaling in HIV-1 infection of dendritic cells," *Current Opinion in HIV and AIDS*, vol. 6, no. 5, pp. 348–352, 2011.

[41] S. R. Walsh, N. Bhardwaj, and R. T. Gandhil, "Dendritic cells and the promise of therapeutic vaccines for human immunodeficiency virus (HIV)-1," *Current HIV Research*, vol. 1, no. 2, pp. 205–216, 2003.

[42] A. R. Stacey, P. J. Norris, L. Qin et al., "Induction of a striking systemic cytokine cascade prior to peak viremia in acute human immunodeficiency virus type 1 infection, in contrast to more modest and delayed responses in acute hepatitis B and C virus infections," *Journal of Virology*, vol. 83, no. 8, pp. 3719–3733, 2009.

[43] J. Rychert, D. Strick, S. Bazner, J. Robinson, and E. Rosenberg, "Detection of HIV gp120 in plasma during early HIV infection is associated with increased proinflammatory and immunoregulatory cytokines," *AIDS Research and Human Retroviruses*, vol. 26, no. 10, pp. 1139–1145, 2010.

[44] K. Kedzierska and S. M. Crowe, "Cytokines and HIV-1: interactions and clinical implications," *Antiviral Chemistry and Chemotherapy*, vol. 12, no. 3, pp. 133–150, 2001.

[45] L. Fantuzzi, F. Belardelli, and S. Gessani, "Monocyte/macrophage-derived CC chemokines and their modulation by HIV-1 and cytokines: a complex network of interactions influencing viral replication and AIDS pathogenesis," *Journal of Leukocyte Biology*, vol. 74, no. 5, pp. 719–725, 2003.

[46] A. Albini, S. Ferrini, R. Benelli et al., "HIV-1 Tat protein mimicry of chemokines," *Proceedings of the National Academy of Sciences of the United States of America*, vol. 95, no. 22, pp. 13153–13158, 1998.

[47] M. Giovanna Quaranta, E. Tritarelli, L. Giordani, and M. Viora, "HIV-1 Nef induces dendritic cell differentiation: a possible mechanism of uninfected CD4(+) T cell activation," *Experimental Cell Research*, vol. 275, no. 2, pp. 243–254, 2002.

[48] D. Guha, P. Nagilla, C. Redinger, A. Srinivasan et al., "Neuronal apoptosis by HIV-1 Vpr: contribution of proinflammatory molecular networks from infected target cells," *Journal of Neuroinflammation*, vol. 9, article 138, 2012.

[49] J. K. Yamamoto, F. Barre-Sinoussi, and V. Bolton, "Human alpha- and beta-interferon but not gamma–suppress the *in vitro* replication of LAV, HTLV-III, and ARV-2," *Journal of Interferon Research*, vol. 6, no. 2, pp. 143–152, 1986.

[50] W. Chen and J. Royer William E., "Structural insights into interferon regulatory factor activation," *Cellular Signalling*, vol. 22, no. 6, pp. 883–887, 2010.

[51] P. M. Pitha, "Multiple effects of interferon on the replication of human immunodeficiency virus type 1," *Antiviral Research*, vol. 24, no. 2-3, pp. 205–219, 1994.

[52] W. Hou, X. Wang, L. Ye et al., "Lambda interferon inhibits human immunodeficiency virus type 1 infection of macrophages," *Journal of Virology*, vol. 83, no. 8, pp. 3834–3842, 2009.

[53] S. D. Barr, J. R. Smiley, and F. D. Bushman, "The interferon response inhibits HIV particle production by induction of TRIM22," *PLoS Pathogens*, vol. 4, no. 2, Article ID e1000007, 2008.

[54] E. Martinelli, C. Cicala, D. Van Ryk et al., "HIV-1 gp120 inhibits TLR9-mediated activation and IFN-α secretion in plasmacytoid dendritic cells," *Proceedings of the National Academy of Sciences of the United States of America*, vol. 104, no. 9, pp. 3396–3401, 2007.

[55] L. A. Zaritsky, L. Gama, and J. E. Clements, "Canonical type I IFN signaling in simian immunodeficiency virus-infected macrophages is disrupted by astrocyte-secreted CCL2," *Journal of Immunology*, vol. 188, no. 8, pp. 3876–3885, 2012.

[56] V. Cobos Jimenez, T. Booiman, S. W. de Taeye et al., "Differential expression of HIV-1 interfering factors in monocyte-derived macrophages stimulated with polarizing cytokines or interferons," *Scientific Reports*, vol. 2, article 763, 2012.

[57] N. Yan, A. D. Regalado-Magdos, B. Stiggelbout, M. A. Lee-Kirsch, and J. Lieberman, "The cytosolic exonuclease TREX1 inhibits the innate immune response to human immunodeficiency virus type 1," *Nature Immunology*, vol. 11, no. 11, pp. 1005–1013, 2010.

[58] A. Lepelley, S. Louis, M. Sourisseau et al., "Innate sensing of HIV-infected cells," *PLoS Pathogens*, vol. 7, no. 2, Article ID e1001284, 2011.

[59] T. B. H. Geijtenbeek, "Host DNase TREX1 hides HIV from DNA sensors," *Nature Immunology*, vol. 11, no. 11, pp. 979–980, 2010.

[60] G. Clerzius, J.-F. Gélinas, and A. Gatignol, "Multiple levels of PKR inhibition during HIV-1 replication," *Reviews in Medical Virology*, vol. 21, no. 1, pp. 42–53, 2011.

[61] H. Park, M. V. Davies, J. O. Langland et al., "TAR RNA-binding protein is an inhibitor of the interferon-induced protein kinase PKR," *Proceedings of the National Academy of Sciences of the United States of America*, vol. 91, no. 11, pp. 4713–4717, 1994.

[62] T. P. Chendrimada, R. I. Gregory, E. Kumaraswamy et al., "TRBP recruits the Dicer complex to Ago2 for microRNA processing and gene silencing," *Nature*, vol. 436, no. 7051, pp. 740–744, 2005.

[63] A. Gatignol, S. Laine, and G. Clerzius, "Dual role of TRBP in HIV replication and RNA interference: viral diversion of a cellular pathway or evasion from antiviral immunity?" *Retrovirology*, vol. 2, article 65, 2005.

[64] L. Endo-Munoz, T. Warby, D. Harrich, and N. A. J. McMillan, "Phosphorylation of HIV Tat by PKR increases interaction with TAR RNA and enhances transcription," *Virology Journal*, vol. 2, article 17, 2005.

[65] S. R. Brand, R. Kobayashi, and M. B. Mathews, "The Tat protein of human immunodeficiency virus type 1 is a substrate and inhibitor of the interferon-induced, virally activated protein kinase, PKR," *Journal of Biological Chemistry*, vol. 272, no. 13, pp. 8388–8395, 1997.

[66] J.-F. Fonteneau, M. Larsson, A.-S. Beignon et al., "Human immunodeficiency virus type 1 activates plasmacytoid dendritic cells and concomitantly induces the bystander maturation of myeloid dendritic cells," *Journal of Virology*, vol. 78, no. 10, pp. 5223–5232, 2004.

[67] J. A. Martinson, A. Roman-Gonzalez, A. R. Tenorio et al., "Dendritic cells from HIV-1 infected individuals are less responsive to toll-like receptor (TLR) ligands," *Cellular Immunology*, vol. 250, no. 1-2, pp. 75–84, 2007.

[68] J. C. Tilton, M. M. Manion, M. R. Luskin et al., "Human immunodeficiency virus viremia induces plasmacytoid dendritic cell activation in vivo and diminished alpha interferon production in vitro," *Journal of Virology*, vol. 82, no. 8, pp. 3997–4006, 2008.

[69] C. Lehmann, M. Lafferty, A. Garzino-Demo et al., "Plasmacytoid dendritic cells accumulate and secrete interferon alpha in lymph nodes of HIV-1 patients," *PloS ONE*, vol. 5, no. 6, Article ID e11110, 2010.

[70] J. E. Ho, S. G. Deeks, F. M. Hecht et al., "Initiation of antiretroviral therapy at higher nadir $CD4^+$ T-cell counts is associated with reduced arterial stiffness in HIV-infected individuals," *AIDS*, vol. 24, no. 12, pp. 1897–1905, 2010.

[71] J.-P. Herbeuval, A. Boasso, J.-C. Grivel et al., "TNF-related apoptosis-inducing ligand (TRAIL) in HIV-1-infected patients and its in vitro production by antigen-presenting cells," *Blood*, vol. 105, no. 6, pp. 2458–2464, 2005.

[72] M. Lichtner, C. Marañón, P.-O. Vidalain et al., "HIV type 1-infected dendritic cells induce apoptotic death in infected and uninfected primary $CD4^+$ T lymphocytes," *AIDS Research and Human Retroviruses*, vol. 20, no. 2, pp. 175–182, 2004.

[73] A. W. Hardy, D. R. Graham, G. M. Shearer, and J.-P. Herbeuval, "HIV turns plasmacytoid dendritic cells (pDC) into TRAIL-expressing killer pDC and down-regulates HIV coreceptors by Toll-like receptor 7-induced IFN-α," *Proceedings of the National Academy of Sciences of the United States of America*, vol. 104, no. 44, pp. 17453–17458, 2007.

[74] N. J. Megjugorac, H. A. Young, S. B. Amrute, S. L. Olshalsky, and P. Fitzgerald-Bocarsly, "Virally stimulated plasmacytoid dendritic cells produce chemokines and induce migration of T and NK cells," *Journal of Leukocyte Biology*, vol. 75, no. 3, pp. 504–514, 2004.

[75] G. Penna, M. Vulcano, S. Sozzani, and L. Adorini, "Differential migration behavior and chemokine production by myeloid and plasmacytoid dendritic cells," *Human Immunology*, vol. 63, no. 12, pp. 1164–1171, 2002.

[76] G. Alter, N. Teigen, B. T. Davis et al., "Sequential deregulation of NK cell subset distribution and function starting in acute HIV-1 infection," *Blood*, vol. 106, no. 10, pp. 3366–3369, 2005.

[77] G. Alter, T. J. Suscovich, M. Kleyman et al., "Low perforin and elevated SHIP-1 expression is associated with functional anergy of natural killer cells in chronic HIV-1 infection," *AIDS*, vol. 20, no. 11, pp. 1549–1551, 2006.

[78] M. L. LaBonte, P. F. McKay, and N. L. Letvin, "Evidence of NK cell dysfunction in SIV-infected rhesus monkeys: impairment of cytokine secretion and NKG2C/C2 expression," *European Journal of Immunology*, vol. 36, no. 9, pp. 2424–2433, 2006.

[79] U.-C. Meier, R. E. Owen, E. Taylor et al., "Shared alterations in NK cell frequency, phenotype, and function in chronic human immunodeficiency virus and hepatitis C virus infections," *Journal of Virology*, vol. 79, no. 19, pp. 12365–12374, 2005.

[80] D. Mavilio, G. Lombardo, A. Kinter et al., "Characterization of the defective interaction between a subset of natural killer cells and dendritic cells in HIV-1 infection," *Journal of Experimental Medicine*, vol. 203, no. 10, pp. 2339–2350, 2006.

[81] A. De Maria, M. Fogli, P. Costa et al., "The impaired NK cell cytolytic function in viremic HIV-1 infection is associated with

a reduced surface expression of natural cytotoxicity receptors (NKp46, NKp30 and NKp44)," *European Journal of Immunology*, vol. 33, no. 9, pp. 2410–2418, 2003.

[82] M. P. Martin, Y. Qi, X. Gao et al., "Innate partnership of HLA-B and KIR3DL1 subtypes against HIV-1," *Nature Genetics*, vol. 39, no. 6, pp. 733–740, 2007.

[83] G. Alter, M. P. Martin, N. Teigen et al., "Differential natural killer cell-mediated inhibition of HIV-1 replication based on distinct KIR/HLA subtypes," *Journal of Experimental Medicine*, vol. 204, no. 12, pp. 3027–3036, 2007.

[84] M. T. M. Vossen, E. M. Westerhout, C. Söderberg-Nauclér, and E. J. H. J. Wiertz, "Viral immune evasion: a masterpiece of evolution," *Immunogenetics*, vol. 54, no. 8, pp. 527–542, 2002.

[85] A. Ahmad and R. Ahmad, "HIV's evasion of host's NK cell response and novel ways of its countering and boosting anti-HIV immunity," *Current HIV Research*, vol. 1, no. 3, pp. 295–307, 2003.

[86] K. L. Collins and D. Baltimore, "HIV's evasion of the cellular immune response," *Immunological Reviews*, vol. 168, pp. 65–74, 1999.

[87] G. B. Cohen, R. T. Gandhi, D. M. Davis et al., "The selective downregulation of class I major histocompatibility complex proteins by HIV-1 protects HIV-infected cells from NK cells," *Immunity*, vol. 10, no. 6, pp. 661–671, 1999.

[88] T. Swigut, A. J. Iafrate, J. Muench, F. Kirchhoff, and J. Skowronski, "Simian and human immunodeficiency virus Nef proteins use different surfaces to downregulate class I major histocompatibility complex antigen expression," *Journal of Virology*, vol. 74, no. 12, pp. 5691–5701, 2000.

[89] J. Nattermann, H. D. Nischalke, V. Hofmeister et al., "HIV-1 infection leads to increased HLA-E expression resulting in impaired function of natural killer cells," *Antiviral Therapy*, vol. 10, no. 1, pp. 95–107, 2005.

[90] M. R. Zocchi, A. Rubartelli, P. Morgavi, and A. Poggi, "HIV-1 tat inhibits human natural killer cell function by blocking L-type calcium channels," *Journal of Immunology*, vol. 161, no. 6, pp. 2938–2943, 1998.

[91] A. Poggi, R. Carosio, G. M. Spaggiari et al., "NK cell activation by dendritic cells is dependent on LFA-1-mediated induction of calcium-calmodulin kinase II: inhibition by HIV-1 Tat C-terminal domain," *Journal of Immunology*, vol. 168, no. 1, pp. 95–101, 2002.

[92] L. Azzoni, R. M. Rutstein, J. Chehimi, M. A. Farabaugh, A. Nowmos, and L. J. Montaner, "Dendritic and natural killer cell subsets associated with stable or declining $CD4^+$ cell counts in treated HIV-1-infected children," *Journal of Infectious Diseases*, vol. 191, no. 9, pp. 1451–1459, 2005.

[93] J. Richard, S. Sindhu, T. N. Q. Pham, J.-P. Belzile, and É. A. Cohen, "HIV-1 Vpr up-regulates expression of ligands for the activating NKG2D receptor and promotes NK cell-mediated killing," *Blood*, vol. 115, no. 7, pp. 1354–1363, 2010.

[94] M. Douaisi, S. Dussart, M. Courcoul, G. Bessou, R. Vigne, and E. Decroly, "HIV-1 and MLV Gag proteins are sufficient to recruit APOBEC3G into virus-like particles," *Biochemical and Biophysical Research Communications*, vol. 321, no. 3, pp. 566–573, 2004.

[95] V. Zennou, D. Perez-Caballero, H. Göttlinger, and P. D. Bieniasz, "APOBEC3G incorporation into human immunodeficiency virus type 1 particles," *Journal of Virology*, vol. 78, no. 21, pp. 12058–12061, 2004.

[96] R. S. Harris, K. N. Bishop, A. M. Sheehy et al., "DNA deamination mediates innate immunity to retroviral infection," *Cell*, vol. 113, no. 6, pp. 803–809, 2003.

[97] B. Mangeat, P. Turelli, G. Caron, M. Friedli, L. Perrin, and D. Trono, "Broad antiretroviral defence by human APOBEC3G through lethal editing of nascent reverse transcripts," *Nature*, vol. 424, no. 6944, pp. 99–103, 2003.

[98] E. N. C. Newman, R. K. Holmes, H. M. Craig et al., "Antiviral function of APOBEC3G can be dissociated from cytidine deaminase activity," *Current Biology*, vol. 15, no. 2, pp. 166–170, 2005.

[99] M. Marin, K. M. Rose, S. L. Kozak, and D. Kabat, "HIV-1 Vif protein binds the editing enzyme APOBEC3G and induces its degradation," *Nature Medicine*, vol. 9, no. 11, pp. 1398–1403, 2003.

[100] X. Yu, Y. Yu, B. Liu et al., "Induction of APOBEC3G ubiquitination and degradation by an HIV-1 Vif-Cul5-SCF complex," *Science*, vol. 302, no. 5647, pp. 1056–1060, 2003.

[101] A. Mehle, B. Strack, P. Ancuta, C. Zhang, M. McPike, and D. Gabuzda, "Vif overcomes the innate antiviral activity of APOBEC3G by promoting its degradation in the ubiquitin-proteasome pathway," *Journal of Biological Chemistry*, vol. 279, no. 9, pp. 7792–7798, 2004.

[102] S. de Silva and L. Wu, "TRIM5 acts as more than a retroviral restriction factor," *Viruses*, vol. 3, no. 7, pp. 1204–1209, 2011.

[103] T. Pertel, S. Hausmann, D. Morger et al., "TRIM5 is an innate immune sensor for the retrovirus capsid lattice," *Nature*, vol. 472, no. 7343, pp. 361–365, 2011.

[104] C. Aiken and S. Joyce, "Immunology: TRIM5 does double duty," *Nature*, vol. 472, no. 7343, pp. 305–306, 2011.

[105] B. D. Kuhl, R. D. Sloan, D. A. Donahue, T. Bar-Magen, C. Liang, and M. A. Wainberg, "Tetherin restricts direct cell-to-cell infection of HIV-1," *Retrovirology*, vol. 7, article 115, 2010.

[106] S. J. D. Neil, S. W. Eastman, N. Jouvenet, and P. D. Bieniasz, "HIV-1 Vpu promotes release and prevents endocytosis of nascent retrovirus particles from the plasma membrane," *PLoS Pathogens*, vol. 2, no. 5, article e39, 2006.

[107] L. Rong, J. Zhang, J. Lu et al., "The transmembrane domain of BST-2 determines its sensitivity to down-modulation by human immunodeficiency virus type 1 Vpu," *Journal of Virology*, vol. 83, no. 15, pp. 7536–7546, 2009.

[108] B. Jia, R. Serra-Moreno, W. Neidermyer Jr. et al., "Species-specific activity of SIV Nef and HIV-1 Vpu in overcoming restriction by tetherin/BST2," *PLoS Pathogens*, vol. 5, no. 5, Article ID e1000429, 2009.

[109] F. Zhang, S. J. Wilson, W. C. Landford et al., "Nef proteins from simian immunodeficiency viruses are tetherin antagonists," *Cell Host and Microbe*, vol. 6, no. 1, pp. 54–67, 2009.

[110] R. Triboulet, B. Mari, Y.-L. Lin et al., "Suppression of MicroRNA-silencing pathway by HIV-1 during virus replication," *Science*, vol. 315, no. 5818, pp. 1579–1582, 2007.

[111] D. P. Bartel, "MicroRNAs: genomics, biogenesis, mechanism, and function," *Cell*, vol. 116, no. 2, pp. 281–297, 2004.

[112] K. W. Witwer, J. M. Sisk, L. Gama, and J. E. Clements, "MicroRNA regulation of IFN-β protein expression: rapid and sensitive modulation of the innate immune response," *Journal of Immunology*, vol. 184, no. 5, pp. 2369–2376, 2010.

[113] A. Gupta, P. Nagilla, H.-S. Le et al., "Comparative expression profile of miRNA and mRNA In primary peripheral blood

mononuclear cells infected with human immunodeficiency virus (HIV-1)," *PloS ONE*, vol. 6, no. 7, Article ID e22730, 2011.

[114] G. Sun, H. Li, X. Wu et al., "Interplay between HIV-1 infection and host microRNAs," *Nucleic Acids Research*, vol. 40, no. 5, pp. 2181–2196, 2012.

[115] J. M. Sisk, J. E. Clements, and K. W. Witwer, "miRNA profiles of monocyte-lineage cells are consistent with complicated roles in HIV-1 restriction," *Viruses*, vol. 4, no. 10, pp. 1844–1864, 2012.

[116] Y. Bennasser, S.-Y. Le, M. Benkirane, and K.-T. Jeang, "Evidence that HIV-1 encodes an siRNA and a suppressor of RNA silencing," *Immunity*, vol. 22, no. 5, pp. 607–619, 2005.

[117] A. Narayanan, K. Kehn-Hall, C. Bailey, and F. Kashanchi, "Analysis of the roles of HIV-derived microRNAs," *Expert Opinion on Biological Therapy*, vol. 11, no. 1, pp. 17–29, 2011.

12

Factors Affecting Adherence to Antiretroviral Treatment in Harari National Regional State, Eastern Ethiopia

Habtamu Mitiku,[1] Tekabe Abdosh,[2] and Zelalem Teklemariam[1]

[1] *Department of Medical Laboratory Sciences, College of Health and Medical Sciences, Haramaya University, P.O. Box 235, Harar, Ethiopia*

[2] *College of Health and Medical Sciences, Haramaya University, School of Medicine, P.O. Box 235, Harar, Ethiopia*

Correspondence should be addressed to Habtamu Mitiku; habtemit@gmail.com

Academic Editors: D. Aunis, J. Poudrier, and K. Yoder

Background. The efficacy of antiretroviral treatment (ART) depends on strict adherence to the regimen, but many factors have been identified for nonadherence. *Method.* To identify the factors for non-adherence to ART, a cross-sectional study was conducted on people living with human immunodeficiency virus (HIV) and attending the ART service at Hiwot Fana and Jugal hospitals; it was done from October to December, 2010. Adherence was defined as taking 95% of the prescribed doses in the week before the survey. Data were collected using a standard interview questionnaire and were analyzed using SPSS Version 16. *Result.* Among the 239 study participants, the magnitude of adherence to ART in the week before interview was 87%. The main reasons for nonadherence were forgetting (47.2%), traveling (18.9%), and being busy doing other things (15.1%). There was not any independent predicator identified for adherence to ART. *Conclusion.* Compared to other similar studies in Ethiopia, in this study a high adherence rate was found. Forgetfulness was the most common reason for the nonadherence. Therefore, the ART counseling needs to give emphasis to using memory aids. In addition, a further study on adherence rate and its determinants with multiple adherence measurements is recommended.

1. Background

HIV/AIDS is the greatest health problem in the world. At the end of 2009, for example, an estimated 33.3 million people were living with HIV, 2.6 million people were newly infected, and 1.8 million lost their lives due to AIDS. Sub-Saharan Africa carries 68% of the global total HIV burden (22.5 million people), which is an inordinate share [1].

ART increases the length, quality of life, and productivity of the people living with HIV (PLWH) by improving survival and decreasing the incidence of opportunistic infections through reduction of the viral load and increase of the level of CD_4 cells [2]. Cognizing this, the government of Ethiopia has done a lot to introduce the treatment [3]. It was first offered in July 2003 through 12 government hospitals on a copayment basis. In early 2005, 211.000 men, women, and children needed ART but only 16,400 received it. In January 2005, free ART through the Global Fund, World Bank, and US President's Emergency Plan for AIDS Relief (PEPFAR) became available in 22 hospitals [4]. There were 497 ART centers serving 167.271 HIV/AIDS patients in October 2009 [5].

The effectiveness of ART relies on a strict adherence to it. In other words, loose obedience, or non obedience to ART can result in inadequate viral suppression, immunologic failure, rapid disease progression, and the development of drug resistance [6, 7]. To avoid the emergence of the resistant strains of the virus, World Health Organization (WHO) recommends at least 95% of adherence to ART [8]. Based on these facts, the importance of adhering to ART has been widely publicized and accepted as a critical element in the success of ART.

However, many of the reported adherence rates are below the recommendation. Among the patients in Soweto, South Africa, the magnitude of adherence was 88% [9]; in a community setting in Atlanta [10], twenty percent of the participants missed at least one dose of ART. In Ethiopia, an adherence rate of 83% was reported in two hospitals of Oromiya Regional State [11], 88.3% in Yirgalem Hospital [12], and 81.2% in three hospitals in Addis Ababa [13].

The commonly identified factors for nonadherence are forgetfulness, poor understanding of the relationship between nonadherence and disease progression, side effects of drugs, alcohol and drug abuse, poor social support, poor health provider-patient relationships, being away from home, fear of disclosure, educational level, and others [12–15]. We, therefore, aimed at determining the level of adherence and identifying the factors that are related to nonadherence to ART among the patients attending at ART units in Harari National Regional State, eastern Ethiopia.

2. Methods

2.1. Study Area, Design, and Period. The study was done in Harari National Regional State. It is found in eastern Ethiopia, and it is 525 km from Addis Ababa. In the region, ART was started in 2005, and there were 1876 people on ART in 2009 (Harari National Regional State Health Report). A cross-sectional study was conducted in the ART units of Hiwot Fana Hospital and Jugal Hospital from October to December, 2010. The PLWH who were attending at the ART unit of either hospital, who were more than 18 years old, who had taken antiretroviral medication at least for one month, and who gave their signed consent to participate in the study, were included.

2.2. Sample Size and Sampling Techniques. In this study the sample size was calculated by using the 0.83 proportion of adherence in the two hospitals of Oromiya Regional Sate [11], 5% margin of error, and 95% confidence interval. Then, 10% nonresponse rate was added. The total sample size was 239. This was allotted to the hospitals proportionally to their monthly average client flow. Finally, by using a systematic sampling method, we selected 160 and 79 ART unit clients from Hiwot Fana Hospital and Jugal Hospital, respectively.

2.3. Data Collection. The data were collected using a structured questionnaire. The questionnaire contained different variables such as sociodemographic characteristics, social support, information related to personal life, alcohol/substance use, treatment side effects, patient self-report for treatment adherence, patient reported reasons for nonadherence, and others. The participants' CD_4 T-cell count before starting and the most recent CD_4 count after starting ARV drugs were retrieved from their ART follow-up records in the hospitals. Nurses who were trained on ART but not currently working in the ART units collected the data.

2.4. Data Analysis. The data were analyzed using SPSS Version 16 software. Adherence to ART in the previous seven days of the interview was measured by the self-report about taking pills. The self-reported dose adherence was defined as a respondent's self-report whether any antiretroviral medication had been skipped in the previous seven days. A respondent was said to be adherent if he/she took ≥95% of the prescribed doses in the previous week. The comparison of those who were adherent (≥95% of their doses of ART medication taken) and nonadherent (≤95% of their doses of ART medication taken) was carried out with various variables. The predicators of adherence were assessed using bivariate logistic regression model. Chi-square test was used to assess the difference between CD_4 count before starting and the most recent CD_4 count after starting ARV drugs. 95% confidence interval with P value ≤ 0.05 was considered as statistically significant. Since no predicator variables were found statistically significant with outcome variable using bivariate logistic regression model, multivariate logistic regression model was not employed to identify the independent predictor of adherence (outcome variable).

2.5. Ethical Considerations. Ethical clearance was obtained from Haramaya University Colleges of Health and Medical Sciences Institutional Research and Ethical Review Committee. All the participants were given an explanation about the objective of the study and their right to participate or not to participate in the study. Those who gave their signed written consent participated. ART follow-up records were retrieved by the nurses working in the ART units, and personal information of the participants was kept confidential.

3. Results

3.1. Sociodemographic Information. Of the 239 study participants, 73.6% were female, 72.4% were between 20 and 39 years of age, 42.7% were married, and 87.4% were literate (Table 1). Their average age was 35 ± 8.69 years with a range of 20 to 69.

3.2. Factors Related to Personal Life and Social Support. About 92.1% and 7.9% of the participants were ≤5 years and >5 years on ART, respectively, with a mean duration of 3 years (range of 1 month to 7 years). Almost all of the respondents (98.3%) took ≤5 pills per day, with a mean of 2.8 pills. About 17.2% of the participants used active substances (Table 2).

Many of the participants (70.7%) lived with other people (spouse, children, parents, siblings, other relatives, and friends). About 47.3% of them had financial, psychological, and physical support from their families. Only 14.2% had financial, psychological, physical, and other support from outside their families (friends, nongovernmental organizations, community-based organizations, religious based organizations, governmental facilities, and others). Many participants had disclosed their HIV status to their family or others (78.7%). They had known their HIV status for a mean of 5 years, with a range of 3 months to 17 years. Of the 73.2% of the participants who had children, 13.4%, 83.3%, and 3.3% of their children were seropositive, seronegative, and not aware of their serostatus, respectively (Table 2).

3.3. Adherence Rate of ART. Two hundred eight (87%) of the participants had taken >95% of their prescribed ARV drugs for the past 7 days. Almost similar adherence rate was observed among males (85.7%) and females (87.5%).

Table 1: Adherence rate by sociodemographic characteristics of the study participants at Hiwot Fana and Jugal hospitals, 2010.

Sociodemographic variable	Adherence status		Total	COR (95 CI)
	Adhered number (%)	Not adhered number (%)		
Sex				
Male	54 (85.7)	9 (14.3)	63 (26.4)	1.00
Female	154 (87.5)	22 (12.5)	176 (73.6)	1.17 (0.51, 2.69)
Age				
20–30	77 (92.8)	6 (7.2)	83 (34.7)	1.00
31–39	77 (85.6)	13 (14.4)	90 (37.7)	0.36 (0.08, 1.63)
40–49	40 (81.6)	9 (18.4)	49 (20.7)	0.79 (0.20, 3.13)
≥50	14 (82.4)	3 (17.6)	17 (7)	1.05 (0.25, 4.44)
Marital status				
Married	86 (84.3)	16 (15.7)	102 (42.7)	1.00
Single	37 (90.2)	4 (9.8)	41 (17.2)	1.49 (0.51–4.35)
Divorced	45 (88.2)	6 (11.8)	51 (21.3)	0.87 (0.22, 3.47)
Widowed	40 (88.9)	5 (11.1)	45 (18.8)	1.07 (0.30, 3.76)
Educational level				
High school and above	78 (90.7)	8 (9.3)	86 (36)	1.00
Regular school 1–8	99 (86.1)	16 (13.9)	115 (48.1)	1.58 (0.64, 3.87)
Able to read and write	7 (87.5)	1 (12.5)	8 (3.3)	1.40 (0.15, 12.8)
Unable to read and write	24 (80)	6 (20)	30 (12.6)	2.44 (0.77, 7.72)
Occupation				
Employed	178 (88.1)	24 (11.9)	202 (84.5)	1.00
Unemployed	30 (81.1)	7 (18.9)	37 (15.5)	1.73 (0.69, 4.37)
Income				
00	40 (97.6)	1 (2.4)	41 (17.2)	1.00
≤500	102 (87.9)	14 (12.1)	116 (48.5)	5.49 (0.69, 43.1)
Do not know*	66 (80.5)	16 (19.5)	82 (34.3)	

*66 participants do not know their average monthly income and are not included in income analysis.
COR: crude odds ratio.
CI: confidence interval.

Table 2: Adherence rate by social support, HIV status disclosure, and substance abuse. Duration of ART treatment and pill burden of the study participants at Hiwot Fana and Jugal hospitals, 2010.

Variable	Adherence status		Total number (%)	COR (95 CI)
	Adhered number (%)	Not adhered number (%)		
Substance abuse				
No	170 (85.9)	28 (14.1)	198 (82.8)	1.00
Yes	38 (92.7)	3 (7.3)	41 (17.2)	0.48 (0.14, 1.66)
Duration				
≤5 year	192 (87.3)	28 (12.7)	220 (92.1)	1.00
>5 years	16 (84.2)	3 (15.8)	19 (7.9)	0.78 (0.21, 2.84)
Support from family				
Yes	98 (86.7)	15 (13.3)	113 (47.3)	1.00
No	110 (87.3)	16 (12.7)	126 (52.7)	1.05 (0.49, 2.23)
Support from others				
Yes	30 (88.2)	4 (11.8)	34 (14.2)	1.00
No	178 (86.8)	27 (13.2)	205 (85.8)	0.88 (0.29, 2.69)
Disclosure of serostatus				
Yes	164 (87.2)	24 (12.8)	188 (78.7)	1.00
No	44 (86.3)	7 (13.7)	51 (21.3)	0.92 (0.37, 2.28)

COR: crude odds ratio.
CI: confidence interval.

Higher adherence rate was observed in the age group of 20–30 years (92.8%). However, adherence rate was not statistically associated with sex (COR: 1.17; 95 CI: 0.51, 2.69) and age group (COR: 1.46; 95 CI: 0.98, 2.17) (Table 1).

Higher adherence rate (90.2%) was observed among singles compared to married study participants (84.3%). The respondents who had high school and above education were more adhered (90.7%) than those who were illiterate (80%). However, there was no statistically significant association between the adherence rate and the marital status and the educational level of the study participants. Higher adherence rate, 88.1% and 97.6%, was observed among employed and study participant's earning ≥500 birr per month, respectively. But no significant statistical association was found between the adherence rate, the occupational status (COR: 1.731; 95 CI: 0.69, 4.37), and the economic status (COR: 5.49; 95 CI: 0.69, 43) of the study participants (Table 1).

Adherence rate of 86.7% was reported among patients who had support from their family while 88.2% adherence rate reported among patients who had support from friends, governmental facilities, nongovernmental organizations, community-based organizations, and religious organizations. Adherence rate of 87.2% and 86.3% was reported among patients who disclosed their serostatus for families, friends, and others and who did not disclose their serostatus, respectively. About 92.7% and 85.9% adherence rates were reported by patients who were using active substances and who were not using active substances, respectively. Social support, disclosure of serostatus, and substance abuse did not have significant influence on the adherence rate of the participants (Table 2).

Adherence rate of 87.3% and 84.2% was reported by the respondents who took the treatment for ≤5 and >5 years, respectively. About 86.5% and 100% adherence rates were reported by the study participants who took ≤5 and >5 pills per day, respectively. Neither the number of years on treatment nor the pill uptake per day had a significant influence on adherence rate of the participants (Table 2).

The CD_4 counts of, before starting ART, 224 (93.3%) participants were found, and 164 (73.2%) of them had CD_4 count <200 cells/mm^3, with a mean of 155.6 cells/mm^3. The most recent CD_4 counts of 207 (86.6%) participants were surveyed, and only 17 (8.2%) of them had CD_4 count <200 cells/mm^3, with a mean of 443.3 cells/mm^3. A significant increase in CD_4 cell count was observed after the initiation of the treatment ($P < 0.01$) (Table 3).

3.4. Reasons for Nonadherence. Few participants (13%) did not adhere to ART. The average number of doses missed in the past 7 days was 1.3. Some missed the treatment due to forgetting (47.2%), some due to travelling (18.9%), and few due to being busy (15.1%) (Figure 1).

3.5. Side Effects of ART Reported by the Respondents. Many of the participants (73.3%) reported one or more side effects of ARV drugs. The most common side effects reported were fatigue or loss of energy (26.4%) and numbness of tingling in hands and feet (25.1%) (Figure 2). All most equal adherence rate, 73% and 74.2%, was reported by the study participants who reported one or more treatment side effects and who did not, respectively. There was no significant association between the adherence rate and the presence or absence of treatment side effects (COR: 0.94; 95 CI: 0.39, 2.23).

Table 3: CD_4 cell count before and after initiation of ART treatment among the study participants at Hiwot Fan and Jugal hospitals, 2010.

CD_4 count	Before treatment No. (%)	After treatment No. (%)	P value
<200 cell/mm^3	164 (73.2)	17 (8.2)	
200–499 cells/mm^3	57 (25.4)	121 (58.5)	<0.01
≥500 cells/mm^3	3 (1.3)	69 (33.3)	

4. Discussion

The adherence rate in the study area was 87%. This was comparable with the one found in Yirgalem Hospital (88.3%) [12] and Soweto, South Africa, (88%) [9]. But it was higher than the rate reported from Oromiya Regional State (83%) [11], Addis Ababa (81.2%) [13], and other developing countries (ranges from 40% to 70%) [14, 16]. The difference might be due to activists which have been undertaken to improve the ART service by governmental organizations and NGOs working in the area.

Tablet burden can often affect any medication adherence. A previous study explained that the fundamental challenge to ART is the complexity regimen, which may include >20 pills per day [14]. Due to the advancement in ART drugs, the daily dose is being reduced [17]. The participants in this study reported that they took a maximum of 7 pills per day; this may have contributed to the high rate of their adherence [11, 13].

Age, sex, and marital status did not significantly affect the adherence rate of the participants. This is also reported by other studies elsewhere [16, 18, 19]. The income of the participants did not significantly affect their adherence. This may be due to the fact that ARV treatment has been given free of charge in Ethiopia since 2005 through the Global Fund, World Bank, and US President's Emergency Plan for AIDS Relief (PEPFAR) [4]. Low economic status was not a predictor of adherence for patients with fully subsidized therapy [12, 17, 20]. A study conducted on Myanmar migrants living in Thailand also showed that free-of-charge treatment strongly improves a long-term regular ART adherence [21].

Like the report by Cauldbeck et al. and Amberbir et al. [17, 20], in this study, although the adherence rate of the respondents increased with an increase in their educational level, there was no significant association between the adherence rate and the educational level. Better educated generally have access to information and are more likely to make better informed decisions [22]. Verbal instructions to patients who are illiterate seem equally as effective as written instructions which are given to all patients [17].

Studies showed that support from family and others supporting PLWH were predictors of ART adherence [14, 19, 20]. In this study, 47.3% of the respondents had family support while only 14.2% had support from friends, community,

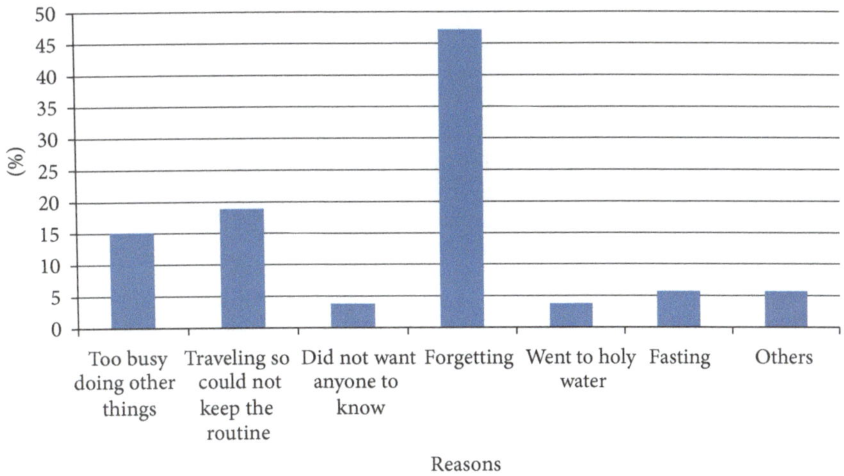

FIGURE 1: Reasons for missing ART medications by study participant in Hiwot Fana and Jugal hospital, 2010.

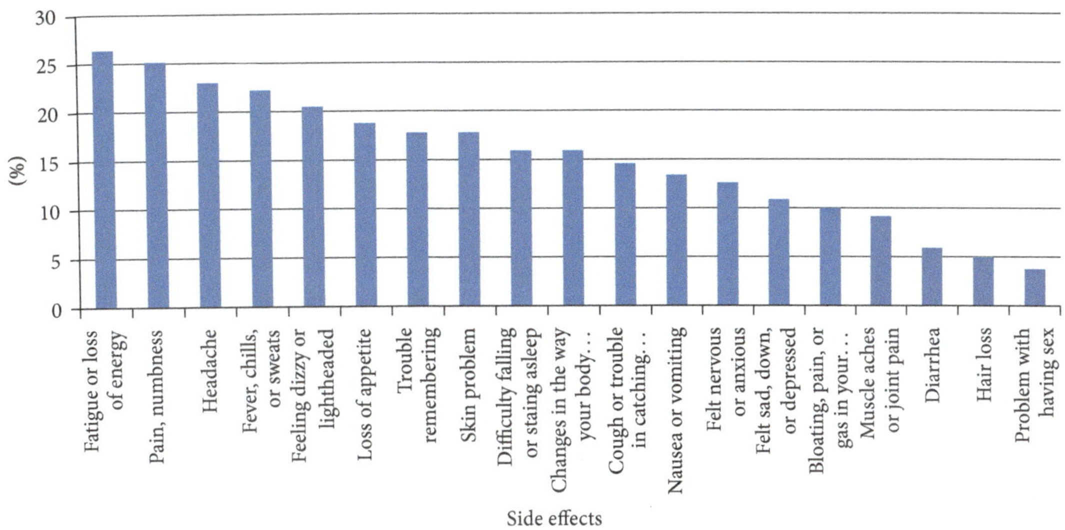

FIGURE 2: Side effects of ART reported by study participants in Hiwot Fana and Jugal Hospitals, 2010.

government, NGOs, and other groups supporting PLWH. And those study participants who had family support less adhered to the treatment than those who had no family support. Even though patients have family support they may miss the dose in working places and other places outside home. This implicates that family support alone is not a factor to increase the uptake of ARV; support from friends, community, government, NGOs, and other groups supporting PLWH also needs to be emphasized.

The respondents' adherence rate was inversely proportional to the length of time they had been on ART. That is, the longer they were on ART, the lesser they adhered. A similar trend was found from studies done in Africa, in the early therapy, before they develop the long term adverse effects of the therapy, HIV positives adhere more because they experience a dramatic increase in their health status [23].

The study participants who disclosed their HIV serostatus adhered to the treatment (87.2%) more than those who did not disclose (66.3%). The latter were likely to have a frequent treatment interruption due to the fact that tablets must be hidden and therefore not be taken in the presence of others [23]. So encouraging voluntary HIV status disclosure in a community with access to ART may help to decrease stigma and improve adherence.

Those that experience side effects from their medications are known to be risk patients for nonadherence to ART [14]. But this was not found to have a significant influence on adherence in this study. This may be due to the mildness of the side effects reported. Those experiencing milder side effects such as skin rash or skin discolorations, fatigue, headache, and fever were more adherent to ART than those experiencing more severe side effects such as metabolic effects (CNS toxicity, sever hepatic necrosis, and renal toxicity) [17].

Forgetfulness, traveling, and being too busy were the most common reasons for poor adherence to medications in this study. Similar reasons were reported in studies conducted in

Adama and Jimma hospitals [11] and Yirgalem Hospital [12], Ethiopia, and in Kenya [18].

There is no gold standard for measuring adherence, and our measurement of adherence is only based on patients' report on missed doses; this may be subjected to social desirability and recall bias, and literature showed that patients tend to overestimate adherence [24]. So the small overall number of nonadherent patients could have interfered with a significance of the statistical difference found.

5. Conclusion

In general, in this study relatively a higher adherence rate was reported compared to other studies in Ethiopia. Forgetfulness was the most common reasons for poor adherence to the medication.

A study conducted in southwest Ethiopia showed that patients who use memory aids were three times more likely to be adherent than those who did not [20]. Therefore, adherence counseling and health information dissemination need to include strategies to minimize forgetfulness using memory aids such as pill boxes, written schedule, and watch bell. In addition, a further study on adherence rate and its determinants with multiple adherence measurements to resolve the barriers to adherence is also recommended.

Conflict of Interests

All the authors declare that they have no conflict of interests associated with the publication of this paper.

Authors' Contribution

Habtamu Mitiku and Zelalem Teklemariam equally contributed to this paper.

Acknowledgments

The authors acknowledge Haramaya University research and publication office for budget allocation and all the participants for their willingness to participate in this study. Thier thanks also extend to Haramaya University, Institutional Review Board, Harar Campus for giving the ethical clearance and to Ms. Muna Abdela for helping in data entry. They also thank all individuals who have in one way or another contributed to the completion of this research.

References

[1] UNAIDS, "Joint United Nations Programme on HIV/AIDS (UNAIDS) Global report," *UNAIDS report on the global AIDS epidemic*, 2010.

[2] R. S. Hogg, B. Yip, C. Kully et al., "Improved survival among HIV-infected patients after initiation of triple-drug antiretroviral regimens," *CMAJ*, vol. 160, no. 5, pp. 659–665, 1999.

[3] Y. Tadios and G. Davey, "Antiretroviral treatment adherence and its correlates in Addis Ababa, Ethiopia," *Ethiopian Medical Journal*, vol. 44, no. 3, pp. 237–244, 2006.

[4] Panos Global AIDS Program, *Antiretroviral Drugs for All? Obstacles to Access to HIV/AIDS: Treatment Lessons from Ethiopia Haiti, India, Nepal and Zambia*, 2006, http://www.panosaids.org/.

[5] AIDS Resource Center, Federal HIV/AIDS Prevention and Control Office, *HIV Care and ART Update in Ethiopia*, http://www.etharc.org/.

[6] D. R. Bangsberg, F. M. Hecht, E. D. Charlebois et al., "Adherence to protease inhibitors, HIV-1 viral load, and development of drug resistance in an indigent population," *AIDS*, vol. 14, no. 4, pp. 357–366, 2000.

[7] C. C. Carpenter, D. A. Cooper, M. A. Fischl et al., "Antiretroviral therapy in adults: updated recommendations of the International AIDS Society-USA Panel," *JAMA*, vol. 283, pp. 381–390, 2000.

[8] V. E. Stone, J. W. Hogan, P. Schuman et al., "Antiretroviral regimen complexity, self-reported adherence, and HIV patients' understanding of their regimens: Survey of women in the HER study," *Journal of Acquired Immune Deficiency Syndromes*, vol. 28, no. 2, pp. 124–131, 2001.

[9] J. B. Nachega, D. M. Stein, D. A. Lehman et al., "Adherence to antiretroviral therapy in HIV-infected adults in Soweto, South Africa," *AIDS Research and Human Retroviruses*, vol. 20, no. 10, pp. 1053–1056, 2004.

[10] S. C. Kalichman, B. Ramachandran, and S. Catz, "Adherence to combination antiretroviral therapies in HIV patients of low health literacy," *Journal of General Internal Medicine*, vol. 14, no. 5, pp. 267–273, 1999.

[11] M. Awel, "Antiretroviral adherence and its detriments among people living with HIV/AIDS on highly active antiretroviral therapy in two hospitals of ormoyia regional state," *Ethiopia. Ethiopian Public Health Association (EPHA) extract from EPHA—sponsored Master Thesis on HIV/AIDS exrtarct*no. 4, 9–19, 2008.

[12] E. Markos, A. Worku, and G. Davey, "Adherence to ART in PLWHA at Yirgalem hospital, South Ethiopia," *The Ethiopian Journal of Health Development*, vol. 22, no. 2, pp. 174–179, 2008.

[13] Y. Tadios and G. Davey, "Antiretroviral treatment adherence and its correlates in Addis Ababa, Ethiopia," *Ethiopian Medical Journal*, vol. 44, no. 3, pp. 237–244, 2006.

[14] D. R. Bangsberg, F. M. Hecht, E. D. Charlebois et al., "Adherence to protease inhibitors, HIV-1 viral load, and development of drug resistance in an indigent population," *AIDS*, vol. 14, no. 4, pp. 357–366, 2000.

[15] J. T. Parsons, E. Rosof, and B. Mustanski, "Patient-related factors predicting HIV medication adherence among men and women with alcohol problems," *Journal of Health Psychology*, vol. 12, no. 2, pp. 357–370, 2007.

[16] K. Peltzer, N. Friend-Du Preez, S. Ramlagan, and J. Anderson, "Antiretroviral treatment adherence among HIV patients in KwaZulu-Natal, South Africa," *BMC Public Health*, vol. 10, article 111, 2010.

[17] M. B. Cauldbeck, C. O'Connor, M. B. O'Connor et al., "Adherence to anti-retroviral therapy among HIV patients in Bangalore, India," *AIDS Research and Therapy*, vol. 6, article 7, 2009.

[18] N. C. Talam, P. Gatongi, J. Rotich, and S. Kimaiyo, "Factors affecting antiretroviral drug adherence among HIV/AIDS adult patients attending HIV/AIDS clinic at Moi Teaching and Referral Hospital, Eldoret, Kenya," *East African journal of public health*, vol. 5, no. 2, pp. 74–78, 2008.

[19] J. I. Campbell, A. L. Ruano, B. Samayoa, D. L. Estrado Muy, E. Arathoon, and B. Young, "Adherence to antiretroviral therapy in

an Urban, free-care HIV clinic in Guatemala City, Guatemala," *Journal of the International Association of Physicians in AIDS Care*, vol. 9, no. 6, pp. 390–395, 2010.

[20] A. Amberbir, K. Woldemichael, S. Getachew, B. Girma, and K. Deribe, "Predictors of adherence to antiretroviral therapy among HIV-infected persons: a prospective study in Southwest Ethiopia," *BMC Public Health*, vol. 8, article 265, 2008.

[21] N. Han, W. Phoolcharoen, and U. Perngparn, "Antiretroviral drug taking in HIV positive among Myanmar migrants in central area of Thailand," *Journal of Health Research*, vol. 23, supplement, pp. 33–36, 2009.

[22] P. O. Erah and J. Arute, "Adherance of HIV/AIDS patients to antiretroviral therapy in a tertiary health facility in Benin City," *African Journal of Pharmacy and Pharmacology*, vol. 2, no. 7, pp. 145–152, 2008.

[23] E. J. Mills, J. B. Nachega, I. Buchan et al., "Adherence to antiretroviral therapy in sub-Saharan Africa and North America: a meta-analysis," *Journal of the American Medical Association*, vol. 296, no. 6, pp. 679–690, 2006.

[24] M. A. Chesney, "Factors affecting adherence to antiretroviral therapy," *Clinical Infectious Diseases*, vol. 30, no. 2, pp. S171–S176, 2000.

Differences in Serum Levels of Magnesium, Phosphate, and Albumin for HAART-Experienced and HAART-Naïve Female Patients Attending Parirenyatwa Opportunistic Infections Clinic in Harare, Zimbabwe

Denise Mudzinge,[1] Tinashe Kenny Nyazika,[2]
Tawanda Jonathan Chisango,[3] and Danai Tavonga Zhou[1]

[1] Department of Medical Laboratory Sciences, College of Health Sciences, University of Zimbabwe, P.O. Box A 178, Harare, Zimbabwe
[2] Department of Chemical Pathology, College of Health Sciences, University of Zimbabwe, P.O. Box A 178, Harare, Zimbabwe
[3] Biotechnology Department, Chinhoyi University of Technology, P.O. Box 2274, Chinhoyi, Zimbabwe

Correspondence should be addressed to Danai Tavonga Zhou; danaizh@yahoo.co.uk

Academic Editors: V. C. Bond and A. Tanuri

Antiretroviral therapy inhibits HIV replication, maintains health, and preserves life. However, both antiretroviral therapy and HIV infection have been reported to have short- and long-term effects on bone metabolism. A cross-sectional study was performed to compare serum bone profiles in HIV positive patients on highly active antiretroviral therapy and compare them to therapy-naïve patients. Serum levels of calcium, magnesium, phosphate, and albumin were measured in 40 female participants on highly active antiretroviral therapy, recruited sequentially from Parirenyatwa Opportunistic Infections Clinic, Harare, Zimbabwe. The 40 women were matched for age with 40 antiretroviral therapy-naïve women. Magnesium, phosphate, and albumin levels were significantly higher in the therapy-naïve than in therapy-experienced patients. There was no statistically significant difference in calcium levels of the two groups of women. Evidence from this study suggests that highly active antiretroviral therapy lowers levels of magnesium, phosphate, and albumin but has no effect on levels of serum calcium.

1. Introduction

Zimbabwe is in sub-Saharan Africa which is at the epicenter of the human immune deficiency virus (HIV) epidemic. According to UNAIDS the prevalence of HIV in Zimbabwe has decreased to about 1 in 10 adults (2012) from a high one of almost 1 in 4 in 2002 [1]. While the decline is commendable HIV infection still remains a major problem in Zimbabwe with 14.3% of adults being HIV positive [2].

The high disease burden of HIV has necessitated a rapid increase in the use of highly active antiretroviral therapy (HAART). As of 2012, over 476 thousand HIV-infected Zimbabweans were on HAART compared to only 8000 in 2003 [1]. In the Zimbabwe National Program, first line drug combinations include a dual combination of tenofovir/TDF/disoproxil fumarate (Gilead Sciences, USA); a nucleoside reverse transcriptase inhibitor (NRTI) and lamivudine/3TC/2,3 dideoxy-3-thiacytidine (GlaxoSmithKline and Pfizer, UK), an NRTI and a triple combination of tenofovir, lamivudine with nevirapine/XR/viramune (Boehringer Ingelheim, USA) a non-nucleoside reverse Transcriptase inhibitor (NNRTI) [3, 4]. In the event of treatment failure the patients are treated with second line drugs including zidovudine/AZT (Company) an NRTI; didanosine/DDI/Videx (Bristol-Myers Squibb Co, USA), an NRTI together with lopinavir and ritonavir; protease inhibitors (PIs) also known as kaletra/aluvia (Abbot Laboratories) [3].

HAART has reduced both the morbidity and mortality of HIV-infected people due to AIDS. However HAART is reported to have adverse side effects, one of which is bone mineralization. Changes in serum levels of biochemical markers of bone metabolism have been shown elsewhere in experimental and clinical studies [5–7]. A number of studies from various parts of the world have reported that HAART may have effects on bone metabolism via vitamin D [8] and/or parathyroid hormone [9]. This has been linked to the greater risk of developing fractures in HIV-infected patients on HAART. Evidence has also been shown in some studies linking current use of HAART to low levels of vitamin D: calcidiol (25-hydroxycholecalciferol) [10]. Calcidiol is most commonly determined in measurements of vitamin D status because of its longer half-life than the active form of vitamin D: calcitriol (1,25 cholecalciferol) [11].

Osteopenia and osteoporosis are conditions involving the weakening of bones which differ in the degree to which bones weaken [12]. Osteopenia and osteoporosis are common manifestations in HAART-experienced patients and are both due to low bone mineral density [13]. In a recent study of a large number of HIV-infected participants, 53.7% of the patients had osteopenia whilst 26.8% had osteoporosis [14, 15]. WHO recommends use of bone mineral density as a marker of bone disorders like osteopenia and osteoporosis [16]. Phosphorus, calcium, and magnesium have a role in bone metabolism. Calcium and phosphate combine together to form hydroxyapatite the inorganic part of bone. Magnesium is an intracellular component of bone cells [17]. A number of studies such as the one by De Socio et al. have reported changes in bone density accompanied by changes in serum levels of phosphate and alkaline phosphate in HIV-infected participants before and after antiretroviral therapy [18, 19].

A European study showed that Tenofovir increases bone turnover and decreases bone mineral density in treated HIV-infected adults [20]. Results in a US study showed that protease inhibitors increase the incidence of osteopenia and osteoporosis in men [21].

Tenofovir, a drug recently introduced to Zimbabwe's First line treatment, has been associated with osteomalacia, low serum levels of phosphate, and elevated alkaline phosphate in a Swiss study [22]. A Nigerian study provided evidence for an elevation in albumin levels due to HAART [6]. This is in contradiction to Southern India study that showed that 84% of patients on ART had low levels of albumin (<28 g/L) as compared to ART naïve patients [23].

There is no published evidence for the bone effect of prescribed first and second lines HAART regimens on Zimbabweans. The objective of this study was to provide evidence of changes in serum bone profiles, if any, in a Zimbabwean population of women using currently prescribed HAART regimens and compare them to a similar group of HIV-infected women who are not yet on HAART (Table 2). The broad objective was to find a noninvasive and cheap method of detecting changes in bone metabolism in HIV-infected and HAART-experienced patients in our resource-limited settings.

2. Materials and Methods

2.1. Study Site. Parirenyatwa Group of Hospitals is a group of public and teaching hospitals found in the capital city of Zimbabwe. The group of hospitals are referral hospitals servicing casualties from Harare City Centre and its environs, together with referred cases from a number of clinics around Harare and other Zimbabwean provinces and districts. The clientele attending the Parirenyatwa Opportunistic Infections (OI) Clinic, the site of our study, is diverse in terms of geographical location, but many are from low-income groups. Those participants who were on HAART were taking a combination of tenofovir, lamivudine and nevirapine for the first line treatment and zidovudine, didanosine, and lopinavir/ritonavir for second line treatment. We sequentially recruited 40 HIV-infected women, aged 18 to 40 years who had been on first line HAART for more than 6 months and consented to be part of our study. 40 HIV-infected women who were HAART-naïve were matched for age with the 40 consenting HAART-experienced women. All the women had no evidence of critical illness at the time of the study.

2.2. Ethical Considerations. Permission to work with the Parirenyatwa OI Clinic was sought from the Clinical Director of Parirenyatwa Group of Hospitals, whilst ethical clearance was given by the Joint Research Ethics Committee of the Parirenyatwa Group of Hospitals and University of Zimbabwe (JREC) after they were satisfied that the research protocol was ethically sound. Participants gave written consent after being informed fully about their role, risks, and benefits in the study and being satisfied that their identities would be protected using anonymous numerical identifiers on all documents and specimen containers.

2.3. Sample Size Calculation. Consider

$$N = \left[\frac{(Z_{\alpha/2} + Z_1 - \beta)^2}{(p_1 - p_2)^2}\right] [p_1 (1 - p_1) + (1 - p_2)], \quad (1)$$

where n = minimum sample size, z = test statistic (at 5%), p_1 = proportion with desired characteristic (0.05), $Z_{\alpha/2} = 1.96$, $Z_1 - \beta$, $p_1 = 0.63$, $p_2 = 0.28$,

- $n = ((1.96 + 0.84)^2/(0.63 - 0.84)^2)(0.63(1 - 0.63) + 0.28(1 - 0.28)) = 27.14 = 28$,
- Final n = 28 + Refusal Rate (Refusal Rate = 15% of n),
- $n = 28 + 12.17 = 40.17$.

Therefore overall minimum sample size = 80 (40 on HAART and 40 HAART-naïve).

2.4. Data and Sample Collection. Demographic data was obtained from the patients and clinic records (Table 1). Blood was drawn into plain tubes by a phlebotomist at the clinic during patients' routine visits. Serum was aliquoted into 2 mL cryotubes and stored at −20°C for up to 20 days.

2.5. Sample Analysis. Serum samples were thawed once at room temperature, and analysis was carried out on a BS120 Mindray Chemistry analyzer. The chemistry analyzer was calibrated, and then controls and samples were assayed for total calcium, magnesium, phosphate, and albumin. Corrected

TABLE 1: Demographic data of 80 female participants.

Characteristic	HAART+ (N = 40)	HAART-naïve (N = 40)	P value, significant difference
Mean age/years	24.4 (5.0)	24.1 (5.2)	0.05, NS
Time since diagnosis of HIV/years	8.8 (2.6)	7.5 (2.6)	<0.05, significant difference
Gravidae/number of pregnancies	3.8 (0.6)	3.5 (0.6)	<0.05, significant difference
Para/number of surviving children	2.2 (1.2)	2.3 (1.2)	>0.05, NS
Income/average per month in USD	62.2 (11.1)	62.0 (10.5)	>0.05, NS

TABLE 2: Comparison of serum bone profiles of female patients on HAART and before HAART.

	HAART+	HAART-naïve	P value, significance
Mean total calcium (mmol/L)	6.92	8.4	
Standard deviation for mean total calcium	0.024	0.03	
Standard error for mean total calcium	0.18	0.202	
95% confidence interval	1.67	1.969	P = 0.23, no significant difference
Mean magnesium (mmol/L)	3.00	4.32	
Standard deviation for mean magnesium	0.021	0.029	
Standard error for mean magnesium	0.158	0.193	
95% confidence interval	0.692	0.99	P = 0.033, significant difference
Mean phosphate (mmol/L)	5.27	12.49	
Standard deviation for mean phosphate	0.23	0.36	
Standard error for mean phosphate	1.696	2.41	
95% confidence interval	0.865	3.31	P = 0.015, significant difference
Mean albumin (mg/dL)	2.87	3.24	
Standard deviation for mean albumin	0.6	0.82	
Standard error for mean albumin	4.42	5.44	
95% confidence interval	2.75	3.08	P = 0.023, significant difference

calcium was calculated for participants with low albumin levels.

3. Results

The mean assayed values for the female patients on HAART (together with the normal reference ranges) were: total calcium 6.92 mg/dL (reference range 8.80–9.50 mg/dL), Magnesium 1.78 mg/dL (Reference Range 1.46–2.68 mg/dL), Phosphate 5.10 mg/dL (reference range 1.80–5.10 mg/dL) and Albumin 2.87 mg/dL (reference 2.80–5.30 mg/dL). The means of the HAART-naïve women were; Total calcium 8.40 mg/dL, Magnesium 2.55 mg/dL, Phosphate 5.10 mg/dL and Albumin 3.25 mg/dL.

4. Conclusion

There was no significant difference between total calcium levels in patients on HAART and HAART-naïve patients. However, the values of calcium for the two groups in our study fall below the normal range. Our results suggest that use of both HIV and HAART may lead to hypocalcaemia. This contradicts with studies done in America where elevation in serum calcium levels in women on antiretroviral therapy including tenofovir was linked to an increase in bone loss [24]. Our results seem to be in agreement with a different set of studies described in India that reported lower levels of the active form of vitamin D (calcitriol), resulting in reduced intestinal calcium absorption. Their report, as we observed, described a decrease in serum calcium levels after HAART initiation [25]. It becomes essential to measure levels of vitamin D in future studies, in order to answer the important question of whether HAART affects bone metabolism via vitamin D.

There were other interesting differences in serum bone profiles of the women in our study. Magnesium and albumin levels were within normal ranges for both groups of women, but the HAART-experienced had lower magnesium and albumin levels than the HAART-naïve patients. Our findings for magnesium do not however agree with two studies: a Brazilian study that showed hypomagnesaemia occurring in 29% of patients on antiretroviral therapy [26] and a study done in Nigeria that showed an elevation in serum albumin, months after antiretroviral therapy initiation [6]. Our results for albumin do correlate with the findings of a study carried out in Southern India, in which serum albumin levels were lower after antiretroviral therapy [23].

Phosphate levels were elevated in HAART-naïve patients, and their levels were above the normal range whilst the HAART-experienced women have on average phosphate levels that fall within normal ranges. Our study contradicts with studies which showed a link between use of tenofovir and hypophosphatemia [27] and studies done in America that showed a decrease in serum phosphate due to reduced renal retention [28].

The results of our study show both expected and unexpected results. It is important to improve this study by increasing the number of study sites, increasing the power by enlarging the sample size, and also measuring the levels of vitamin D (calcidiol or calcitriol). The results of this and future studies will be used to advocate for change in practice in treatment of HIV-infected women on HAART. Clinicians and decision makers may have to consider giving patients on HAART vitamin D supplements to avoid weakening of bones in Zimbabweans on HAART. Another study involving both men and women is also necessary in order to determine what serum bone profiles changes may be happening in men due to HIV infection and/or HAART. Is serum bone profiling a potentially noninvasive, inexpensive method that can be used routinely to detect changes in bone metabolism in the HIV infected patients in our resource-limited setting? This study shows evidence of changes in serum bone profiles. A larger study that also aims to determine association between serum bone profiles and measurement of the WHO gold standard (mineral bone density) may help answer that question.

Conflict of Interests

The authors declare no conflict of interests.

Acknowledgments

The authors would like to thank the University of Zimbabwe, Department of Medical Laboratory Sciences, for funding the research, University of Zimbabwe, Department of Medical Laboratory Sciences technical staff, for assistance and guidance during the practical work, and Parirenyatwa Opportunistic Infections Clinic staff and patients.

References

[1] Global AIDS Response Progress Report, http://www.unaids.org/en/dataanalysis.

[2] The World Factbook, https://www.cia.gov/library/publications/the-world-factbook/fields/2155.html.

[3] National Drug and Therapeutics Policy Advisory Committee, *Guidelines for Antiretroviral Therapy in Zimbabwe*, Ministry of Health and Child Welfare Zimbabwe, Harare, Zimbabwe, 2005.

[4] Stavudine to be phased out, http://www.zbc.co.zw/news-categories/health/9945-stavudine-to-be-phased-out.html.

[5] K. K. A. van Rompay, L. L. Brignolo, D. J. Meyer et al., "Biological effects of short-term or prolonged administration of 9-[2-(phosphonomethoxy)propyl]adenine (tenofovir) to newborn and infant macaques," *Antimicrobial Agents and Chemotherapy*, vol. 48, no. 5, pp. 1469–1487, 2004.

[6] H. O. Olawumi and P. O. Olatunji, "The value of serum albumin in pretreatment assessment and monitoring of therapy in HIV/AIDS patients," *HIV Medicine*, vol. 7, no. 6, pp. 351–355, 2006.

[7] P. Tebas, W. G. Powderly, S. Claxton et al., "Accelerated bone mineral loss in HIV-infected patients receiving potent antiretroviral therapy," *AIDS*, vol. 14, no. 4, pp. F63–F67, 2000.

[8] A. Conesa-Botella, E. Florence, L. Lynen, R. Colebunders, J. Menten, and R. Moreno-Reyes, "Decrease of vitamin D concentration in patients with HIV infection on a non nucleoside reverse transcriptase inhibitor-containing regimen," *AIDS Research and Therapy*, vol. 7, article 40, 2010.

[9] K. E. Childs, S. L. Fishman, C. Constable et al., "Short communication: inadequate vitamin D exacerbates parathyroid hormone elevations in tenofovir users," *AIDS Research and Human Retroviruses*, vol. 26, no. 8, pp. 855–859, 2010.

[10] C. N. Dao, P. Patel, E. T. Overton et al., "Low vitamin D among HIV-infected adults: prevalence of and risk factors for low vitamin D levels in a cohort of HIV-infected adults and comparison to prevalence among adults in the us general population," *Clinical Infectious Diseases*, vol. 52, no. 3, pp. 396–405, 2011.

[11] A. G. Pittas, M. Chung, T. Trikalinos et al., "Systematic review: vitamin D and cardiometabolic outcomes," *Annals of Internal Medicine*, vol. 152, no. 5, pp. 307–314, 2010.

[12] S. Landonio, T. Quirino, P. Bonfanti et al., "Osteopenia and osteoporosis in HIV+ patients, untreated or receiving HAART," *Biomedicine and Pharmacotherapy*, vol. 58, no. 9, pp. 505–508, 2004.

[13] C. Cazanave, M. Dupon, V. Lavignolle-Aurillac et al., "Reduced bone mineral density in HIV-infected patients: prevalence and associated factors," *AIDS*, vol. 22, no. 3, pp. 395–402, 2008.

[14] J. Thomas and S. M. Doherty, "HIV infection—a risk factor for osteoporosis," *Journal of Acquired Immune Deficiency Syndromes*, vol. 33, no. 3, pp. 281–291, 2003.

[15] M. G. A. van Vonderen, P. Lips, M. A. van Agtmael et al., "First line zidovudine/lamivudine/lopinavir/ritonavir leads to greater bone loss compared to nevirapine/lopinavir/ritonavir," *AIDS*, vol. 23, no. 11, pp. 1367–1376, 2009.

[16] The WHO Scientific Group on the Prevention and Management of Osteoporosis (Geneva, Switzerland), *Prevention and Management of Osteoporosis: Report of a WHO Scientific Group*, 2003.

[17] M. F. Fazlini, A. R. Suriah, Y. Zaitun, M. Kandiah, W. S. Chee, Y. M. Chan et al., "Calcium supplementation amongst postmenopausal women: effect on serum calcium, phosphorus and magnesium levels," *International Food Research Journal*, vol. 20, no. 1, pp. 477–480, 2013.

[18] G. V. L. De Socio, G. Fabbriciani, M. Massarotti, S. Messina, E. Cecchini, and B. Marasini, "Hypophosphotemic osteomalacia associated tenofovir: a multidisciplinary approach is required," *Mediterranean Journal of Hematology and Infectious Diseases*, vol. 4, no. 1, 2012.

[19] A. Malik, P. Abraham, and N. Malik, "Acute renal failure and Fanconi syndrome in an AIDS patient on tenofovir treatment—case report and review of literature," *Journal of Infection*, vol. 51, no. 2, pp. e61–e65, 2005.

[20] H.-J. Stellbrink, C. Orkin, J. R. Arribas et al., "Comparison of changes in bone density and turnover with abacavir-lamivudine versus tenofovir-emtricitabine in HIV-infected adults: 48-week results from the ASSERT study," *Clinical Infectious Diseases*, vol. 51, no. 8, pp. 963–972, 2010.

[21] P. Tebas, W. G. Powderly, S. Claxton et al., "Accelerated bone mineral loss in HIV-infected patients receiving potent antiretroviral therapy," *AIDS*, vol. 14, no. 4, pp. F63–F67, 2000.

[22] C. A. Fux, A. Rauch, M. Simcock et al., "Tenofovir use is associated with an increase in serum alkaline phosphatase in the Swiss HIV Cohort Study," *Antiviral Therapy*, vol. 13, no. 8, pp. 1077–1082, 2008.

[23] M. Sundaram, C. N. Srinivas, E. M. Shankar, P. Balakrishnan, S. Solomon, and N. Kumarasamy, "Cofactors for low serum albumin levels among HIV-infected individuals in Southern India,"

Journal of the International Association of Physicians in AIDS Care, vol. 8, no. 3, pp. 161–164, 2009.

[24] M. T. Yin, C. A. Zhang, D. J. McMahon et al., "Higher rates of bone loss in postmenopausal HIV-infected women: a longitudinal study," *Journal of Clinical Endocrinology and Metabolism*, vol. 97, no. 2, pp. 554–562, 2012.

[25] M. Muthuraj, "Serum zinc, calcium and albumin levels in pulmonary tuberculosis patients co-Infected with HIV," *Global Journal of Biotechnology & Biochemistry*, vol. 5, no. 1, pp. 27–35, 2010.

[26] M. S. Biagioni Santos, A. C. Seguro, and L. Andrade, "Hypomagnesemia is a risk factor for nonrecovery of renal function and mortality in AIDS patients with acute kidney injury," *Brazilian Journal of Medical and Biological Research*, vol. 43, no. 3, pp. 316–323, 2010.

[27] S. L. Day, H. A. Leake Date, A. Bannister, M. Hankins, and M. Fisher, "Serum hypophosphatemia in tenofovir disoproxil fumarate recipients is multifactorial in origin, questioning the utility of its monitoring in clinical practice," *Journal of Acquired Immune Deficiency Syndromes*, vol. 38, no. 3, pp. 301–304, 2005.

[28] B. Fernandez-Fernandez, A. Montoya-Ferrer, A. B. Sanz, M. D. Sanchez-Nino, M. C. Izquierdo, J. Poveda et al., "Tenofovir nephrotoxicity: 2011 update," *AIDS Research and Treatment*, vol. 2011, Article ID 354908, 11 pages, 2011.

Utilization of Modern Contraceptives among HIV Positive Reproductive Age Women in Tigray, Ethiopia: A Cross Sectional Study

Yemane Berhane,[1] Haftu Berhe,[2] Gerezgiher Buruh Abera,[2] and Hailemariam Berhe[2]

[1] *Axum College of Nursing, Tigray, Ethiopia*
[2] *Department of Nursing, College of Health Sciences, Mekelle University, Ethiopia*

Correspondence should be addressed to Gerezgiher Buruh Abera; gbamsc2002@gmail.com

Academic Editors: E. M. Fenyo and C. Wejse

Background. HIV infected women in sub-Saharan Africa are at substantial risk of unintended pregnancy and sexually transmitted infections. In developing countries including Ethiopia counseling and provision of modern contraceptives of choice to HIV infected women including those on antiretroviral therapy (ART) is an important strategy to prevent unintended pregnancies and sexually transmitted infections. Little is known about the existing practices and utilization of modern contraceptives among HIV positive reproductive age women attending ART units. *Objective.* The aim of this study was to assess utilization of modern contraceptives and associated factors among HIV positive reproductive age women attending ART units in zonal hospitals of Tigray region, North Ethiopia. *Method.* Institution based cross-sectional study was conducted by interviewing 364 HIV positive reproductive age women in all zonal hospitals of Tigray region using systematic sampling technique. Structured and pretested questionnaire was used to obtain information from the respondents. Descriptive, bivariate, and multivariate methods were used to analyze utilization of modern contraceptives and the factors associated with it. *Result.* Three hundred sixty-four subjects participated with a response rate of 99.2%. The mean age of the respondents was 31.9 ± 6.5 (SD) years. About 46% of participants utilized modern contraceptives, 59.9% out of them used dual method. However, a significant proportion of the respondents (46%) reported that they wished to have a desire for children. Being secondary education and higher (AOR: 2.85; 95% CI: 1.17–6.95) and currently on HAART (AOR: 3.23; 95% CI: 1.49–7.01) they were more likely to utilize modern contraceptive. But those women who were $\geq$25 years old, house wives, single, divorced, or widowed were less likely to utilize modern contraceptive. *Conclusion.* Results of this study revealed that the number of respondents who were ever heard of modern contraceptives was high. However, modern contraceptive utilization was still low. Additional efforts are needed to promote modern contraceptive utilization in general and dual method use in particular among HIV positive reproductive age women.

1. Introduction

At the Alma-Ata conference (1978), Family Planning services were highlighted as one of the basic and important strategies for reducing high risk pregnancies that often occurred too early, too late, and too frequent and also as a way to improve child heath. Family planning programs have helped women worldwide to avoid millions of unintended pregnancies often associated with high risk abortions since the 1960s [1].

In many countries, PMTCT programs focus on antenatal HIV testing and provision of ARV prophylaxis to HIV infected women and their newborns. However, these three components constitute just one of the four pillars for PMTCT, the remaining being primary HIV prevention in women of child-bearing age, family planning (FP) for the prevention of unwanted pregnancies, and care and treatment for HIV infected women and their HIV affected children. HIV/AIDS has had devastating effects and is currently a common complication of pregnancy in Ethiopia [2].

Counseling and provision of contraception of choice to HIV infected women including those on ART is an important strategy to prevent unintended pregnancies among HIV positive women who would rather wish to delay pregnancy or stop child bearing altogether. Dual function contraceptives that simultaneously prevent HIV transmission as well as unwanted pregnancies might be the most appropriate contraceptive method for women living with HIV/AIDS [3].

Contraception can be provided either within the treatment programs or by active referral to routine family planning providers. This would reduce number of pregnancies among HIV positive women and reduce the number of HIV infected infants. The other benefit of contraception is that it averts HIV infection in infants at a lower cost compared to other PMTCT interventions. Indeed the prevention of unintended pregnancies among women living with HIV is one of the World Health Organization (WHO) four elements of comprehensive approach to prevent mother-to-child transmission of HIV [4–7].

The Millennium Development Goals, adopted in New York in 2000, promote universal education and gender equality, maternal and child health, and prevention and treatment for HIV/AIDS [8].

Provision of comprehensive reproductive health care is central to attaining these goals Worldwide, as many as one-third of the 357,000 annual maternal deaths are attributable to unintended pregnancies; the majority of these mortalities occur in low- and middle-income countries [9–11]. Enhanced access to family planning services particularly modern contraceptives, in sub-Saharan Africa, would result in marked reductions in unintended pregnancies and unsafe abortions, a projected 69% decrease in maternal deaths, and a 57% decrease in newborn deaths [10].

In addition to substantial risks of dying from pregnancy complications, women in sub-Saharan Africa are also at increased risk of HIV infections. Providing safe, effective contraception to HIV infected women who desire it has also been identified by the World Health Organization as a primary strategy for prevention of pediatric infections [12].

Ethiopia is one of the countries most severely affected by HIV/AIDS pandemic. According to the 2007 single point HIV prevalence estimate of Ethiopia for the year 2010, the average adult female HIV prevalence was 2.9%. Out of the total HIV positive populations in the country, 717,669 were females, of which 90,311 HIV positive pregnant women. For Tigray according to 2007 single point HIV prevalence estimate, the total adult female HIV prevalence for 2010 was 3.7%. There were 7,073 HIV positive pregnant women [2, 12, 13]. Utilization of modern contraceptives among HIV positive reproductive age women ever enrolled in ART units, in Tigray region, is among those essential and critical issues which need study in wide range, but little is known about.

2. Methodology

2.1. Setting. The study was carried out in all zonal hospitals of ART units in Tigray region. Tigray region is the Northern most National Regional state of Ethiopia. The region covers about 50,000 square kilometers. The total population of Tigray projected based on 2007 statistical census agency is about 4.3 million of which 82.6% are rural and 51% are female. According to the 2003 (EFY) Health and Health Related Indicators published by FMOH, Tigray has 14 hospitals (1 referral, 6 zonal, and 7 district hospitals), 209 health centers, and 572 health posts that give health service coverage of 83% [14]. Currently there are about 6500 HIV positive women enrolled in the ART units of the zonal hospitals. An institution based cross-sectional study design was conducted, and it was conducted from May to December, 2012.

The source population was all HIV positive women of reproductive age (15–49 years) attending ART units, and the study population was sampled HIV positive women of reproductive age (15–49 years) attending ART clinics.

The sample from each hospital was allocated proportionally to the number of clients on ART at each institution. The sample size for the study was determined by assuming prevalence of modern contraceptive utilization (P) to be 59% from the study conducted in Lusaka, Zambia among HIV infected women [15], a confidence level of 95% (CI), and marginal error of 5% (d) giving a sample size of 372.

Based on evidences obtained from the respective zonal hospitals, the source population was 2970. So population correction was used to get the corrected finite sample size that was 331. To compensate for nonresponse rate 10% of the sample was added =33; finally a total of 364 HIV positive women were sampled for the study. The total sample size was proportionally allocated to all zonal hospitals based on the number of client flow rate on 3 weeks prior to the study. Systematic random sampling technique was used to select eligible participants from each hospital ART units.

Structured and pretested questionnaire was used to obtain information from the respondents. The tool consists of demographic, socioeconomic characteristics, information on contraceptive utilization, and associated factors. An exit interview was conducted during the regular working hours by the trained nurses. We also had conducted a medical record review to confirm HAART history and to obtain clinical data (WHO stage of disease and CD4 cell count). Six degree holder nurses were supervising the data collection in the respective hospitals.

The dependent variable was utilization of modern contraceptives, and the independent variables were demographic characteristics, fertility related factors, socio-economic factors, HIV related factors, duration on ART and ART status, drug side effects, contraceptive service integration, WHO clinical stage of disease, disclosure, and partners HIV status.

Contraceptive utilization: sexually active respondents who responded positively after being asked whether they utilized modern contraceptive in the last one month.

Modern methods: including pills, IUD, injectables, implants and male and female condoms (excluding lactational amenorrhoea, rhythm, and withdrawal).

Consistent condom use: use of male or female condom during every sexual intercourse.

Dual contraceptive methods: utilization of any hormonal or permanent modern contraceptive method along with male or female condom.

Integration of contraceptive services: referred to a report from participants who received a contraceptive method in a spot with the ART services.

To maintain the data quality, the data collectors and supervisors were trained in the methods, objectives, confidentiality, and other technical aspects of the study before data collection commenced. The questionnaire was first prepared in English, translated into the local language (Tigrigna), and then translated back to English. The questionnaire was pretested in 5 percent of the participants in Wukro hospital a week before the commencement of the main research. Completed questionnaire was cross-checked daily for inconsistencies and completeness.

The data was coded, entered, edited, and analyzed using SPSS version 16.0 for windows. Binary logistic regression was used to test the significance of associations. Important associations (odds ratio, confidence intervals, and P value) were also calculated furthermore, multi-co-linearity diagnostics and interaction of variables were tested by the use of logistic regression model.

Ethical clearance and approval was obtained from Mekelle University College of the Health Sciences; Permission was also secured from Tigray Regional Health Bureau and from the six zonal hospitals. Participation was on a voluntary basis after informed verbal consent, and responses were kept confidential.

3. Result

A total of 364 subjects participated with a response rate of 99.2%. Overall, 315 (87.3%) of the respondents were from the urban area. The mean age of the respondents was 31.9 ± 6.5 (SD) years. Approximately, 55 percent of the participants were in the age group of 25 to 34 years. Three hundred thirty-two (92%) were from orthodox religion and 338 (93.6%) were ethnically Tigrians. In terms of educational status, 87 (24.2%) were illiterate. Over 43% were currently married, and the majority (71.5%) had primary level of education or less. Over half, 195 (54%), were unemployed, and the majority of the respondents, 171 (47.40%), reported earning less than or equal to 500 ETB a month (Table 1).

TABLE 1: Sociodemographic characteristics of HIV positive reproductive age women attending ART units (n = 361), zonal hospitals, Tigray, North Ethiopia, 2012.

Variables	Frequency (N)	Percentage (%)
Age		
15–24	36	10
25–34	197	54.5
≥35	128	35.5
Education		
Illiterate	87	24.2
Read and write	85	23.5
Primary (1–8)	86	23.8
Secondary education (9 and above)	103	28.5
Religion		
Orthodox	332	92
Muslim	22	6.1
Others	7	2
Marital status		
Married	156	43.2
Single	33	9.1
Divorced/separated	121	33.5
Widowed	51	14.2
Occupation		
House wife	111	30.7
Daily laborer	84	23.3
Government employee	101	28
Private employee	65	18
Monthly house hold income		
0–500	171	47.4
501–1500	140	38.8
1501–2500	35	9.7
≥2501	15	4.1
Residence		
Urban	315	87.3
Rural	46	12.7

Results of this study revealed that 100% of the study subjects ever heard at least one modern contraceptive. Three hundred sixty one women have practiced sex-one month prior to data collection. Less than half, 167 (46.3%), were currently using a modern contraceptive method. The most commonly used method, 100 (59.9%), was dual contraceptives. Overall, 29.3% of the respondents reported using hormonal methods only (injectables, pill, and Norplant; 22.7%, 4.2%, and 2.4% resp.). IUDs were not reported by any respondent. Out of the dual or condom only users 109 (92.4%) reported utilizing condom consistently. Current use of modern FP methods was the highest, 68 (40.7%) among the women with secondary and above level education. In this study married women were found to be using modern contraceptives the most 110 (65.9%).

The main reason women choose current method was health professionals advice, 54 (32.3%), easy to use, 44 (26.3%), and perceived less side effects, 29 (17.4%).

About half of modern contraceptive users (49.7%) got the service within the ART clinic. A substantial number of women, 194 (53.7%), were not currently utilizing any modern method. Among those who did not use modern contraceptives, 95 (49%) stated their reason as fear of drug interaction. However, 235 (65.1%) of the participants were intended to continue or use in the future (Table 2).

Overall, it was found that 166 (46%) of all participants wanted to have more children, and considerable proportion of women (79.8%) have at least one child. Out of the women that were using modern contraceptives, 49.1% had 2-3 children followed by one or no living children. Among the women who did not desire having more children, 56.3% (94) were currently using modern methods. With regards to their partner's serostatus, 161 (85.5%) were aware of their partner's serostatus (153 (82.3%) seropositive and 6 (3.2%) seronegative). The rest, 27 (14.5%) did not know about their partner's HIV status. The median time since first HIV diagnosis was

TABLE 2: Current utilization of modern contraceptives among HIV positive reproductive age women attending ART units, zonal hospitals, Tigray, North Ethiopia, 2012.

Variables	Frequency (N)	Percentage (%)
Ever heard of modern Contraceptives (N = 361)		
Yes	361	100
No	0	0
Total	**361**	**100**
Type of method ever heard		
Pill	43	11.9
Injectables	11	5.3
Male condom only	05	1.4
Dual methods	78	21.6
Any greater than or equal two methods	216	59.8
Total	**361**	**100**
Reason to choose method (N = 167)		
Health professionals advice	54	32.3
Perceived less side effects	29	17.4
Observed friends experience	18	10.8
Easy to use	44	26.3
Agreement with partner	2	1.2
Effectiveness	20	12
Total	**167**	**100**
Reasons for not to use contraceptives (N = 194)		
Fear of drug interaction	95	26.3%
Trying pregnancy	78	21.6%
Partner does not want contraceptive	18	5%
Others	3	0.8%
Total	**194**	**53.7%**

3.00 years, ranging from 0.1 to 9.9 years. More than half (68.7%) had recent CD4 counts >250 cells/mm^3 (mean recent CD4 = 376.8 (SD = 147.7)) with the mean duration on ART of 3.4 years ± 1.86 (SD). Nearly 60% of women were in WHO stage of disease I or II and 92% had disclosed their HIV status to their regular partner. Two hundred and twenty-four (81.4%) participants were currently on HAART while 67 (18.6%) were not. One hundred forty-four (86.2%) of women on HAART utilize modern methods. A large number of participants 212 (58.7%) had been concerned about side effects of method choice like irregular bleeding, infertility and vomiting. 41% of those who have no or only one child had utilized modern contraceptives (Table 3).

In Bivariate analysis, women were less likely to report modern contraceptive use if house wives, single, divorced, or widowed. Conversely, secondary or higher education attended, and those who had a monthly income of 1501–2500 ETB, being counseled for contraceptive, those with a CD4 count ≤250 cells/mm^3 and currently on HAART had increased odds of contraceptive use. The results from the multivariable logistic regression modeling revealed that independent predictors of modern contraceptive utilization for HIV positive women of reproductive age in zonal hospitals, Tigray region, were age, occupation, educational status, and currently on HAART. Therefore, women 25–34 years old (AOR: 0.30; 95% CI: 0.12–0.79), ≥35 years old (AOR: 0.31; 95% CI: 0.11–0.87), and house wives (AOR: 0.4; 95% CI: 0.17–0.93) had lower odds of using modern contraception. The odds of using modern contraception were higher among women with secondary education and higher attended (AOR: 2.85; 95% CI: 1.17–6.95). Similarly, those women currently on HAART were 3.23 times more likely to utilize modern methods (AOR: 3.23; 95% CI: 1.49–7.01). There were no significant independent associations between contraceptive use and counseling for contraceptive, house hold monthly income, and CD4 cell count in adjusted analyses (Table 4).

4. Discussion

This study attempted to assess utilization of modern contraceptives and associated factors among HIV positive reproductive age women. Overall, less than half (46.3%) of HIV positive reproductive age women in this study (86.2% ART experienced and 13.8% pre-ART) reported modern contraceptive use which was higher than the modern contraceptive prevalence rate in Tigray region irrespective of HIV status (21.2%) [16]. The higher uptake of family planning among this population might be due to high injectables and condom use rates and due to time deference. But, still congruent with the national target for CPR in the general population (44%) to achieve MDGs by 2015 though the prevalence of modern contraceptive in HIV positive women is expected to become higher than the general population to avert vertical and horizontal transmission of the virus [17]. Similarly, our finding was higher than that of the study done in Addis Ababa (28%) [18] and Rwanda (31%) [19], but in line with the report on contraceptive utilization in Malawi (46%) [20]. In contrary, the study has found that current use of modern contraceptive methods was lower than that from findings of a study done in Asela hospital, Oromia, Ethiopia, which is estimated at 76.5% [21]. This variation might be due to high desire for children, 46% in this study. The current finding is also lower than findings from Mbarara, Uganda (85%) [22], Lesotho (82–86%) [23], Lusaka, Zambia (59.2%) [20]. The possible reason for this might be due to geographical variation.

Even though modern contraceptive methods were widely available at free cost in ART treatment units and/or hospitals, more than half were not using any modern methods. While the Ethiopian AIDS Control Program National guidelines advocate for dual family planning methods to prevent HIV/STI transmission and unintended pregnancies for HIV positive individuals, only (59.9%) women reported dual method use in this study. But this finding was higher than that of the study finding in Lusaka, Zambia [20]. The possible difference might be due to geographic and time variations and study design used.

Out of the dual method/condom users, about 70% of women utilize condom consistently which is broadly in line with a study done in Soweto, South Africa [24]. Use of only

TABLE 3: Fertility, HIV, and clinical related factors among HIV positive reproductive age women, zonal hospital, Tigray, North Ethiopia, 2012.

Variables	Modern contraceptive utilization	
	Yes (%)	No (%)
Desire for children		
Yes	73 (43.7%)	93 (47.9%)
No	94 (56.3%)	101 (52.1%)
Partner's serostatus ($N = 186$)		
Negative	6 (4.2%)	0
Positive	117 (83%)	36 (80%)
Unknown	18 (12.8%)	9 (20%)
Discuss with partner about contraceptive ($N = 186$)		
Yes	133 (94.3%)	42 (93.3%)
No	8 (5.7%)	3 (6.7%)
HIV disclosure to regular partner		
Yes	127 (90.1%)	44 (97.8%)
No	14 (9.9%)	1 (2.2%)
Side effects ($N = 212$)		
Irregular bleeding	63 (60.6%)	67 (62%)
Vomiting	12 (11.6%)	11 (10.2%)
Infertility	25 (24%)	26 (24.1%)
Others	4 (3.8%)	4 (3.7%)
Counseling service for contraceptive		
Yes	165 (98.8%)	183 (94.3%)
No	2 (1.2%)	11 (5.7%)
Current HAART use		
Yes	144 (86.2%)	150 (77.3%)
No	23 (13.8%)	44 (22.7%)
Years since on ART2		
0.1–2.0 years	29 (20.1%)	57 (38%)
≥2.1 years	115 (79.9%)	93 (62%)
WHO clinical stage		
1/2	99 (59.3%)	117 (60.3%)
3/4	68 (40.7%)	77 (39.7%)

hormonal contraceptive was found to be low (Depo provera (22.7%) followed by pills (4.2%) and only 2.4% reported use of Norplant). IUDs only were not reported by any respondent. This finding is congruent with EDHS report in Tigray region, irrespective of HIV status [25]. Similar results were also found in a survey done in Uganda [21].

In the study area, the most common reason for method choice was health professional's advice (32.3%). This finding is consistent with some studies elsewhere in Ethiopia [25, 26].

The study revealed that considerable proportion of women respondents (65.1%) have intention to use or continue to use modern contraceptive utilization. This finding is higher than that of the study done in Gondar university hospital [27]. This might be related to the fact that large numbers of women attending ART units have improved their awareness through time on contraceptive utilization due to frequent counseling services.

To date, published experiences and data on provision of contraception services within HIV care clinics were limited. Yet this remains one of the most promising options for providing family planning for HIV positive women and deserves particular attention. This study showed that among those currently using a contraceptive method, 98.8% of women had been counseled on family planning methods and only 49.7% were provided at the antiretroviral treatment clinic. Though the finding is higher than that of a study done in Mombasa, Kenya [28], this entails the need to integrate family planning and other reproductive health services with the general ART service and may be one of the problems to meet reproductive health care needs of these women. Service integration offers options for preventing unintended pregnancies to HIV positive clients (using/not using ART), and as a part of PMTCT services.

Access to ARV is increasing in developing countries and enables HIV positive individuals to live longer and healthier lives. For instance, studies from industrialized countries suggest that ARV is associated with changes towards unsafe sex [29]. However, results from developing nations have been mixed [30, 31]. Conversely, increased contact with health care professionals to receive treatment may encourage positive

TABLE 4: Bivariate and multivariate analyses of variables associated with contraceptive use among HIV positive women (aged 15–49 years), attending ART units in zonal hospitals, Tigray, (N = 361) North Ethiopia, 2012.

Variable	Utilize contraceptive Yes (%)	No (%)	Crude OR (95% CI)	Adjusted OR (95% CI)	P-value
Educational status					
Illiterate	29 (17.4%)	58 (29.9%)	1	1	
Read and write	39 (23.3%)	46 (23.7%)	1.70 (0.92, 3.14)	1.45 (0.66, 3.15)	
Primary (1–8)	31 (18.6%)	55 (28.4%)	1.13 (0.60, 2.11)	0.92 (0.41, 2.09)	
Secondary and above (grade 9 and above)	68 (40.7%)	35 (18.0%)	3.89 (2.12, 7.11)*	2.85 (1.17, 6.95)**	0.02
Occupation 2					
Government employee	66 (39.5%)	35 (18.0%)	1	1	
Daily laborer	35 (21%)	49 (25.3%)	0.38 (0.21, 0.69)*	0.98 (0.43, 2.27)	
House wives	38 (23.8%)	73 (37.6%)	0.28 (0.16, 0.49)*	0.4 (0.17, 0.93)**	0.034
Private employee	28 (16.8%)	37 (19.1%)	0.40 (0.21, 0.76)*	0.51 (0.23, 1.12)	
Age group (years)					
15–24	19 (11.4%)	17 (8.8%)	1	1	
25–34	97 (58.1%)	100 (51.5%)	0.87 (0.43, 1.77)	0.3 (0.12, 0.79)**	0.015
≥35	51 (30.5%)	77 (39.7%)	0.59 (0.28, 1.2)	0.31 (0.11, 0.87)**	0.026
Grouped monthly income (ETB)					
≤500	67 (40.1%)	104 (53.6%)	1	1	
501–1500	69 (41.3%)	71 (36.6%)	1.5 (0.96, 2.37)*	1.38 (0.77, 2.48)	
1501–2500	22 (13.2%)	13 (6.7%)	2.6 (1.24, 5.57)*	1.98 (0.76, 5.19)	
≥2501	9 (5.4%)	6 (3.1%)	2.3 (0.79, 6.84)*	2.43 (0.66, 8.96)	
Counseling service for contraceptive					
Yes	165 (47.4%)	183 (52.6%)	4.96 (1.08, 22.7)*	5.07 (0.71, 36.1)	
No	2 (15.4%)	11 (84.6%)	1	1	
Grouped CD4					
≤250 cells/mm^3	63 (37.7%)	50 (25.8%)	1.74 (1.1, 2.73)*	0.94 (0.50, 1.75)	
>250 cells/mm^3	104 (62.3%)	144 (74.2%)	1	1	
Current HAART use					
Yes	144 (86.2%)	150 (77.3%)	1.84 (1.06, 3.20)*	3.23 (1.49, 7.01)**	0.003
No	23 (13.8%)	44 (22.7%)	1	1	

*Statistical significance in COR, **statistical significance in AOR, OR: odds ratio, CI: confidence interval, and 1: reference.

changes in sexual behavior. This study revealed that women receiving HAART were 3.23 times more likely to report contraceptive use than pre-ART women. Our finding, indicating significantly higher prevalence of contraceptive use among HAART users compared with pre-ART women is broadly consistent with recent findings from Uganda, Mbarara and Soweto, South Africa [18, 22]. The reasons for higher contraceptive prevalence among HAART users were not directly explored in this study. However, an important possible reason for the observed differences is that women receiving HAART have more regular contact with health care professionals as a function of the clinical follow-up. During these regular clinic visits, reproductive and sexual health issues are raised, and the opportunity to discuss and commence use of contraception is presented. In general, ART provides opportunity to discuss FP and other RH matters. Hence receiving ART was associated with increased contraceptive utilization among the study participants which may indirectly informs us about the effectiveness of the HIV prevention program in the hospitals. In contrast to this, a study in Ghana showed that participants receiving HAART were significantly less likely to utilize contraceptives [32].

Although not statistically significant, half of the women who have concern about side effects of methods were not utilizing contraceptives. Studies elsewhere in Africa showed that concerns about side effects and inconveniences were by far the most prominent reasons for low utilization or discontinuation of modern contraceptives among women [33, 34].

HIV status disclosure to regular partner was not associated with use of contraception in either Bivariate or multivariable analyses. This is in contrast to a recent study in Uganda that showed that the lack of HIV disclosure was associated with lower odds of use of modern contraceptives among HIV women enrolled in HIV clinics in Uganda [35].

Sociodemographic factors (age, education, and occupation) were associated with contraception use. This study noted that women attending secondary education and higher had increased odds of contraceptive use, similar to findings reported from some African countries [33–36]. The higher the level of education, the more they appreciate the advantages of contraceptive use compared to those without education. The possible reason might be in this study is that most secondary education and higher attended women were married (currently with their regular partner) so frequent sexual contact may predispose them to unintended pregnancy and STIs. Individuals with more education might have higher levels of HIV/AIDS knowledge and are less likely to have stigma towards HIV/AIDS, thus enabling them to easily change risky sexual behavior. Additionally, individuals with higher education might be able to seek and accept information that would help protect their partners and themselves from HIV and STI transmission and re-infection. This finding is in line with the Ethiopian family planning guideline report which declared that women education increases FP use, improves communication with partner, and advance women's status in the community [16].

Younger age was associated with increased contraceptive use, though the desire for future children is high in this age group. This finding is in line with study done in Mbarara, Uganda and Zambia, Lusaka [20, 22]. House wives were less likely to utilize modern contraceptive as compared to government employees in this study. Similar findings were found from a study done in Southern Nation Nationalities and People's Region, Mexico, and Ghana [36]. This might be due to the effect of husband's reproductive health decision making power that could overwhelm the effect of women's financial and domestic decision making autonomy on couple's family planning use. On the other hand, a significant proportion of the respondents (46%) reported that they wished to have a desire for children which is in line with a study done in Addis Ababa (44.7%) [26].

5. Limitations of the Study

(i) First, the cross-sectional study design makes it difficult to determine the direction of causality.

(ii) Second, there is a risk of social desirability bias whereby HIV positive women may over-report their contraceptive use because of pressure from health workers and community members to practice protected sex.

6. Conclusion

Modern contraceptive method heard among the participants in this study population is high; however, modern contraceptive utilization was still low. Dual method use was about 60%. Use of certain long-term contraceptive methods available in the hospitals, such as implants and IUDs, was low.

Likelihood (chances) of being current user of modern contraceptives by a woman increased with the increase in education level, being daily laborer, being government employee, and ART experience/being on HAART. Old age was associated with reduction in odds (chances) of being current user of modern contraceptives. High number of current family planning users and some others intended future modern contraceptive use. Moreover, a significant proportion of the respondents (46%) reported that they wished to have a desire for children.

(i) As countries plan improvement strategies to enhance contraception uptake among HIV infected reproductive age women, additional efforts are needed to promote modern contraceptive utilization in general and dual method use in particular.

(ii) Investing in women education better to be strengthened.

(iii) Regional health bureau should consider resource mobilization and address issues of demand together with stakeholders for promoting and strengthening the FP and other reproductive health issues.

(iv) Health care providers who are assigned in ART clinics should consider implications for preventing vertical and heterosexual transmission of HIV, the need for appropriate counseling for contraceptives, and the importance of HARRT use.

(v) Hospital managers and clinical officers need to consider integration of family planning with ART services.

(vi) Further exploration (magnitude of unwanted pregnancy) among HIV positive reproductive age women is recommended.

References

[1] World Health Organization, *Sexual and Reproductive Health of Women Living with HIV/AIDS*, 2006.

[2] Ethiopia MOH, Single point HIV prevalence estimate, Tigray, 2007.

[3] IMAP, *Statement on Dual Protection Against Unwanted Pregnancy and Sexual Transmitted Infections Including HIV*, IPPF International Medical Advisory Panel, 2000.

[4] *Strategic Approaches To the Prevention of HIV Infection in Infants*, World Health Organization (WHO), Morges, Switzerland, 2002.

[5] S. A. Cohen, "the role of contraception in preventing HIV, Hiding in plain sight," *Guttmacher Policy Review*, vol. 11, no. 1, pp. 2–5, 2008.

[6] USAID Issue Brief. Adding family planning to PMTCT sites increases the benefits of PMTCT, 2003.

[7] M. D. Sweat, K. R. O'Reilly, G. P. Schmid, J. Denison, and I. De Zoysa, "Cost-effectiveness of nevirapine to prevent mother-to-child HIV transmission in eight African countries," *AIDS*, vol. 18, no. 12, pp. 1661–1671, 2004.

[8] United Nations, "Millennium development goals," http://www.un.org/millenniumgoals/.

[9] World Health Organization, *Trends in Maternal Mortality: 1990 to 2008*, World Health Organization, Geneva, Switzerland, 2010.

[10] Guttmacher Institute, *Facts on Investing in Family Planning and Maternal and Child Heath*, Guttmacher Institute, New York, NY, USA, 2010.

[11] D. Hubacher, I. Mavranezouli, and E. McGinn, "Unintended pregnancy in sub-Saharan Africa: magnitude of the problem and potential role of contraceptive implants to alleviate it," *Contraception*, vol. 78, no. 1, pp. 73–78, 2008.

[12] World Health Organization, *PMTCT Strategic Vision 2010–2012*, World Health Organization, Geneva, Switzerland, 2010.

[13] *Trends in Demographic and Reproductive Health Indicators in Ethiopia*, Macro International, Calverton, Md, USA, 2007.

[14] "Back ground of Tigray region," 2012, http://en.wikipedia.org/wiki/TigrayRegion.

[15] C. J. Carla, M. S. Li, C. K. Matoba et al., "Modern contraceptive and dual method use among HIV infected women in Lusaka, Zambia," *Infectious Diseases in Obstetrics and Gynecology*, vol. 2011, Article ID 261453, 8 pages, 2011.

[16] EDHS Preliminary Report Central Statistical Agency, MEASURE DHS, ICF Macro, Addis Ababa, Ethiopia, 2011.

[17] *National Guideline For Family Planning Services in Ethiopia*, Ministry of Health, 2011.

[18] Z. Girum, *Unmet Reproductive Health Care Needs and Occurrence of Unintended Pregnancy among HIV Positive Women in Antiretroviral Treatment Units in Addis Ababa*, 2011.

[19] E. B. Delvaux, "Pregnancy desires and contraceptive knowledge and use among PMTCT," *International Center For AIDS Care and Treatment Programs*, vol. 23, no. 1, pp. 19–26, 2009.

[20] I. F. Hoffman, F. E. A. Martinson, K. A. Powers et al., "The year-long effect of HIV-positive test results on pregnancy intentions, contraceptive use, and pregnancy incidence among Malawian women," *Journal of Acquired Immune Deficiency Syndromes*, vol. 47, no. 4, pp. 477–483, 2008.

[21] T. Largesse, *Assessment of Fertility Desire and Family Planning Utilization Among HIV Positive People Who Are on Antiretroviral Treatment, Grey Literature*, 2011.

[22] I. Andia, A. Kaida, M. Maier et al., "Highly active antiretroviral therapy and increased use of contraceptives among HIV-positive women during expanding access to antiretroviral therapy in Mbarara, Uganda," *The American Journal of Public Health*, vol. 99, no. 2, pp. 340–347, 2009.

[23] T. Adair, "Unmet need for contraception among HIV-positive women in Lesotho and implications for mother-to-child transmission," *Journal of Biosocial Science*, vol. 41, no. 2, pp. 269–278, 2009.

[24] A. Kaida, F. Laher, S. A. Strathdee et al., "Contraceptive use and method preference among women in Soweto, South Africa: the influence of expanding access to HIV care and treatment services," *PLoS ONE*, vol. 5, no. 11, Article ID e13868, 2010.

[25] Central Statistical Agency, Ethiopia and ORC Macro, *Ethiopia Demographic and Health Survey (EDHS) 2005*, Central Statistical Agency, Calverton, Maryland, USA; ORC Macro, Addis Ababa, Ethiopia, 2006.

[26] T. Wesenyelesh, *Fertility Desire and Family Planning Demand Among HIV Positive Men and women in Follow Up Care, Grey Literature*, 2011.

[27] L. Tesfaye, M. Admassu, A. Getachew, and H. R. Sharma, "Fertility desires and family planning demand among HIV-positive clients in follow-up care at antiretroviral treatment unit in Gondar university hospital, Ethiopia," *Vulnerable Children and Youth Studies*, vol. 7, no. 1, pp. 20–35, 2012.

[28] A. Sarna, S. Luchters, K. Shikely et al., "Fertility preferences and family planning experiences among ART clients in Mombasa, Kenya," in *Linking Reproductive Health, Family Planning, and HIV/AIDS in Africa*, Addis Ababa, Ethiopia, October 2006.

[29] L. Myer, R. J. Carter, M. Katyal, P. Toro, W. M. El-Sadr, and E. J. Abrams, "Impact of antiretroviral therapy on incidence of pregnancy among HIV-infected women in Sub-Saharan Africa: a cohort study," *PLoS Medicine*, vol. 7, no. 2, Article ID e1000229, 2010.

[30] L. Myer, C. Morroni, and K. Rebe, "Prevalence and determinants of fertility intentions of HIV-infected women and men receiving antiretroviral therapy in South Africa," *AIDS Patient Care and STD'S*, vol. 21, no. 4, pp. 278–285, 2007.

[31] A. Sarna, S. M. F. Luchters, S. Geibel et al., "Sexual risk behaviour and HAART: a comparative study of HIV-infected persons on HAART and on preventive therapy in Kenya," *International Journal of STD and AIDS*, vol. 19, no. 2, pp. 85–89, 2008.

[32] N. M. Ncube, J. Akunna, F. Babatunde et al., "Sexual risk behavior among HIV-positive persons in Kumasi, Ghana," *Ghana Medical Journal*, vol. 46, no. 1, pp. 27–33, 2012.

[33] S. Dabral and S. L. Malik, "Demographic study of Gujjars of Delhi: IV, Kap of family planning," *Journal of Human Ecology*, vol. 16, no. 4, pp. 231–237, 2004.

[34] G. Bizuneh, S. Solomon, and M. Yilma, "Unmet need and evaluation of program options to meet unmet need for contraception in Ethiopia: further analysis of the 2000 and 2005," Ethiopia Demographic and Health Survey, 2008, http://www.measuredhs.com/pubs/pdf/FA62/FA62.pdf.

[35] R. K. Wanyenze, N. M. Tumwesigye, R. Kindyomunda et al., "Uptake of family planning methods and unplanned pregnancies among HIV-infected individuals: a cross-sectional survey among clients at HIV clinics in Uganda," *Journal of the International AIDS Society*, vol. 14, no. 1, article 35, 2011.

[36] C. B. Polis, R. H. Gray, T. Lutalo et al., "Trends and correlates of hormonal contraceptive use among HIV-infected women in Rakai, Uganda, 1994–2006," *Contraception*, vol. 83, no. 6, pp. 549–555, 2011.

15

Nonadherence Factors and Sociodemographic Characteristics of HIV-Infected Adults Receiving Antiretroviral Therapy in Nnamdi Azikiwe University Teaching Hospital, Nnewi, Nigeria

Ijeoma Okoronkwo,[1] Uchenna Okeke,[1,2] Anthonia Chinweuba,[1] and Peace Iheanacho[1]

[1] *Department of Nursing Sciences, University of Nigeria, Enugu Campus, Enugu, Nigeria*
[2] *Nursing Services Department, Nnamdi Azikiwe University Teaching Hospital, Nnewi, Nigeria*

Correspondence should be addressed to Ijeoma Okoronkwo; ijeoma.okoronkwo@unn.edu.ng

Academic Editors: Z. Banki, X. Burbano, and A. Corbett

Adherence to treatment instructions with antiretroviral therapy (ART) is very crucial for successful treatment outcome. However, sticking to treatment instructions pose-great challenges to HIV/AIDS patients. This cross-sectional study was on HIV infected adults attending ART clinic in Nigeria to explore nonadherence factors in relation to their socioeconomic characteristics. Validated structured questionnaire was administered to 221 participants. Results showed a high nonadherence rate of 85.1%. The commonest occurring factors of non-adherence were forgetfulness (53.8%), busy schedule (38.8%), side effects of drugs (31.9%), and stigma (31.9%). Males were more likely to complain from busy schedule, feeling healthy, fear of partner disclosure, long waiting period, and long term regimen. Patients with no formal education were more likely to attribute non-adherence to poor communication, side effects of drugs, and stigma. Employed patients seemed to miss their drugs more than the unemployed and artisans. The high non-adherence rate has serious implications for the control of HIV in infected individuals and management of HIV in general. Nurses should intensify efforts on patient education and counseling.

1. Introduction

HIV/AIDS is one of the major public-health problems worldwide, affecting mostly people who are at the most productive stage of life. Out of the estimated 34 million people living with HIV/AIDS globally as at the end of 2010, 68% reside in Sub-Saharan Africa [1]. Nigeria has an HIV prevalence of 4.1% and currently an estimated 3.6 million people are living with HIV/AIDS [2] which puts Nigeria as the second country with the largest number of people living with HIV (PLWH) after South Africa.

The development and availability of antiretroviral therapy (ART) became a turning point in the control and prevention of the epidemic. With the success of ART in improving the quality of life of PLWH and reducing morbidity and mortality, HIV has become a chronic manageable disease [3]. Studies have shown a correlation between higher levels of adherence and improved virological and clinical outcomes [4, 5]. However, ensuring that PLWH receive, and adheres to their highly active ART poses a challenge to the treatment efficacy [6].

In Nigeria ART was commenced (i.e., combining at least 3 drugs from various classes of ART into a cocktail that produces a dramatic reduction in viral load and allows immune suppression) in 2002 and coverage stood at 359,181 in 2010 [2]. Adherence to ART according to Carter [7] refers to timely intake of the right dose of prescribed pills through the right route while observing dietary restrictions. Some available methods for measuring adherence have been reported to include self-reports (through interviews, surveys, and diaries), pill counts, clinical assessments, prescription refills, and directly observed therapy (DOT) [8, 9]. Getting clients to take drugs daily is one of the greatest challenges for effective ART as missing few doses can lead to drug resistance. World Health Organization [10] observes that patients with long term illness have problems with adhering to treatment instructions. It therefore becomes pertinent that treatment instructions are strictly adhered to in order to optimize ART effectiveness.

In Nigeria, there are designated health facilities that run daily retroviral clinics as well as provide free ART. This study was conducted in one of such facilities where PLWH are treated principally with two groups of drugs classified as "first line" and "second line". The first line, which is the focus of this study, is presented as "combipak" containing three drugs—Zidovudine + Lamivudine + Nevirapine. The combination is administered one tablet each, twice daily. Patients are followed up on monthly appointments. In line with WHO's [11] revised ART guideline for resource constrained settings, highly active antiretroviral therapy is initiated on all patients with CD4 + T cell count below 350 cells/μL, regardless of symptom. On each appointment, CD4 + T cell count is repeated and adherence to drug is ascertained by pill count of the previous supply. Effort is made through counseling to retain each client on the first line drugs due to their benefits because the second line drugs have more side effects. Various health care providers—including clinical psychologists—are involved in client counseling to encourage adherence.

However, it is often observed that some of these patients still fail to adhere to their treatment regimen. These patients return to the clinic for followup looking very ill with their drugs supply unexhausted. Various authors have observed that many PLWH do not adhere strictly to their treatment regimen [8, 9, 12], which according to Carter [7] might involve missing a drug in a combined therapy or a dose of the combined therapy, improper medication timing, and/or not taking the correct dose of any of the drugs.

Various factors have been identified as posing challenges to adherence such as forgetfulness, side effects of the drugs, illiteracy, and stigmatization [12–14]. In addition, Agu et al. [15] and Bello [16] identified high pill burden, ART-associated and travel costs, being female, single, high educational status, lack of knowledge, negative perception towards ART medication, and nonavailability of drugs at treatment site as other possible factors. There is paucity of research on how these factors become manifested on a population with diverse sociodemographic characteristics. This study investigated factors affecting non-adherence to ART among adult HIV-infected patients attending the ARV clinic of a hospital in southeast Nigeria and related these to their sociodemographic characteristics.

2. Methods

2.1. Research Design and Study Participants. A cross-sectional descriptive survey was conducted at the adult retroviral clinic of the Nnamdi Azikiwe University Teaching Hospital, Nnewi, southeast Nigeria. This centre is one of the designated free HIV retroviral outpatient clinics in the country. Two hundred and twenty-one adult HIV-infected patients were consecutively recruited into the study based on the inclusion criteria of: adult patients willing to participate and those who have been on ART for at least 3 months. Each patient that attended the ART outpatient clinic and who met the inclusion criteria was approached by one of the researchers; the purpose of the study, his/her role in the study, and the implication of his/her involvement were explained before a signed consent to participate was obtained.

The minimum sample size of 221 was determined using the statistical formula of Fisher for calculating sample size: $Nf = N/1 + (N)/(n)$, where $N = Z^2 pq/d^2$ and n = estimated study population [17]. Average monthly attendance of HIV-infected adults from hospital records was 1,680.

2.2. Data Collection. The instrument used for this study was ART non-adherence and socio-demographic characteristics questionnaire (ARTNa-SDCQ) developed by the researchers based on the literature review. The questionnaire contained two sections. Section A was on sociodemographic data of respondents; section B contained four close-ended questions on: the duration of time a patient had been taking drugs; whether; ever missed drugs; how often drugs were missed and reasons for non-adherence (for those who admitted ever missing drugs, with eighteen possible options). Adherence was defined in this study as having taken at least 95% of the total prescribed pills at the prescribed dosing intervals as recommended by WHO [10]. This was determined by left-over pill count and self-report. Respondents were required to select as many options as they felt were contributory to not taking their drugs as prescribed. The factors were grouped as client, institutional, and medication related.

The reliability of the instrument was established by pilot testing it in an outstation ART clinic similar in characteristics to the study population. Twenty adult HIV-infected patients attending the ART clinic who met the study inclusion criteria were used. Data obtained were subjected to Cronbach's alpha test. An alpha of 0.72 and a standardized item (inter item) coefficient of 0.85 were obtained.

2.3. Ethical Considerations. The study was approved by the Research Ethical Committee of Nnamdi Azikiwe University Teaching Hospital, Nnewi, where the study was to be conducted. Permission was obtained from the management of the ARV clinic. Subsequently, each prospective respondent was approached by any of the researchers and the purpose and demands of the study were explained. They were informed that participation was voluntary and were assured of anonymity and confidentiality of information before informed consent was obtained.

Copies of the questionnaire were administered directly to the consenting patients and left-over pills were counted by the researcher to corroborate patient's response. Any patient with more than 5% left over (i.e., more than 3 pills) of each drug was considered nonadhering. Data were collected on each clinic day before the routine clinic activities commenced. This was to reduce patients' distractions in form of going for CD4 count check and other laboratory investigations. The researchers assisted those who needed help to complete the questionnaire. Data collection continued on subsequent

Table 1: Factors of nonadherence and relationship with respondents' sex.

Reasons for nonadherence	n (%)	Female $n = 126$ (67%)	Male $n = 62$ (33%)
Personal factors			
Forgetfulness	101 (66)	68 (54.0)	33 (53.2)
Busy schedule	73 (47.7)	47 (37.3)	26 (41.9)
Feeling healthy	30 (16.0)	20 (15.9)	10 (16.1)
Ignorance of consequences	33 (21.6)	19 (15.1)	14 (22.6)
Poverty	12 (6.4)	7 (5.6)	5 (8.1)
Do not feel like taking drugs	38 (24.8)	25 (19.8)	13 (21.0)
No confidence in the treatment	17 (9.0)	9 (7.1)	8 (12.9)
Fear of partner disclosure	29 (15.4)	16 (12.7)	13 (21.0)
Provider/institutional factors			
Poor communication	63 (41.2)	49 (38.9)	14 (22.6)
Judgmental attitude of provider	20 (13.1)	11 (8.7)	9 (14.5)
Lack of trust and confidentiality	42 (27.5)	25 (19.8)	17 (27.4)
Long waiting period	38 (24.8)	20 (15.9)	18 (29.0)
Unavailability of drugs	13 (6.9)	6 (4.8)	7 (11.3)
Drug related factors			
Side effects of drugs	60 (39.2)	48 (38.1)	12 (19.4)
Stigma	60 (17.7)	38 (30.2)	22 (35.5)
Frequency of taking drugs	27 (39.2)	14 (11.1)	13 (21.0)
Long term regimen	41 (26.8)	23 (18.3)	18 (29.0)
Quantity of drugs to be taken	16 (8.5)	9 (7.1)	7 (11.3)
Mean ± SEM of sex		25.22 ± 4.16	14.39 ± 1.69
Unpaired t-test result			
t_{cal}		2.414	
Df		34	
95% confidence interval		1.708 to 19.96	
P value		0.0213*	
Are means significantly different? ($P < 0.05$)		Yes	

Note. Percentage was calculated based on proportion of nonadherent groups.
*The scores are statistically significantly different ($P < 0.05$).

clinic days until the sample size was reached and this lasted for one month.

2.4. Data Analysis. Data collected on demographic characteristics and adherence to drugs were analyzed descriptively. Responses to factors responsible for non-adherence were categorized into three groups: client, institutional, and medication related factors. The relationship between respondents' demographic characteristic, and their reasons for non-adherence to drugs were analyzed inferentially using GraphPad Prism 5.20 statistical package. t-test for unpaired data was used to analyze the relationship between respondents' adherence to ART and their demographic characteristics of sex and marital status, while analysis of variance (ANOVA) was employed to establish the relationship with their age, educational qualification, and employment status at $P \leq 0.05$.

3. Results

3.1. Sociodemographic Characteristics. Of the 221 respondents, 188 (85.1%) indicated that they missed taking their drugs as prescribed in the preceding month while only 33 (14.9%) claimed they had never missed. Of the 188 patients that admitted non-adherence, 86 (45.7%) have been on ART for less than one year and 72 (38.3%) were on drugs between one year and 2.5 years, while the remaining 30 (16.0%) maintained the intake beyond 2.5 years and up to 5 years.

3.2. Factors of Nonadherence and Relationship with Respondents' Sex. Out of the 188 patients on ART who indicated they had missed taking their drugs as prescribed in the preceding month, 126 (67.0%) were females while 62 (33.0%) were males (see Table 1). The majority of 101 (53.7%) of the respondents, identified forgetfulness as a factor of non-adherence, the rate of which was almost the same for both sexes (females = 54%, and males = 53.2%). There was significant difference in the means of responses on the non-adherence factors identified by male and female patients on ART. At 95% CI and df = 34, the unpaired t_{cal} was 2.414 and $P = 0.0213$. The mean ± SEM of gender in relation to the factors was 25.22 ± 4.16 for the females and 14.39 ± 1.69 for the males. Except for forgetfulness, poor communication and side effects of drugs

Table 2: Factors of nonadherence and relationship with respondents' age.

Reasons for nonadherence	n (%)	20–29 $n = 59$ (31.4%)	30–39 $n = 74$ (36.4%)	40–49 $n = 55$ (29.2%)
Personal factors				
Forgetfulness	101 (53.7)	27 (45.8)	42 (56.8)	32 (58.2)
Busy schedule	73 (38.8)	16 (27.1)	28 (37.8)	29 (52.7)
Feeling healthy	30 (15.9)	1 (1.6)	15 (20.3)	14 (25.4)
Ignorance of consequences	33 (17.5)	14 (23.7)	13 (17.6)	6 (10.9)
Poverty	12 (6.4)	4 (6.8)	6 (8.1)	2 (3.6)
Do not feel like taking drugs	38 (20.2)	20 (33.9)	16 (21.6)	2 (3.6)
No confidence in the treatment	17 (9.0)	4 (23.7)	9 (12.2)	4 (7.2)
Fear of partner disclosure	29 (15.4)	7 (11.9)	18 (24.3)	4 (7.2)
Provider/institutional factors				
Poor communication	63 (33.5)	22 (37.3)	24 (38.1)	17 (30.9)
Judgmental attitude of provider	20 (10.6)	8 (13.6)	8 (32.4)	4 (7.2)
Lack of trust and confidentiality	42 (22.3)	14 (23.7)	20 (27.0)	8 (14.5)
Long waiting period	38 (20.2)	15 (25.4)	17 (44.7)	6 (10.9)
Unavailability of drugs	13 (6.9)	4 (6.8)	5 (23.0)	4 (7.2)
Drug related factors				
Side effects of drugs	60 (31.9)	18 (30.5)	21 (28.4)	21 (38.2)
Stigma	60 (31.9)	20 (33.9)	23 (31.1)	17 (30.9)
Frequency of taking drugs	27 (14.36)	14 (23.7)	10 (13.5)	3 (5.4)
Long term regimen	41 (21.8)	19 (32.2)	15 (20.3)	7 (12.7)
Quantity of drugs to be taken	16 (8.5)	9 (15.2)	6 (8.1)	1 (1.8)
ANOVA summary result				
F		2.440		
Df		2		
P value		0.0973		
Are means significantly different? ($P < 0.05$)		No		

were identified by higher percentages of females than the males; more males than females identified the rest of the items.

3.3. Factors of Nonadherence and Relationship with Respondents' Age. There was no definite pattern in the responses based on age (see Table 2). However, forgetfulness (58.2%) and busy schedule (52.7%) were most frequent among respondents aged 40–49 years. Respondents aged 30–39 were nonadherent due to institutional factors of long waiting periods (44.7%) and poor communication (38.1%). Respondents aged 20–29 years (33.9%) were the highest in non-adherence because they simply "do not feel like taking drugs" and are "ignorant of the consequences" (23.7%). ANOVA results with df = 53 showed no significant difference in non-adherence factors among the groups ($F = 2.440$ and $P = 0.0973$).

3.4. Factors of Nonadherence and Relationship with Respondents' Marital Status. One hundred and seven (56.9%) of the respondents were married, while the remaining 81 (43.1%) were single (never married, divorced, or widowed). Many of the items had close responses from the groups (see Table 3). However, respondents who were single 31 (38.3%) were more nonadhering due to poor communication by care providers than the married patients 32 (29.9%). Similarly, the single respondents did not adhere to the ART regimen due to stigma 35 (43.2%) and long-term regimen of drug intake 25 (30.9%). Mean ± SEM of the reported non-adherence factors for both groups were similar (single = 19.00 ± 2.69; married = 20.61 ± 3.071). Unpaired t-test of the data at 95% CI and df = 34 showed t_{cal} as 0.3948 and $P = 0.6955$. Overall, there was no significant difference in non-adherence factors identified by the married and single adult HIV-infected patients on ART.

3.5. Factors of Nonadherence and Relationship with Respondents' Educational Status. The majority of the respondents had some formal education. Seventy-seven, 52, and 28 had secondary, higher and primary education, respectively, while 31 had none (see Table 4). All categories of the respondents attributed their non-adherence to forgetfulness. In addition, those that had higher education (55.8%) and those with no formal education (51.6%) identified busy schedule. Also, those with no formal education failed to adhere to their ART due to poor communication (61.3%), side effects of drugs (58.1%), stigma (54.8%), and lack of trust and confidentiality (38.7%). Results of ANOVA at df = 71 showed a significant difference in non-adherence factors and respondents' educational status ($F = 4.839$ and $P = 0.0041$).

TABLE 3: Factors of nonadherence and relationship with respondents' marital status.

Reasons for nonadherence	n (%)	Single $n = 81$ (43.1%)	Married $n = 107$ (56.9%)
Personal factors			
Forgetfulness	101 (53.7)	43 (51.9)	58 (54.2)
Busy schedule	73 (38.8)	32 (39.5)	41 (38.3)
Feeling healthy	30 (15.9)	14 (17.3)	16 (15.0)
Ignorance of consequences	33 (17.5)	17 (21.0)	16 (15.0)
Poverty	12 (6.4)	5 (6.2)	7 (6.5)
Do not feel like taking drugs	38 (20.2)	17 (21.0)	21 (19.6)
No confidence in the treatment	17 (9.0)	7 (8.6)	10 (9.4)
Fear of partner disclosure	29 (15.4)	10 (12.4)	19 (17.8)
Provider/institutional factors			
Poor communication	63 (33.5)	31 (38.3)	32 (29.9)
Judgmental attitude of provider	20 (10.6)	10 (12.4)	10 (9.4)
Lack of trust and confidentiality	42 (22.3)	19 (23.5)	23 (21.5)
Long waiting period	38 (20.2)	20 (24.7)	18 (16.8)
Unavailability of drugs	13 (6.9)	6 (7.4)	7 (6.5)
Drug related factors			
Side effects of drugs	60 (31.9)	31 (38.3)	29 (27.1)
Stigma	60 (31.9)	35 (43.2)	25 (23.4)
Frequency of taking drugs	27 (14.36)	13 (16.1)	14 (13.1)
Long term regimen	41 (21.8)	25 (30.9)	16 (15.0)
Quantity of drugs to be taken	16 (8.5)	7 (8.6)	9 (8.4)
Mean ± SEM of marital status		19.00 ± 2.69	20.61 ± 3.07
Unpaired t-test result			
t_{cal}		0.3948	
Df		34	
95% confidence interval		−9.910 to 6.688	
P value		0.6955	
Are means significantly different? ($P < 0.05$)		No	

3.6. Factors of Nonadherence and Relationship with Respondents' Employment Status. Employed respondents 92 (48.9%) were more likely to miss their drugs when compared with the artisans 95 (29.3%) and unemployed groups 41 (21.8%). Table 5 shows that employed respondents identified, among others, forgetfulness 49 (53.3%), busy schedule 42 (45.6%), and side effects of drugs 38 (41.3%) as their factors of nonadherence. Artisans and the unemployed had lower scores for most of the items. Analysis of variance (ANOVA) of the data showed a significant difference in non-adherence factors and respondents employment status (df = 53; F = 9.525; $P = 0.0003$).

4. Discussion

The rate of nonadherence to antiretroviral drugs among patients receiving ART in Nnamdi Azikiwe University Teaching Hospital, Nnewi, as shown in this study was rather high as only 14.9% (33) of the subjects indicated that they have never missed their medication. This is particularly significant considering that the method of data collection was self-report. Although previous studies had noted that some PLWH do not adhere strictly to their treatment regimen [8, 9] the rate in the present study was rather much higher than what was reported in similar studies. For instance, Igwegbe et al. [8] had worked in the same locality, though among pregnant women and found about 21.7% being nonadherent. However, the findings of Uzochukwu et al., [12] which reported a non-adherence rate of 75%, were closer to that of the present study. The consequence of this level of non-adherence is worrisome both for the individual and the entire population because of the virological outcomes. A possible explanation for this finding is the fact that the method used was self-report. According to Uzochukwu et al., [12] a common limitation of this method in assessing adherence is its subjectivity. For example the patient may say what he feels that may help him get the desired attention from his doctor or what he thinks will impress the doctor.

4.1. Socio-Demographic Variables and Factors of Nonadherence. With regard to gender and factors of non-adherence, it was noticed that more males than females were more likely to complain of factors like busy schedule, fear of partner disclosure, long waiting period, ignorance of consequences,

Table 4: Factors of nonadherence and relationship with respondents' educational status.

Reasons for nonadherence	n (%)	No formal $n = 31$ (16.5)	Primary $n = 28$ (14.9)	Secondary $n = 77$ (41.0)	Higher $n = 52$ (27.6)
Personal factors		20 (64.5)	15 (53.6)	36 (46.7)	30 (57.7)
Forgetfulness	101 (53.7)				
Busy schedule	73 (38.8)	16 (51.6)	10 (35.1)	18 (23.4)	29 (55.8)
Feeling healthy	30 (15.9)	6 (19.3)	4 (14.3)	12 (15.6)	8 (15.4)
Ignorance of consequences	33 (17.5)	7 (22.6)	5 (17.9)	17 (22.1)	4 (7.7)
Poverty	12 (6.4)	3 (9.7)	2 (7.1)	4 (5.2)	3 (5.8)
Do not feel like taking drugs	38 (20.2)	8 (25.8)	6 (21.4)	15 (19.5)	9 (17.3)
No confidence in the treatment	17 (9.0)	4 (12.9)	3 (10.7)	6 (7.8)	4 (7.7)
Fear of partner disclosure	29 (15.4)	6 (19.3)	4 (14.3)	13 (16.9)	6 (11.5)
Provider/institutional factors					
Poor communication	63 (33.5)	19 (61.3)	5 (17.9)	20 (26.0)	19 (36.5)
Judgmental attitude of provider	20 (10.6)	4 (12.9)	2 (7.1)	7 (9.1)	7 (13.5)
Lack of trust and confidentiality	42 (22.3)	12 (38.7)	7 (25.0)	12 (15.6)	11 (21.1)
Long waiting period	38 (20.2)	6 (19.3)	7 (25.0)	14 (18.2)	11 (21.1)
Unavailability of drugs	13 (6.9)	3 (9.7)	2 (7.1)	5 (6.5)	3 (5.8)
Drug related factors					
Side effects of drugs	60 (31.9)	18 (58.1)	4 (14.3)	16 (20.8)	22 (42.3)
Stigma	60 (31.9)	17 (54.8)	9 (32.1)	18 (23.4)	16 (30.8)
Frequency of taking drugs	27 (14.36)	5 (16.1)	2 (7.1)	10 (13.0)	10 (19.2)
Long term regimen	41 (21.8)	8 (25.8)	8 (28.6)	15 (19.5)	10 (19.2)
Quantity of drugs to be taken	16 (8.5)	4 (12.9)	3 (10.7)	5 (6.5)	4 (7.7)
ANOVA summary result					
F		4.839			
Df		3			
P value		0.0041**			

**The scores are statistically significantly different ($P < 0.05$).

long term regimen, and stigma. However, more females than males seemed to be non-adherent due to forgetfulness, poor communication, and side effects of drugs. These findings are not quite in agreement with those of Wasti et al., [14] where women were generally found to be more nonadherent than men. Busy schedule and forgetfulness will likely work together to affect non-adherence. Ignorance of consequences of non-compliance is a high risk for non-adherence. Good communication promotes access to care and adherence to ART. With effective communication, patients must be made aware that ART is a lifelong treatment [9]. This suggests the need for adequate client communication and assessment of understanding. Health care providers need to spend sufficient time in adherence counseling at every visit.

Concerning the relationship between non-adherence factors and age, the 40–49 years age group was the most nonadherent due to forgetfulness. Social responsibilities tend to increase with age and this may probably have been the case with this e eldest group in this study. Patients aged 20–29 years were most frequently nonadherent because they did not feel like taking drugs. The findings also interestingly showed that the same group reported ignorance of the consequences of their non-adherence more than the other two groups. However, statistical analysis did not show any significant variation in the factors of non-adherence as a result of age.

There was also no significant difference in non-adherence factors between the married and the single respondents. This finding is not consistent with that of Agu et al. [15] and Bello [16]. Nevertheless single patients seemed to be more non-adhering due to poor communication by care providers than the married. Similarly, they were also likely to be more nonadhering due to stigma and long term regimen. This finding could be explained by the extent of social support the patient has. Married clients, especially those whose spouses are either seropositive or are aware of their HIV status, are likely to have people who support and encourage them and this can enhance adherence on the long term as well as reduce stigma.

Educational status had a significant influence on some of the factors associated with non-adherence although no definite pattern was shown. Forgetfulness was common to all the categories. However, those with higher education

TABLE 5: Factors of nonadherence and relationship with respondents' employment status.

Reasons for nonadherence	n (%)	Employed $n = 92$ (48.9)	Unemployed $n = 41$ (21.8)	Artisan $n = 55$ (29.3)
Personal factors				
Forgetfulness	101 (53.7)	49 (53.3)	23 (56.1)	29 (52.7)
Busy schedule	73 (38.8)	42 (45.6)	14 (34.1)	17 (30.9)
Feeling healthy	30 (15.9)	13 (14.1)	8 (19.5)	9 (16.4)
Ignorance of consequences	33 (17.5)	18 (19.6)	6 (14.6)	9 (16.4)
Poverty	12 (6.4)	7 (7.6)	3 (7.3)	2 (3.6)
Do not feel like taking drugs	38 (20.2)	17 (18.5)	10 (24.4)	11 (20.0)
No confidence in the treatment	17 (9.0)	10 (10.9)	4 (9.8)	3 (5.4)
Fear of partner disclosure	29 (15.4)	13 (14.1)	9 (21.9)	7 (12.7)
Provider/institutional factors				
Poor communication	63 (33.5)	31 (33.7)	22 (53.7)	10 (18.2)
Judgmental attitude of provider	20 (10.6)	9 (9.8)	6 (14.6)	5 (9.1)
Lack of trust and confidentiality	42 (22.3)	23 (25.0)	7 (17.1)	12 (21.8)
Long waiting period	38 (20.2)	17 (18.5)	11 (26.8)	10 (18.2)
Unavailability of drugs	13 (6.9)	6 (6.5)	4 (9.8)	3 (5.4)
Drug related factors				
Side effects of drugs	60 (31.9)	38 (41.3)	13 (21.7)	9 (16.4)
Stigma	60 (31.9)	31 (33.7)	14 (34.1)	15 (27.3)
Frequency of taking drugs	27 (14.36)	14 (15.2)	7 (17.1)	6 (10.9)
Long term regimen	41 (21.8)	26 (28.3)	4 (9.8)	11 (20.0)
Quantity of drugs to be taken	16 (8.5)	9 (9.8)	4 (9.8)	3 (5.4)
ANOVA summary result				
F		9.525		
Df		2		
P value		0.0003***		

***The scores are statistically significantly different ($P < 0.05$).

were more likely than the other groups to attribute their non-adherence to busy schedule. Patients with no formal education were more likely to attribute non-adherence to poor communication, side effects of drugs, stigma, and lack of trust and confidentiality. Although Agu et al. [15] and Bello [16] had earlier identified higher educational status as a factor of non-adherence, the findings of our study did not show any correlation of educational status with non-adherence. However, education obviously plays a considerable role in understanding and communication of information between parties.

The results further showed that employed patients were more likely to cite forgetfulness, busy schedule, and stigma as reasons for non-adherence than the unemployed and artisans. This finding was statistically significant. The possible explanation is that their jobs kept them busy making them forget their drugs. Also the fact of working in an employed job may heighten their fear of stigma since they spend a good chunk of their time in the company of other people in their places of work; this may contribute to their forgetfulness. Stigma will not make them bring out their drugs in the office. Fear of stigma in the place of work may also be due to fear of losing their jobs if their HIV statuses are known.

On the basis of the foregoing, in-depth one-on-one counseling will most likely help clients to resiliently withstand sigma, accept their condition, and adapt more positively to the challenges of the illness and prolonged drug use. Again, follow-up of patients on ART will most likely help to reduce factors of non adherence like forgetfulness, ignorance, and lack of confidence in treatment.

5. Conclusion

Non-adherence was found to be high among the respondents in this study and several factors were cited as reasons. More information, education, and communication campaigns targeted at the general public are required to eliminate or reduce stigma to the barest minimum. This will help to improve adherence for those who might have the need to take their medications outside their homes, such as those in paid employments. Policies should be made and rules should be enforced to protect the rights of PLWH in the work place as well as prevent any form of discrimination against them. Health care providers need to spend sufficient time in adherence counseling at every visit emphasizing eating before drugs intake to minimize side effects. Strategies to automatically remind patients at due medication times such as setting alarms will be invaluable to reduce forgetfulness. Further studies are required to determine particular drugs which clients find most problematic.

Conflict of Interests

All the authors declare that they have no conflict of interests with the publication of this paper.

Acknowledgments

The authors acknowledge the management of Nnamdi Azikiwe University Teaching Hospital, Nnewi, for giving them the ethical approval to conduct this research. They are also grateful to the consultant and nurses in charge of the ARV clinic for their cooperation throughout the period of study. The authors equally appreciate the participants for their willingness to participate in this study.

References

[1] UNAIDS, "Joint United Nations Programme on HIV/AIDS (UNAIDS) World AIDS Day report," 2011.

[2] National Agency for the control of AIDS (NACA), "Update on the HIV/AIDS epidemic response inNigeria," 2011, http://www.naca.gov.ng/index2.php .

[3] O. O. Oguntibeju, "Quality of life of people living with HIV and AIDS and antiretroviral therapy," *HIV/AIDS-Research and Palliative Care*, vol. 4, pp. 117–124, 2012.

[4] P. R. Harrigan, R. S. Hogg, W. W. Y. Dong et al., "Predictors of HIV drug-resistance mutations in a large antiretroviral-naive cohort initiating triple antiretroviral therapy," *Journal of Infectious Diseases*, vol. 191, no. 3, pp. 339–347, 2005.

[5] C. Orrell, D. R. Bangsberg, M. Badri, and R. Wood, "Adherence is not a barrier to successful antiretroviral therapy in South Africa," *AIDS*, vol. 17, no. 9, pp. 1369–1375, 2003.

[6] R. M. Granich, C. F. Gilks, C. Dye, K. M. De Cock, and B. G. Williams, "Universal voluntary HIV testing with immediate antiretroviral therapy as a strategy for elimination of HIV transmission: a mathematical model," *The Lancet*, vol. 373, no. 9657, pp. 48–57, 2009.

[7] M. Carter, "Adherence. Information series for HIV positive people. NAM," 2005, http://www.aidsmap.com/Adherence/cat/1464/.

[8] A. O. Igwegbe, J. O. Ugboaja, and L. A. Nwajiaku, "Prevalence and determination of non adherence to antiretroviral therapy among HIV positive pregnant women in Nnewi, Nigeria," *International Journal of Medicine and Medical Sciences*, vol. 2, no. 8, pp. 238–245, 2010.

[9] A. W. Nyambura, *Factors that influence non-adherence to antiretroviral therapy among HIV/AIDS patients in central province, Kenya [Ph.D. thesis]*, 2009, http://www.who.int/hiv/ .

[10] World Health Organization (WHO), *Adherence to HIV Treatment*, World Health Organization, Geneva, Switzerland, 2004.

[11] World Health Organization (WHO), *Rapid Advice: Antiretroviral Therapy for HIV Infection in Adults and Adolescents*, World Health Organization, Geneva, Switzerland, 2009.

[12] B. S. C. Uzochukwu, O. E. Onwujekwe, A. C. Onoka, C. Okoli, N. P. Uguru, and O. I. Chukwuogo, "Determinants of non-adherence to subsidized anti-retroviral treatment in southeast Nigeria," *Health Policy and Planning*, vol. 24, no. 3, pp. 189–196, 2009.

[13] E. Monjok, A. Smesny, I. B. Okokon, O. Mgbere, and E. J. Essien, "Adherence to antiretroviral therapy in Nigeria: an overview of research studies and implications for policy and practice," *HIV/AIDS*, vol. 2, pp. 69–76, 2010.

[14] S. P. Wasti, P. Simkhada, J. Randall, J. V. Freeman, and E. van Teijlingen, "Factors influencing adherence to antiretroviral treatment in Nepal: a mixed-methods study," *PLoS ONE*, vol. 7, no. 5, Article ID e35547, 2012.

[15] K. A. Agu, O. Okojie, R. G. King et al., "Medication adherence and risk factors for non-adherence among patients taking highlyactive retroviral therapy," *West African Journal of Pharmacy*, vol. 22, no. 1, 2011.

[16] S. I. Bello, "HIV patients'adherence to antiretroviral therapy in Sobi Specialist Hospital, Ilorin, Nigeria," *Journal of Advanced Scientific Research*, vol. 2, no. 3, pp. 52–57, 2011.

[17] M. O. Araoye, *Research Methodology with Statistics for Health and Social Sciences*, Nathadex Publishers, Awka, Nigeria, 2003.

Early Atherosclerosis in HIV Infected Subjects on Suppressive Antiretroviral Treatment: Role of Osteoprotegerin

Alessandra D'Abramo, Claudia D'Agostino, Alessandra Oliva, Marco Iannetta, Gabriella D'Ettorre, Francesco Vullo, Massimo Mancone, Maria Rosa Ciardi, Claudio Maria Mastroianni, and Vincenzo Vullo

Department of Public Health and Infectious Diseases, "Sapienza" University of Rome, Viale del Policlinico 155, 00161 Rome, Italy

Correspondence should be addressed to Alessandra D'Abramo; alessandra.dabramo@libero.it

Academic Editors: H. C. Mwandumba and J. Poudrier

Cardiovascular disease is increased in HIV-infected patients. Cytokines such as osteoprotegerin are implicated in atherosclerosis. The aim of our study was to evaluate the role of osteoprotegerin in the development and progression of atherosclerosis in HIV infected subjects on suppressive antiretroviral treatment. We enrolled 76 patients; 35 HIV infected men on suppressive Highly Active Antiretroviral Therapy with Framingham score <10%; 21 HIV negative individuals matched for age, gender, and Framingham score, and 20 subjects with Framingham score >10% as control groups. HIV positive subjects underwent echocardiography, electrocardiography, and heart multidetector computed tomography, whereas in HIV negative subjects, tomography was only performed in case of any abnormalities either in echocardiography or electrocardiography. In HIV positive patients, computed tomography showed stenosis in 51.4% of the subjects. Osteoprotegerin plasma levels were higher in HIV-infected patients than those in healthy controls but lower than in HIV negative subjects with Framingham score >10%. Higher osteoprotegerin plasma levels were found in HIV positive patients with grade I stenosis than in patients with grade II/III stenosis. In conclusion, in HIV infected subjects with Framingham score <10%, osteoprotegerin plasma concentrations are associated with atherosclerosis, in particular at the early stage of the process.

1. Introduction

Cardiovascular disease (CVD) is an emerging and significant cause of morbidity and mortality in HIV-infected patients [1]. HIV itself and antiretroviral drugs may contribute to the increased risk of CVD. In addition to traditional risk factors (age, smoking, dyslipidemia, and diabetes), chronic viral infection, immune activation, and inflammation play a central role in vascular damage and endothelial dysfunction [2]. Proinflammatory cytokines such as interleukin (IL)-6 and IL-1 are associated with development and progression of atherosclerosis [3–7]; furthermore, new soluble markers including osteoprotegerin (OPG) have been shown to be involved in this process. The OPG/RANK (receptor activator of NF-kappaB)/RANKL (receptor activator of NF-kappaB ligand), member of TNF superfamily, is a key regulatory system in bone remodelling by regulating development and activation of osteoclasts [8–11]. Recent studies showed the implication of the OPG/RANKL system in vascular disease, especially in vascular calcification, atherosclerosis and plaque formation [12–15]. There are few data about the relationship between OPG and cardiovascular disease in HIV infection; thus, the role of OPG is not yet well established. The aim of our study was to evaluate the role of OPG in the development and progression of atherosclerosis in HIV infected subjects on suppressive antiretroviral treatment.

2. Materials and Methods

2.1. Ethics Statement. The study protocol designed according to the Helsinki Declaration II was approved by the local ethics committee. All the patients gave written informed consent to participate.

2.2. Patients. We recruited 76 patients from the Department of Public Health and Infectious Disease and the Department of Cardiovascular, Respiratory, Nephrologic and Geriatric Sciences of "Sapienza" University of Rome (Italy). Thirty-five were HIV-infected men on Highly Active Antiretroviral Therapy (HAART) since 48 weeks with undetectable viremia (<37 copies/mL) and low cardiovascular diseases risk defined by a Framingham score <10%. Subjects with diagnosis of metabolic syndrome (waist circumference: men >102 cm and women >88 cm, triglycerides ≥150 mg/dL, HDL cholesterol: men <40 mg/dL and women <50 mg/dL, blood pressure: ≥130/85 mm Hg or use of medication for hypertension, and fasting glucose ≥100 mg/dL or use of medication for hyperglycemia) were excluded [16]. As control groups we enrolled 21 HIV negative individuals matched for age, gender, and Framingham score and 20 HIV negative additional subjects with Framingham score >10%. For each patient we collected medical and family history, lifestyle, smoking status, antiretroviral therapies, HIV-RNA zenith, and nadir CD4+ cell count. Current lymphocytes T CD4+ and CD8+ cell count were determined by flow cytometric analysis (MACSQuant Analyser Miltenyi Biotec, Germany) and HIV-1 RNA plasma levels were detected by a quantitative reverse polymerase chain reaction (Amplicor HIV monitor; Roche Diagnostic System, Branchburg, NJ version 1.5, l.o.d. 37 copies/mL). Serum glucose; triglycerides; and total cholesterol, high-density lipoprotein cholesterol (HDL), and low-density lipoprotein cholesterol (LDL) were measured in blood samples. Body mass index (BMI) was calculated (kg/m^2) and recorded for each individual. Stress test echocardiography and electrocardiography (ECG) were performed in all patients. Ineligible participants were females, aged <18 years, previous virological failure, recent AIDS-defining illness, coinfected with hepatitis virus, patients with other comorbidities (diabetes mellitus, arterial hypertension, kidney disease, and hormonal dysfunction).

2.3. IL-6 and Osteoprotegerin Detection. IL-6 was measured with an ELISA kit (eBioscience bender MedSystem, Inc Vienna, Austria). The detection limit of assay was 3.1 pg/mL. Osteoprotegerin were measured by ELISA kits (Biomedica Gruppe, Vienna Austria). The detection limit of assay was 0.12 pmol/L.

2.4. Multidetector Computed Tomography (MDTC) and Coronary Angiography (CA). The severity of CVD was evaluated in 35 HIV+ patients using a low-dose prospectively ECG-triggered CT coronary angiography protocol with 64-slice multidetector MDCT scanner (Somatom Definition Siemens medical Solution, Forehheimen, Germany) [17, 18]. MDTC dataset were transferred and analyzed through a dedicated cardiac workstation (Vitrea 2.6, Vital images, USA). For the analysis, the American Heart Association (AHA) coronary arteries segmentation model was adopted and all segments with a diameter ≥1 mm at their origin were included [19, 20]. The degree of luminal stenosis was classified as mild (grade I: 30–49%), moderate (grade II: 50–69%), severe (grade III: 70–99%), or coronary occlusion (grade IV: 100%). A threshold of 50% luminal narrowing in any coronary segment greater than 1.5 mm in diameter was adopted to define clinically significant coronary stenosis. All patients with grade II and III stenosis at MDTC were considered for coronary angiography. This was performed using standard technique with angiograms evaluated by blinded operator to the MDTC results. The decision to perform coronary revascularization was made according to the recently appropriateness criteria [21, 22]. On the other hand, HIV negative subjects underwent MDTC only in case of any abnormalities either in echocardiography or ECG; in the presence of significant stenosis a coronary angiography was set up (Figure 1).

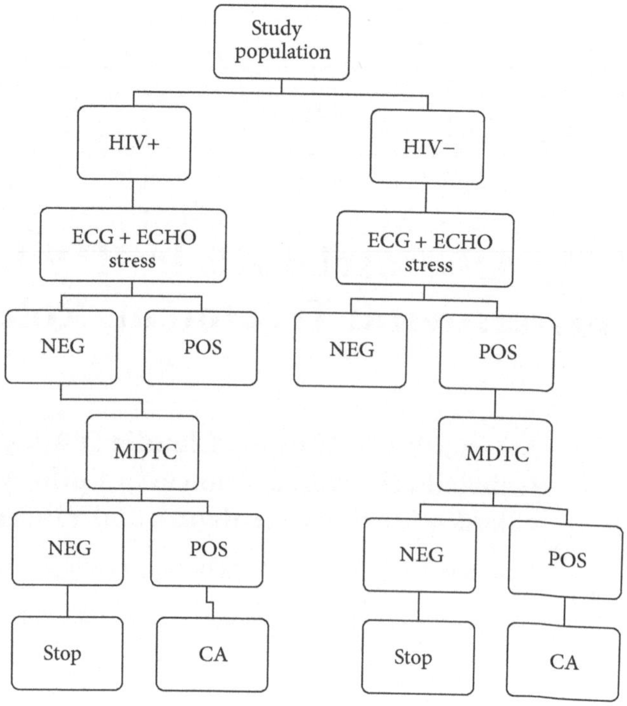

FIGURE 1: Diagnostic flowchart. Picture showing the diagnostic approach to cardiovascular disease.

2.5. Statistical Analysis. Continuous data were analyzed with Student's t test, whereas the nonparametric Mann-Whitney test was applied for values not normally distributed. Pearson correlation coefficient was used for correlations. Linear regression model was tested to evaluate the association between IL-6, OPG, and the grade of stenosis. Data were expressed as median and mean ± standard deviation (SD). A P value of <0.05 was considered statistically significant. Statistical analyses were performed using STATA (version 9) software (STATA Corp. LP, College Station, TX).

3. Results

3.1. Characteristics of the Study Population. General characteristics of the study population are summarized in Table 1. All HIV infected subjects were males with low cardiovascular diseases risk (Framingham score <10%), mean age was 53 ± 8.8 years. 57.1% were not smokers, and BMI mean was

Table 1: Clinical characteristics.

	HIV− (FS < 10%)	HIV+	HIV− (FS > 10%)
Age (M ± SD)	48 ± 9	53 ± 8.8	55 ± 8
Sex	21 M, 0 F	35 M, 0 F	20 M, 0 F
Smoke status (*n*, %)			
no	15 (71%)	20 (57.1%)	6 (30%)
yes	6 (29%)	15 (42.9%)	14 (70%)
CD4+ (mmc) (M ± SD)	770 ± 221	570 ± 341.2	689 ± 197
CD4+ % (M ± SD)	36 ± 9.3	17.3 ± 7.6	33.6 ± 8.7
CD4+ (mmc) nadir (M ± SD)	—	287.7 ± 253.4	—
CD4+ % nadir (M ± SD)	—	12.9 ± 8.7	—
HIV-RNA zenith (cp/mL) (M ± SD)	—	257376.5 ± 346884.8	—
HIV-RNA (cp/mL)	<37	<37	<37
Lipid-lowering therapy			
no	21 (100%)	35 (100%)	12 (60%)
yes	0	0	8 (40%)
Systolic blood pressure (mmHg)	114.8 ± 17.5	117.3 ± 15.5	125.8 ± 18.5
Diastolic blood pressure (mmHg)	81.8 ± 11.4	77.3 ± 12.5	88.3 ± 20.5
Triglycerides (mg/dL) (M ± SD)	113.6 ± 31	178.8 ± 90.2	198.5 ± 82
Cholesterol Total (mg/dL) (M ± SD)	150.3 ± 35.8	200.7 ± 51.7	266.3 ± 48.7
Cholesterol HDL (mg/dL) (M ± SD)	53.2 ± 16.7	41.8 ± 13.6	39.8 ± 12.6
Cholesterol LDL (mg/dL) (M ± SD)	102.5 ± 32.4	133.3 ± 47.2	172.7 ± 42.4
Body mass index (kg/m^2) (M ± SD)	18.7 ± 2.5	20.7 ± 2.4	21.7 ± 2.3
Framingham score	3.2 ± 2.1%	4.1 ± 3.2%	13.4 ± 5.4%

FS: Framingham score; M: mean; SD: standard deviation; HDL: high density lipoprotein; LDL: low density lipoprotein.

20.7 ± 2.4 kg/m^2. Average nadir and current lymphocytes T CD4+ cells count was 287.7 ± 253.45 cell/mmc and 570 ± 341.28 cell/mmc, respectively. The mean plasma concentrations of total cholesterol was 200 ± 51.79 mg/dL, HDL cholesterol was equal to 41.8 ± 13.67 mg/dL, LDL cholesterol was equal to 133.35 ± 47.25 mg/dL, and triglycerides were equal to 178.8 ± 90.22 mg/dL. None of the subjects was receiving lipid-lowering therapy.

3.2. Multidetector Computed Tomography and Coronary Angiography. MDCT examination was successfully and safely performed in all patients. We observed stenosis in 18/35 (51.4%) and no stenosis in 17/35 (48.6%). In patients with stenosis, 5/18 (27.7%) had mild stenosis (i.e., grade I) and 13/18 (72.3%) had grade II stenosis. As expected, no one had grade III stenosis. Among patients with grade II stenosis, 8/13 (61.5%) had 1 vessel and 5/13 (38.5%) 2 vessels coronary disease. All the plaques detected were eccentric and in 10/13 (76.9%) were soft. 13/13 (100%) patients with grade II stenosis at CT underwent CA and 6 (46.1%) underwent a percutaneous coronary intervention with application of 16 drug-eluting stents (Biosensors, Biomatrix DES). Twenty HIV negative subjects with CVD had grade II/III stenosis at MDTC and underwent CA; 8 (40%) underwent a percutaneous coronary intervention with application of 16 drug-eluting stents. Twenty-one HIV negative subjects with Framingham score <10% did not perform MDTC because of the absence of modifications at the echocardiography stress test and ECG.

3.3. Osteoprotegerin and Interleukin-6. Osteoprotegerin (OPG) plasma levels were significantly higher in HIV-infected patients than in healthy controls but lower than those in HIV negative subject with CVD (mean ± SD: 5.79 ± 2.82 versus 3.6 ± 1.7 versus 8.6 ± 4.3 pmol/L; median: 5.6 versus 3.6 versus 7 pmol/L) ($P = 0.001$) (Figure 2). We observed higher OPG plasma levels in HIV positive patients with mild coronary stenosis than in patients with grade II stenosis (mean ± SD 6.1 ± 1.5 versus 5.3 ± 1.7 pmol/L; median: 6.2 versus 5.7 pmol/L) ($P = 0.05$) (Figure 3). Interestingly, even in the 20 HIV negative subjects with CVD, OPG plasma concentration was higher in subjects with grade I stenosis than in subjects with grade II stenosis (9 ± 4.1 versus 8.1 ± 4.9 pmol/L) ($P = 0.2$). We observed negative correlation between OPG plasma levels and total cholesterol ($P = 0.032$) and LDL cholesterol ($P = 0.089$). IL-6 plasma levels were higher in HIV positive subjects than in HIV negative individuals but lower than those in HIV negative subjects with CVD (mean ± SD 60.94 ± 17.55 versus 46.78 ± 9.9 versus 72.85 ± 35.4 pg/mL; median: 58.4 versus 47 versus 61.7 pg/mL) ($P = 0.034$) (Figure 4). We observed a statistical correlation between IL-6 plasma levels and the grade of stenosis in HIV positive patients (63.8 ± 17.7 versus 51.9 ± 13.5 pg/mL) ($P = 0.045$). Moreover, in HIV negative men with CVD the IL-6 mean value was higher in men with grade II/III stenosis than in those with grade I stenosis (71.9 versus 55.1 pg/mL) ($P = 0.244$). We found a positive correlation between IL-6 plasma levels and cholesterol LDL ($P = 0.039$). We did not find any significant correlation between OPG

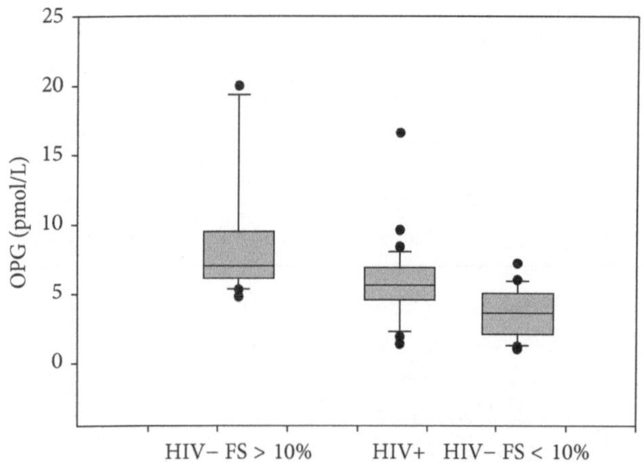

Figure 2: OPG plasma levels. OPG plasma levels were higher in HIV-infected patients than in healthy controls but lower than those in HIV negative subject with Framingham score (FS) >10%. Horizontal bars represent median. Upper and lower whisker mean third quartile +1.5 (Inter Quartile Range, IQR) and first quartile −1.5 (IQR).

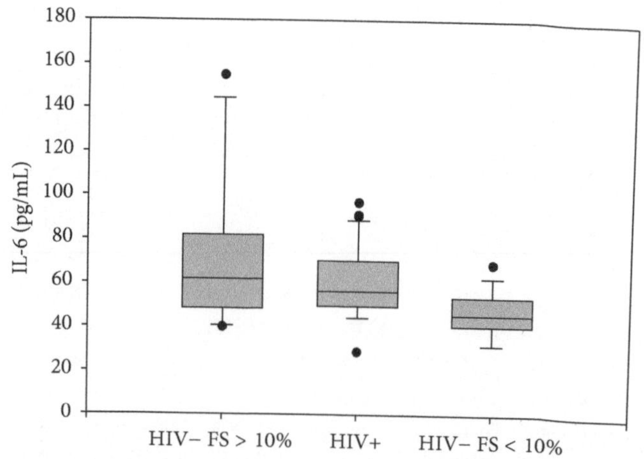

Figure 4: IL-6 plasma levels. IL-6 plasma levels were higher in HIV-infected patients than healthy controls but lower than those in HIV negative subject with Framingham Score (FS) >10%. Horizontal bars represent median. Upper and lower whisker mean third quartile +1.5 (Inter Quartile Range, IQR) and first quartile −1.5 (IQR).

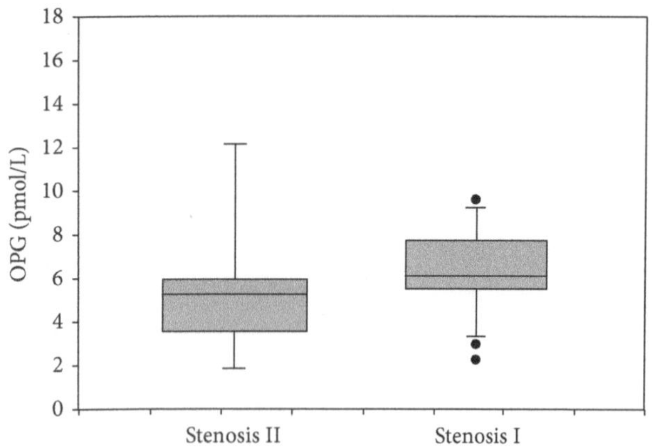

Figure 3: OPG and stenosis. OPG plasma levels in HIV positive patients with grade I stenosis versus patients with grade II stenosis. Horizontal bars represent median. Upper and lower whisker mean third quartile +1.5 (Inter Quartile Range, IQR) and first quartile −1.5 (IQR).

plasma levels, IL-6 plasma levels, and immune-virological parameters.

4. Discussion

HIV infected adults have higher risk of cardiovascular disease than the general population due to an accelerated atherosclerosis process [23]. Several risk factors play an important role in the pathogenesis and progression of atherosclerosis in HIV patients: both HAART toxicity (mitochondrial dysfunction and oxidative stress induced by thymidine analogues or even the accumulation of abnormal laminin A associated with HIV protease inhibitor) and the virus itself induce metabolic disorders, immune activation, and chronic inflammation [24, 25].

In this study, we enrolled 35 HIV infected men on suppressed HAART by at least 48 weeks with Framingham score <10%, 21 HIV negative individuals matched for age, gender, and Framingham score and 20 subjects with Framingham score >10%. We observed an increased prevalence of coronary stenosis in HIV infected patients than in uninfected controls as suggested by the absence of any abnormalities either in echocardiography or ECG in the latter group.

Heart CT scan is an accurate instrument for noninvasive assessment of coronary arteries which can substantially contribute to the diagnosis and management of cardiovascular disease [17]. In fact, it is able to distinguish calcified, partially calcified, and noncalcified plaques to quantify stenosis, their degree, and their extension. Although heart CT is not currently recommended in asymptomatic individuals, it could be considered in patients with low cardiovascular risk because of its ability to early identify small and soft plaques.

It is known that chemokines/cytokines including IL-6 and the OPG/RANK/RANKL system are involved in endothelial dysfunction leading to atherosclerosis development and progression. IL-6 and OPG plasma levels in HIV positive subjects were higher than those in healthy controls.

IL-6 is a proinflammatory and multifunctional cytokine which is secreted by many cell types such as macrophages, T lymphocytes and endothelial cells. Several reports have consistently shown that baseline levels of IL-6 are powerful predictor of cardiovascular events [3, 4, 26]. Our data confirm a correlation between increasing IL-6 plasma levels and severity of coronary stenosis, thus suggesting the proatherogenic role of this cytokine despite HIV-RNA suppression under HAART.

As already known, there is a link between residual HIV replication, inflammation, endothelial dysfunction, and atherosclerosis; residual viral replication, persistent viral expression, and the loss of immunoregulatory cells can induce immune activation and inflammation whose persistence may result in endothelial dysfunction, vascular damage, and atherosclerosis [2].

Furthermore, OPG/RANK/RANKL system, member of TNF superfamily mostly implicated in bone remodelling, is involved in immune and in vascular system. In fact, RANKL, expressed by osteoblast cells and their precursors, activates its receptor, RANK, expressed by osteoclast cells and their precursors, promoting osteoclasts formation, activation, and prolonging osteoclasts survival. The effects of RANKL are blocked by the secretory glycoprotein osteoprotegerin which acts as a decoy receptor for RANKL. Changes in RANKL/OPG ratio are critical in the pathogenesis of bone disease [10].

The relationship between bone and vascular disease is shown; in this contest OPG could be considered as a bridge from bone to vascular system [12, 13]. The role of OPG in cardiovascular disease is still debated. In support of the antiatherosclerotic effect of OPG, recent findings showed an accelerated atherosclerotic lesion progression in OPG deficient mice [27]. Acting as a decoy receptor of RANKL, OPG blocks the RANKL effect by triggering endothelial chemotactic and angiogenic properties, by enhancing monocyte and T cell infiltration and osteogenic differentiation of multipotential vascular mesenchymal cells. On the other hand, OPG might contribute to endothelial dysfunction by blocking the RANKL signalling which is able to activate protective intracellular endothelial pathways such as the nitric oxide synthase pathway and increase the adhesion and migration of inflammatory cells through the endothelium and the activity of metalloproteases [15, 28, 29].

In our study, we found higher OPG plasma levels in HIV positive subjects than in healthy control but lower than those in HIV negative subjects with Framingham score >10% suggesting association between OPG plasma levels and cardiovascular disease. The increased OPG plasma concentration found in HIV positive patients with low cardiovascular risk may suggest that OPG is implicated in the early phase of atherosclerosis development process. Surprisingly, in HIV positive subjects we found that patients with grade I stenosis had higher OPG values rather than patients with grade II stenosis. Instead, in HIV negative patients with severe stenosis OPG plasma levels were higher than in HIV positive men. These apparently conflicting findings could be explained by the different composition and stage of the plaques; in fact, in HIV negative subjects with Framingham score >10% the calcium concentration in the plaque was higher than in HIV positive patients in whom most of the plaques were soft. OPG is expressed in different cell types including endothelial cells and vascular smooth muscle cells which are represented more in soft plaques. In this setting, OPG may indirectly prevent calcification by protecting arterial smooth muscle cells from apoptosis and OPG inactivation may lead to increased calcification which is present in older plaques [26].

Whereas in the bone system, OPG is considered as a counter-regulatory mechanism to protect bone loss; in the vascular system increased, OPG plasma levels may indicate endothelial damage [30–32]. However, further studies investigating the exact role of OPG in atherosclerosis are needed.

5. Conclusion

We showed that OPG plasma concentrations are associated with atherosclerosis in HIV infected subjects with a low Framingham score. OPG plasma measurement could be a useful and noninvasive tool in clinical practice in order to early discriminate subjects at risk of developing atherosclerosis.

Disclosure

The project described was supported by the Department of Public Health and Infectious Disease of "Sapienza" University of Rome.

Conflict of Interests

None of the authors have any conflicts or potential conflicts of interest.

References

[1] A. Hakeem, S. Bhatti, and M. Cilingiroglu, "The spectrum of atherosclerotic coronary artery disease in HIV patients," *Current Atherosclerosis Reports*, vol. 12, no. 2, pp. 119–124, 2010.

[2] B. Coll, S. Parra, C. Alonso-Villaverde et al., "The role of immunity and inflammation in the progression of atherosclerosis in patients with HIV infection," *Stroke*, vol. 38, no. 9, pp. 2477–2484, 2007.

[3] S. W. Worm and P. Hsue, "Role of biomarkers in predicting CVD risk in the setting of HIV infection?" *Current Opinion in HIV and AIDS*, vol. 5, no. 6, pp. 467–472, 2010.

[4] O. Melander, C. Newton-Cheh, P. Almgren et al., "Novel and conventional biomarkers for prediction of incident cardiovascular events in the community," *Journal of the American Medical Association*, vol. 302, no. 1, pp. 49–57, 2009.

[5] G. Biasillo, M. Leo, R. della Bona, and L. M. Biasucci, "Inflammatory biomarkers and coronary heart disease: from bench to bedside and back," *Internal and Emergency Medicine*, vol. 5, no. 3, pp. 225–233, 2010.

[6] M. Guzmán-Fulgencio, J. Medrano, N. Rallón et al., "Soluble markers of inflammation are associated with framingham scores in HIV-infected patients on suppressive antiretroviral therapy," *Journal of Infection*, vol. 63, no. 5, pp. 382–390, 2011.

[7] A. C. Ross, N. Rizk, M. A. O'Riordan et al., "Relationship between inflammatory markers, endothelial activation markers, and carotid intima-media thickness in HIV-infected patients receiving antiretroviral therapy," *Clinical Infectious Diseases*, vol. 49, no. 7, pp. 1119–1127, 2009.

[8] X. Cheng, M. Kinosaki, R. Murali, and M. I. Greene, "The TNF receptor superfamily: role in immune inflammation and bone formation," *Immunologic Research*, vol. 27, no. 2-3, pp. 287–294, 2003.

[9] D. Stejskal, J. Bartek, R. Pastorková, V. Růzicka, I. Oral, and D. Horalík, "Osteoprotegerin, RANK, RANKL," *Biomedical Papers of the Medical Faculty of the University Palacky, Olomouc, Czechoslovakia*, vol. 145, no. 2, pp. 61–64, 2001.

[10] H. L. Wright, H. S. McCarthy, J. Middleton, and M. J. Marshall, "RANK, RANKL and osteoprotegerin in bone biology and disease," *Current Reviews in Musculoskeletal Medicine*, vol. 2, no. 1, pp. 56–64, 2009.

[11] B. F. Boyce and L. Xing, "Functions of RANKL/RANK/OPG in bone modeling and remodeling," *Archives of Biochemistry and Biophysics*, vol. 473, no. 2, pp. 139–146, 2008.

[12] L. C. Hofbauer and M. Schoppet, "Clinical implications of the osteoprotegerin/RANKL/RANK system for bone and vascular diseases," *Journal of the American Medical Association*, vol. 292, no. 4, pp. 490–495, 2004.

[13] S. Kiechl, P. Werner, M. Knoflach, M. Furtner, J. Willeit, and G. Schett, "The osteoprotegerin/RANK/RANKL system: a bone key to vascular disease," *Expert Review of Cardiovascular Therapy*, vol. 4, no. 6, pp. 801–811, 2006.

[14] P. Collin-Osdoby, "Regulation of vascular calcification by osteoclast regulatory factors RANKL and osteoprotegerin," *Circulation Research*, vol. 95, no. 11, pp. 1046–1057, 2004.

[15] A. van Campenhout and J. Golledge, "Osteoprotegerin, vascular calcification and atherosclerosis," *Atherosclerosis*, vol. 204, no. 2, pp. 321–329, 2009.

[16] S. M. Grundy, H. B. Brewer Jr., J. I. Cleeman, S. C. Smith Jr., and C. Lenfant, "Definition of metabolic syndrome: Report of the National Heart, Lung, and Blood Institute/American Heart Association Conference on Scientific Issues Related to Definition," *Circulation*, vol. 109, no. 3, pp. 433–438, 2004.

[17] C. R. Hamilton-Craig, D. Friedman, and S. Achenbach, "Cardiac computed tomography-evidence, limitations and clinical application," *Heart Lung and Circulation*, vol. 21, no. 2, pp. 70–81, 2012.

[18] G. D'Ettorre, M. Francone, M. Mancone et al., "Significant coronary stenosis detected by coronary computed angiography in asymptomatic HIV infected subjects," *Journal of Infection*, vol. 64, no. 1, pp. 82–88, 2012.

[19] M. D. Cerqueira, N. J. Weissman, V. Dilsizian et al., "Standardized myocardial segmentation and nomenclature for tomographic imaging of the heart. A statement for healthcare professionals from the Cardiac Imaging Committee of the Council on Clinical Cardiology of the American Heart Association," *The international journal of cardiovascular imaging*, vol. 18, no. 1, pp. 539–542, 2002.

[20] W. G. Austen, J. E. Edwards, R. L. Frye et al., "A reporting system on patients evaluated for coronary artery disease. Report of the Ad Hoc Committee for Grading of Coronary Artery Disease, Council on Cardiovascular Surgery, American Heart Association," *Circulation*, vol. 5, pp. 15–40, 1975.

[21] S. B. King 3rd, S. C. Smith Jr., D. A. Morrison et al., "Focused update of the ACC/AHA/SCAI, 2005 guideline update for percutaneous coronary intervention: a report of the American College of Cardiology/American Heart Association task force on practice guidelines: 2007 Writing group to review new evidence and update the ACC/AHA/SCAI, 2005 guideline update for percutaneous coronary intervention, writing on behalf of the 2005 writing committee," *Circulation*, vol. 117, pp. 261–295, 2008.

[22] M. R. Patel, G. J. Dehmer, J. W. Hirshfeld, P. K. Smith, and J. A. Spertus, "ACCF/SCAI/STS/AATS/AHA/ASNC appropriateness criteria for coronary revascularization. A Report by the American College of Cardiology Foundation Appropriateness Criteria Task Force, Society for Cardiovascular Angiography and Interventions, Society of Thoracic Surgeons, American Association for Thoracic Surgery, American Heart Association, and the American Society of Nuclear," *Journal of the American College of Cardiology*, vol. 53, no. 6, pp. 530–553, 2009.

[23] J. Lo, S. Abbara, L. Shturman et al., "Increased prevalence of subclinical coronary atherosclerosis detected by coronary computed tomography angiography in hiv-infected men," *AIDS*, vol. 24, no. 2, pp. 243–253, 2010.

[24] M. W. Lorenz, C. Stephan, A. Harmjanz et al., "Both long-term HIV infection and highly active antiretroviral therapy are independent risk factors for early carotid atherosclerosis," *Atherosclerosis*, vol. 196, no. 2, pp. 720–726, 2008.

[25] S. G. Deeks, "Immune dysfunction, inflammation, and accelerated aging in patients on antiretroviral therapy," *Topics in HIV Medicine*, vol. 17, no. 4, pp. 118–123, 2009.

[26] W. Lieb, P. Gona, M. G. Larson et al., "Biomarkers of the osteoprotegerin pathway: clinical correlates, subclinical disease, incident cardiovascular disease, and mortality," *Arteriosclerosis, Thrombosis, and Vascular Biology*, vol. 30, no. 9, pp. 1849–1854, 2010.

[27] B. J. Bennett, M. Scatena, E. A. Kirk et al., "Osteoprotegerin inactivation accelerates advanced atherosclerotic lesion progression and calcification in older $ApoE^{-/-}$ mice," *Arteriosclerosis, Thrombosis, and Vascular Biology*, vol. 26, no. 9, pp. 2117–2124, 2006.

[28] F. Montecucco, S. Steffens, and F. Mach, "The immune response is involved in atherosclerotic plaque calcification: could the RANKL/RANK/OPG system be a marker of plaque instability?" *Clinical & Developmental Immunology*, vol. 2007, Article ID 75805, 8 pages, 2007.

[29] A. Quercioli, G. Luciano Viviani, F. Dallegri, F. MacH, and F. Montecucco, "Receptor activator of nuclear factor kappaB ligand/osteoprotegerin pathway is a promising target to reduce atherosclerotic plaque calcification," *Critical Pathways in Cardiology*, vol. 9, no. 4, pp. 227–230, 2010.

[30] A. Vik, E. B. Mathiesen, J. Brox et al., "Serum osteoprotegerin is a predictor for incident cardiovascular disease and mortality in a general population: The Tromsø Study," *Journal of Thrombosis and Haemostasis*, vol. 9, no. 4, pp. 638–644, 2011.

[31] M. Schoppet, A. M. Sattler, J. R. Schaefer, M. Herzum, B. Maisch, and L. Hofbauer, "Increased osteoprotegerin serum levels in men with coronary artery disease," *Journal of Clinical Endocrinology and Metabolism*, vol. 88, no. 3, pp. 1024–1028, 2003.

[32] J. J. Hwang, J. Wei, S. Abbara, S. K. Grinspoon, and J. Lo, "Receptor activator of nuclear factor-κB ligand (RANKL) and its relationship to coronary atherosclerosis in HIV patients," *Journal of Acquired Immune Deficiency Syndromes*, vol. 61, no. 3, pp. 359–363, 2012.

The Age of Initiation of Drug Use and Sexual Behavior May Influence Subsequent HIV Risk Behavior: A Systematic Review

Patrick Baldwin, Roman Shrestha, Jessica Potrepka, and Michael Copenhaver

University of Connecticut, Department of Allied Health Sciences, 358 Mansfield Road, Unit 2101, Storrs, CT 06269-2101, USA

Correspondence should be addressed to Michael Copenhaver; michael.copenhaver@uconn.edu

Academic Editors: D. Aunis, H. C. Mwandumba, and J. Poudrier

Researchers examining injection drug users (IDUs) in drug treatment have been trying for decades to determine the optimal way to intervene to prevent the transmission and spread of human immunodeficiency virus (HIV) in this population. Although efficacious HIV risk reduction interventions are widely available, questions remain about what specific factors are most related to HIV risk behavior and defined as unprotected sexual activity and/or high risk drug use. This review involved an evaluation of the research literature in order to better understand the association between drug use and sexual behavior debut on HIV risk behavior. Findings suggest that drug use debut and sexual behavior debut may be related to subsequent HIV risk behavior. Evidence to date implies that intervening at an earlier age to assist youth to avoid or delay these high risk behaviors may be an additional means of reducing subsequent HIV risk.

1. Introduction

Globally, an estimated 3 million people who inject drugs are living with HIV, representing roughly one in 10 infections worldwide [1]. An estimated 49,273 individuals in the U.S. were infected with HIV in 2011 and injection drug users (IDUs) remain at high risk for HIV transmission. Since the epidemic began, nearly 182,000 injection drug users with an AIDS diagnosis have died, including an estimated 4,218 in 2010. Of the approximate 32,050 new cases of AIDS reported in 2011, 3,961 were IDU-associated. In 2011, 7.4% of all newly diagnosed cases in adults and adolescents were from IDU-associated behavior [2]. With the high rate of HIV risk in the IDU population, it is even more important to understand the events leading to risk behavior.

Part of the global HIV epidemic involves adolescents who are initiating sexual activity at progressively earlier ages [3] and putting themselves and others at increased risk for HIV infection. A 2011 CDC survey found that 47% of high school students reported having sexual intercourse, 6.2% reported having intercourse before age 13, and an alarming 39.8% reported not using a condom during their last intercourse [4]. The average reported age of first sexual intercourse in the USA is age 14.4, with more males than females (9.0% versus 3.4%, resp.), and more African-American teens than other racial/ethnic groups reporting sexual activity before age 13—highlighting a common racial disparity pattern [4, 5]. Although data exist regarding HIV risk and prevalence rates, questions remain about what factors are most predictive of subsequent HIV risk behavior among adolescents and young adults, and thus what strategies could potentially alter this trajectory.

While research has focused on identifying predictors of risk behaviors in adolescence, the influence of the age of debut, defined as the initiation or the first occurrence of certain behaviors such as substance use and coitus, on later HIV risk outcomes remains largely unexplored in the empirical research literature. Health behavior research to date has examined how the debut of specific risk behaviors among youth is predictive of various negative health outcomes among those individuals later in life as adults [6–15]. For example, early sexual debut has been linked to short-term negative outcomes such as higher levels of depression among adolescents [16] and delinquency [17], as well as longer-term negative outcomes including lowered expectations for pursuing higher education [18, 19], poorer academic performance [20], less consistent contraceptive use [21], unintended pregnancies [14], increasingly risky sexual behaviors [22–35], and likelihood of having multiple partners [36–38]. Conversely, other studies indicate that the delay of sexual initiation tends to be protective of future risk behavior [3, 16, 18, 39].

There are clear parallels between sexual debut and substance use debut in terms of the potential pattern of influences on subsequent health risks. A growing number of studies have also been concerned with the linkage between early onset of drug use and a range of negative health risk outcomes that occur in adulthood. For example, an earlier age of substance use debut is a well-documented risk factor for subsequently developing substance use disorders [13, 40–48], poorer academic performance, and lower academic expectations [48, 49]. Drug use debut and HIV transmission risk behavior have also been tentatively linked in several recent studies [50–55], although this linkage was not the primary focus of these studies.

Like other types of substance use in adolescence, drinking alcohol at an early age remains a serious health concern since it may interfere with brain development and lead to cognitive and behavioral dysfunctions that foster risk taking [56] and later substance use problems [6, 57]. Early onset of alcohol consumption may also tend to establish a pattern of maladaptive coping mechanisms in which alcohol is implemented to manage stress [44]. Furthermore, substance use—particularly heavy drug use—during a critical period of neurobiological development may lead to poorer memory and learning functioning, reduced inhibition, abnormalities in executive functioning and neuronal activation, and alterations in brain structure, as well as a host of other neurocognitive sequelae [58].

In addition to the parallels between drug use debut and sexual debut, numerous studies have highlighted a cooccurrence of both behaviors, linking the debut of one type of behavior to the other, or both, and underscore their complex and often interwoven associations [20, 59–64]. For example, one investigation of Swedish high school students found that teens who reported sexual debuts at age 15 used more tobacco, illicit drugs, and alcohol than their aged-matched inexperienced peers, suggesting a clustering of risk behaviors linked with early sexual initiation [65]. By systematically exploring the relevant literature in the present review, we seek to more clearly elucidate the progression of HIV risk behaviors over time so as to better inform future HIV prevention interventions.

2. Methods

2.1. Selection of Studies. We searched for studies that included quantitative data about sexual debut, drug use debut, and subsequent HIV risk behavior. In conducting this literature review, peer-reviewed studies were included if they met all of the following criteria: (1) identified either age of sexual debut, age of substance use debut, or both; (2) assessed at least one concurrent or subsequent HIV-related substance use or sexual risk behavior as an outcome; and (3) were published in English (see Figure 1).

2.2. Search Strategy. An extensive literature search was conducted in the online database PubMed that included studies from 2001 through December, 2012. Our primary objective was to review scientific data related to the influence of both sexual and substance use debut on subsequent HIV risk behavior. We cross-referenced previous reviews and primary studies for additional citations. In an initial search, both of our domains, drug use debut and sexual debut, were crossed one-at-a-time with consequential HIV risk behavior, using multiple combinations of search terms; see Table 1.

The search was not limited to any particular geographic area or region and there were no restrictions imposed on the age of subject populations. As such, definitions of "early debut" of either risk behavior varied across studies, making preadolescence, adolescence, and young adulthood more useful terms that would ensure coverage of all target groups and encompass a broader age range. Sexual debut was defined as first oral, anal, or vaginal sex. Substance use included all illicit drugs, cannabis, alcohol, and tobacco. HIV risk behavior outcomes included unprotected sexual activities, sexual activities under the influence of drugs and/or alcohol, sex with multiple partners, exchange sex, injection drug use (IDU)—particularly using uncleaned syringes or sharing injection equipment, sex with an IDU partner or partners, STI, pregnancy, and HIV serostatus.

A total of 1,469 articles were retrieved as of December 30, 2012. Thirteen additional articles were found in the reference section of the relevant journal articles. After the removal of 318 duplicated records, 1,164 articles remained for preliminary review. After inspecting study titles and abstracts, we found that 920 records were not directly relevant to the study objectives, leaving 244 records for further, more detailed, review. A full-text copy of this subset of studies was obtained and assessed for inclusion. 187 full-text records were excluded because they did not investigate an association between the variables of interest and behavioral outcomes that constitute HIV risk behaviors. Finally, a total of 57 studies were included for this review (see Figure 1).

3. Findings

3.1. Early Initiation of Sexual Behavior and Concurrent Health Risks. Early initiation of sexual behavior is viewed as a health risk since youth who initiate sexual behavior at an earlier age spend relatively more years at potential risk for HIV and a range of other sexually transmitted diseases versus those who are not sexually active until a later point. One study found that among a sample of female high school students in Nova Scotia, aged 15 to 19, having vaginal intercourse before 15 years was associated with sexual risk-taking behaviours—such as not using a condom, unplanned intercourse due to substance use, having a casual partner, and having multiple sexual partners—at later points in adolescence [78]. Similarly, Pettifor et al. evaluated risk factors related to early coitarche among 7,692 South African youth and found that 18% of males

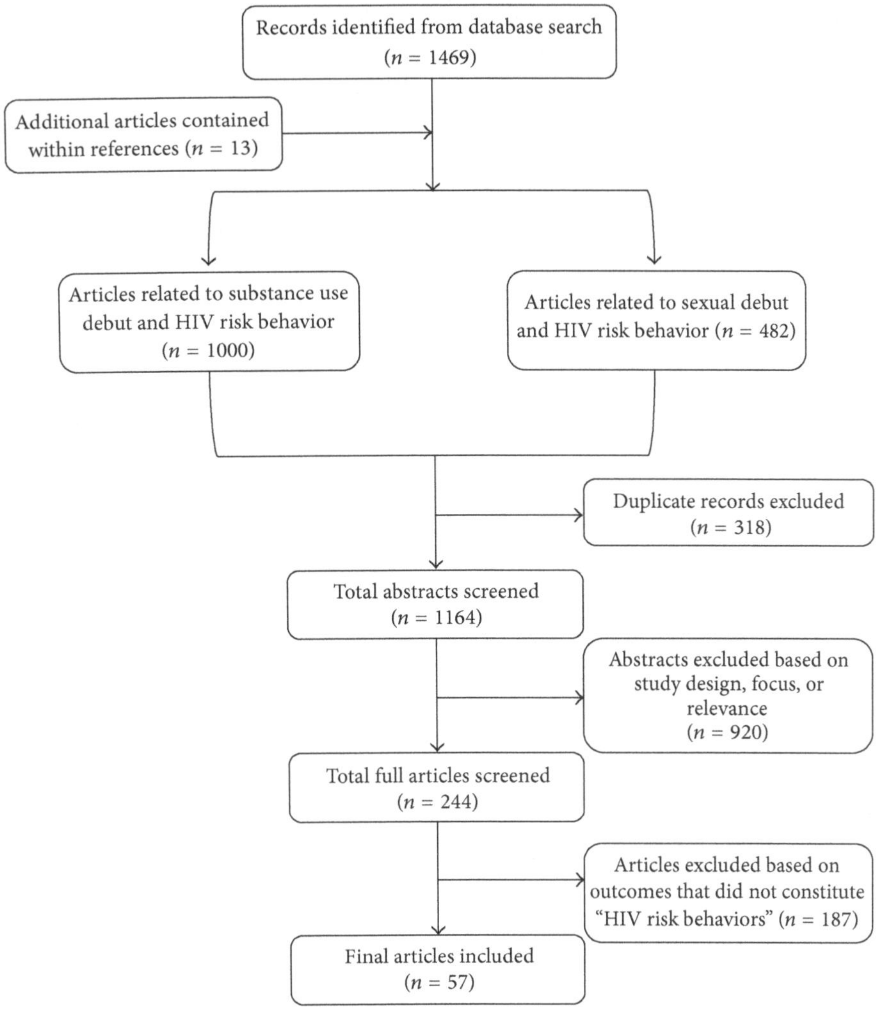

FIGURE 1: Study inclusion flow diagram.

and 8% of females reported sexual debut at age 14 or younger [91], while a cross-sectional study of homeless 13- to 17-year olds in Brazil revealed that one-third of females and two-thirds of males in the sample reported sexual debuts under the age of twelve [68]. An earlier sexual debut was associated with inconsistent condom use [68] and a lack of condom use [91].

Nkansah-Amankra et al. examined data from the Colorado Youth Risk Behavior Surveillance System (2005)—sampling 1,498 adolescents in 29 public schools, grades 9–12—and found an association between patterns of adolescent drug use and high risk sexual behavior [85]. Females in the sample who reported using two illegal substances were 12 times more likely to report early sexual debuts than those reporting no use, while females using three substances were 44 times more likely to report early sexual debuts. Additionally, adolescent binge drinking was also associated with higher odds of having multiple partners. The results suggested that adolescents with drug-use experience had a greater tendency to report being involved in high risk sexual activity and consequently to be at greater risk for contracting and spreading HIV.

In a seven-year cohort study of American Indian teens aged 14–18 living in a Northern Plains community in South Dakota, Mitchell et al. (2007) found that while predictors of early sexual initiation differed by gender, having used alcohol or drugs at sexual debut was a significant predictor of early sexual initiation for both males and females [82] as other researchers have found [20, 62]. Still another investigation showed that young men in rural South Africa reporting sexual debut before age 15 were more likely to not use condoms at first sex and to have had multiple and casual partners than those who had initiated sex at 15 or older [28]. Likewise, a later investigation revealed that sexual debuters aged 16 and younger, particularly males reporting female partners, were more likely to have had multiple sexual partners than later debuters—highlighting a similar, albeit gender-specific, combination of risky behaviors occurring at sexual debut [35].

Thus, there is evidence from diverse samples that, not surprisingly, earlier initiation of sexual behavior among youth is linked with higher levels of concurrent health risk behaviors among these samples. A similar pattern of findings have been identified with regard to health risks associated

Table 1: Search terms and terminology used for retrieval of eligible citations and reports.

"coital" **AND** "debut" **AND** "risk"		
"substance" **AND** "debut" **AND** "HIV"		
"risk behavior" **AND** "initiation" **AND** "subsequent"		
"drug initiation" **OR** "sexual initiation" **AND** "risk" **AND** "HIV"		
"Substance use" **OR** "drug use" **OR** "needle sharing" **OR** "syringe sharing" **OR** "first injection" **OR** "drug initiation" **OR** "IDU"	**AND**	"age of initiation" **OR** "age of debut" **OR** "age of first use" **OR** "early initiation" **OR** "early age" **OR** "age of onset"
"Sexual debut" **OR** "sexual intercourse" **OR** "sexual initiation" **OR** "risky sexual behavior"	**AND**	"subsequent" **OR** "early initiation" **OR** "adolescence" **OR** "early age" **OR** "age of onset" **OR** "age of first use"

with earlier initiation of drug use behavior among youth, as detailed below.

3.2. Initiation of Substance Use and Concurrent Health Risks. Miller et al. explored factors associated with IDU initiation before age 16 among 542 IDUs [81]. Thirty-eight percent of the sample initiated IDU prior to age 16. There was also an association between earlier initiation of injection drug use and the following variables: gender (being female), identifying as a sex worker, using other drugs, and having a history of criminal justice system involvement. Early drinkers more likely to report subsequent alcohol problems, unprotected sexual intercourse, multiple partners, and being drunk or high during sexual intercourse. Likewise, a study conducted in Canada assessed the circumstances surrounding the initiation of injection drug use among 560 street-recruited youth (median age of drug use debut was age 13; median age of IDU debut was age 17) and found a significant association between age of first drug use and history of IDU [74]. A study conducted in Russia assessed 558 IDUs and their non-IDUs sexual partners and found that the initiation of alcohol use at a younger age (mean = 14.2 years) was related to an earlier onset of coitarche (mean = 15.5 years) and a younger age of first drug use (mean = 16.8 years) [6]. Thus, a significant correlation was found between age of first alcohol use and the age at first sexual intercourse as well as the likelihood for having multiple sexual partners and age of initiating injection drug use behavior.

A cross-sectional behavioral survey that evaluated 805 street-based adolescents in the Ukraine reported a pattern of elevated HIV risk stemming from both unprotected sex and injection drug use [100]. Almost 75% of the sample of adolescents had experienced sexual behavior debut before the age of 15. Among those who reported injecting drugs within the past month, 44% had shared needles at least once and reported lower levels of condom use. These studies built on earlier studies in this area by examining health outcomes linked with injection drug use initiation among youth from diverse samples.

Noninjection drug use also shares a strong linkage with early coital debut across a vast ethnic and national landscape. Using data gathered from seven national and three local surveys, the National Campaign to Prevent Teen Pregnancy's Research Task Force found that, compared to delayed sexual activity, early sexual activity among young US teens has been linked to a greater number of sexual partners over time. In addition, these surveys found that sexually experienced youth aged 14 and younger are much more likely to smoke, use drugs and alcohol, and participate in delinquent activities than their inexperienced peers [101], though the precise sequence of behaviors remains uncertain. Other national survey data gathered in the USA show that girls who had begun smoking marijuana by age 14 or cigarettes by age 12 were significantly more likely to be pregnant by age 15, though it is plausible that these predictors were moderated by some common underlying risk factors [66]. In a cross-sectional sample of 15- to 21-year-old male and female vocational students in Thailand, recent cigarette smoking, alcohol consumption, and illicit substance use were all strongly associated with earlier onset of sexual intercourse for males, though whether or not experimentation with drugs predisposed these individuals to engage in risky sexual behavior was unclear [79]. Additionally, a 2009 survey assessing risk behavior of Mississippi public high school students [37] found similar associations between drinking alcohol, smoking cigarettes, and using marijuana or other drugs and early sexual initiation. Black respondents, it was found, were more likely to report early sexual initiation.

3.3. Debut of Risk Behaviors and Subsequent HIV Risk Outcomes. Although the majority of studies examined associations among concurrent health risk variables, we also identified an expanding body of relevant literature that focused on the influence of early risk behaviors (e.g., sexual activity and drug use) on HIV risk behaviors at later points in life. In addition to the lingering effects of early sexual experiences on a wide range of health outcomes discussed earlier [33], early coitus has an association with HIV risk behaviors, specifically, later in life in a range of diverse contexts and populations.

In a large population-based study of over 23,000 Danish men aged 18–45, Buttmann et al. found that those with early sexual debuts (i.e., sexual activity before age 14) were more likely to have subsequently engaged in risky sexual behaviour (i.e., having 8 or more lifetime sexual partners and two or more current partners) than older debuters [22]. This association was also evident in a cross-sectional survey of 15–18-year-old adolescent boys in Tehran; of those who were sexually experienced, about 15% had sexual debuts by age 12, 35% by age 14, and 55% by age 15. Moreover, early sexual debut was a predictor of multiple sexual partners in one's lifetime. A similar pattern was shown in a 3-year longitudinal study of male and female urban minority adolescents in the USA; early initiators (those who had engaged in sex by 7th grade) were more likely than later initiators (those who had abstained by the end of middle school) have reported multiple sex partners, being involved in a pregnancy, forcing a partner to have sex, having frequent intercourse, and having sex while intoxicated or under the influence [30]. The same study, however, noted significant gender differences in these outcomes; early female initiators were four times more likely to be involved in a pregnancy and were half as likely to report consistent condom use versus their male counterparts, while males were more likely than females to report having had at least four sexual partners.

The association between early sexual debut and subsequent risky behavior or HIV infection is also seen in studies with exclusively female samples [70, 75, 97]. One population-based study of nearly 65,000 women in four Nordic countries illustrated that young age of first sexual intercourse was highly associated with reporting risk-taking behaviors. Among the sample of women aged 18 to 45, young age of first intercourse (age 14 or younger) was highly associated with risk-taking behaviors, such as a greater number of lifetime sexual partners, recent partners, and history of STIs [31].

Fatusi and Wang investigated the association between early coital debut and STIs among a nationally representative sample of 15- to 24-year-old males in Nigeria and found that early sexual debut (sexual intercourse before age 16) had a significant independent association with self-reported STIs [26]. In addition, early sexual initiators were significantly more likely to have sex with casual or commercial partners and multiple partners and less likely to use condoms. Having multiple sexual partners, in this case, mediated the association between age of sexual debut and subsequent STI [26]. Similar findings that clearly show a strong association between early sexual debut and subsequent STIs have also been documented in mixed-gender samples [77] and among gay men [29], while the early sexual debut and multiple partners correlation has been shown among South African youth [35]. Another study of 15- to 24-year-old males in South Africa reported findings consistent with the following: those who initiated sex before age 15 were more likely to report no condom use and a casual partner at first sex. Furthermore, early sexual debut was strongly associated with having more than three partners within the past three years, thus placing them at higher risk for HIV and other STIs [28].

In one study, Fuller et al. focused on both sexual and IDU debut behavior and examined the factors associated with injection initiation during adolescence (i.e., age 21 or younger) compared with young adulthood (i.e., older than age 21) among 226 street-recruited IDUs in the Baltimore, MD, area [72]. The overall median age of IDU initiation was age 23 and 40% of the sample reported initiating IDU during adolescence. Those who reported initiating injection drug use during adolescence tended to demonstrate relatively rapid progression to IDU compared to those who initiated injection drug use as adults. Forty-two percent of study participants reported that their sexual debut occurred prior to age fourteen. Those who reported initiating IDU during adolescence were more likely to report having their first sexual experience prior to age 14 as well as having multiple sex partners in the previous six months [72].

In a later study, Fuller et al. evaluated predictors of age of injection drug use initiation and HIV-related risk behaviors among a similar population—144 IDUs in Baltimore, MD [61]. This study reported that race, neighborhood, and educational level were significant predictors of age of injection drug use initiation. In this study, the median age at initiation of IDU was age 21. Fifty-one percent of the participants had initiated IDU during adolescence. Adolescent initiators were twice as likely as young adult initiators to report that their first sexual experience have taken place before they were 14 years of age. Adolescent-initiating IDUs were less likely than adult-initiating IDUs to report high-risk sex and injection behaviors, but more likely to report high-risk networks. Cheng et al. explored risk factors associated with the initiation of injection drug use among 2,231 injectors in Northern Thailand [45]. The analyses indicated that the age of drug initiation was negatively associated with the risk of injection initiation such that the older the age of initiation of any type of drug use, the lower the risk of initiating injection drug use. Likewise, in a study of IDUS in southern Thailand, HIV status was also correlated with an earlier age of injection initiation [90, 95] and injecting at drug debut [90]—underscoring the importance of drug use debut as a salient HIV risk factor.

Muga and colleagues assessed HIV-related outcomes among 1,111 IDUs in Spain and reported that both age of drug use debut and duration of injection drug use were associated with participants contracting HIV [84]. Subramaniam and Stitzer evaluated adolescents (aged 14–18) who reported substance abuse and their subsequent risk for HIV [93]. Approximately half of injection heroin users in the group reported sharing needles or "works" during this particular period of time, leaving them highly susceptible to Hepatitis-C and HIV infection. Forty percent of the total sample population, however, including both opioid- and heroin-users, engaged in HIV risk behaviors such as having multiple sexual partners and always having unprotected sex. Likewise, Parviz et al. focused on drug- and sex-related risk behavior outcomes among 242 IDUs in Pakistan and found that a slightly younger age of first injection (age 25 versus age 28) was associated with subsequent drug-related HIV risk behavior (i.e., receptive needle sharing) [88]. Forty-seven percent of those who participated in the study engaged in receptive needle sharing, 22% had sexual intercourse—of whom only 7% used condoms—and none had cleaned their needles with bleach.

More recently, Dillon et al. explored the associations among age of sexual behavior debut and sexual risk behaviors among 158 predominantly Latina immigrants (mean age: 27.2 years) living in Miami, FL. The following variables were associated with a younger age of sexual behavior debut: a greater number of sexual partners, more frequent sex-related alcohol or drug use, and greater levels of intoxication from alcohol or drugs during sex [25]. Dorjgochoo et al. also examined the associations between various behavioral factors and HIV status among 3,391 sexually active Haitians [69]. The mean age of sexual debut was age 16.5 for females and age 14.6 for males. HIV infection for female participants was associated with years of sexual activity, confirmed/suspected STI in females, and suspected STI in partners or suspicion that partners had outside sexual partners; HIV infection among male participants was associated with drug use and sexual debut with an unknown person. Interestingly, later sexual debut was not protective of HIV infection among women or men in this sample. Moreover, sexual debut after age 16 was positively associated with HIV infection in males. In contrast, Medhi et al. focused on factors associated with HIV serostatus among 426 female sex workers (mean age of 25.7 years) in India and found in a multivariate analysis that HIV-infected status was significantly associated with lifetime injection drug use, initiating sexual intercourse before age 15 and testing positive for one or more STIs [80]. Likewise, Gore-Felton et al. showed in a sample of 16- to 25-year-old male and female IDUs in Russia (mean sexual debut ages 14.84 and 15.50, resp.) that young age of sexual initiation was significantly associated with sexual risk behaviors in the past 30 days for men but not women [73]. This suggests a strong association between young coital debut and subsequent risky sexual and injection drug use behaviors. Taken together, studies from diverse geographic locations and populations suggest that earlier risk behaviors—including sexual activity and drug use—are significantly associated with HIV risk behaviors at later points in life.

4. Discussion

We reviewed studies that included data on the initiation of sexual and drug use behavior and concurrent and subsequent health risk behaviors. Although the majority of studies were cross-sectional and included information linking recent risk behaviors among youth, we also uncovered evidence of a linkage between early initiation of various risk behaviors and health risk behaviors later in life. Not surprisingly, the pattern of outcomes tend to show that the early initiation of sexual behavior and substance use are related to a range of other recent health risks, such as various STIs [26, 27, 33, 67], HIV [75], SUDs such as cannabis use disorders and alcohol use disorders [60, 102], psychiatric disorders including MDD [8], Hepatitis-C and cervical cancer [24], engaging in commercial sex exchange work [26, 71], poor school performance and conduct disorder [52], physical violence [65], receptive needle sharing [86], pregnancy [27, 66], and externalizing disorders [42]. In contrast, the longitudinal associations tend to be less clear cut based on the studies currently available.

The associations between sexual and drug debuts with contemporaneously occurring risk behaviors, as well as those occurring at later points in life, appear to be complex and therefore difficult to precisely capture. In the studies reported to date, it is also difficult to pinpoint the influence of sexual and substance use debuts as other risk factors—that particularly the initiation of drug and/or alcohol use—are often reported to occur concurrently. As indicated above, an early age of sexual initiation is associated with subsequent sexual risk behaviors, but also with subsequent risky drug use behavior [80] and substance use in general [42, 60, 103, 104]. Importantly, both types of risk behavior debuts have been linked to HIV infection [29, 69, 70, 75, 80, 81, 84, 90, 95, 97]. Likewise, the association of an early drug use debut and later risk behavior appears to be multidirectional, as subsequent risky substance use practices (e.g., needle sharing), sexual practices (e.g., multiple partners, transactional sex, lack of condom use), and substance use in general have all been linked. This crossover of risk behavior domains, thus, suggests that early initiation of either type of risk behavior can be associated with the other [6, 24, 25, 27, 31, 37, 49, 63–65, 76, 78–80, 89, 98, 103, 104], and both might operate synergistically (e.g., drinking or illicit drug use coupled with unprotected sex [105]) as part of a tendency toward a generally riskier lifestyle.

The overall influence of earlier initiation of sexual activity tends to be negative but varies significantly across ethnicities and/or geographic location, socioeconomic status, gender [30], and sexual orientation, thus precluding universal generalizations, as might be expected. Despite disagreement among researchers about whether early sexual involvement fits into a larger constellation of generic "problem behaviors" or merely experimentation as a normative part of development [33, 106, 107], theories suggest that sensation-seeking [63, 105], increased feelings of invulnerability, and risk-proneness—or a propensity to be attracted to potentially risky behavior—likely play prominent roles in influencing early sexual debuts [14]. Adolescence, after all, is a period preceding full cognitive development and emotional maturity [108].

The larger cultural contexts in which these behaviors occur must be considered, as sexual and substance use norms and perceptions are often shaped by religious, national/regional, and social values. In many cultures, adolescent sexual activity is increasingly viewed as a normative aspect of developing responsible intimate relationships as teens mature into adulthood, rather than a delinquent behavior like drug use [30, 33, 107]. Consequently, the disparate cultural norms inherent in the vast array of countries, communities, and ethnic subgroups included in this review may be expected to differentially influence the trajectories of subsequent risk behaviors [62].

The age of sexual initiation carries serious implications for STI risk; early sexual debut potentially increases the duration of lifetime sexual exposure, allowing a relatively longer sexual career overall and, hence, more time for individuals with young debuts to accrue sexual partners, especially during adolescence, when relationships are often short in duration and changing sexual partners is more common [22, 26, 31] and risk-proneness is heightened [21]. The importance of considering the nature of and context in which initial sexual experiences occur cannot be overstated, as sexual coercion, sex under the influence, and rape are profoundly different sexual experiences than consensual intercourse within the context of a trusting, intimate relationship, for instance, and have profoundly different implications for influencing future risk behavior [32, 99]. Many studies simply were not designed to disentangle these important qualitative details nor the emotional context surrounding diverse experiences surrounding the first sexual intercourse.

Table 2

Study	Study location	Sample size (N) (sex; age)	Study design	Study population	Summary of findings
Abdala et al., 2012 [6]	St. Petersburg, Russia	$N = 558$ (M,F; 18–58)	Cross-sectional	IDUs and non-IDUs sexual partners of IDUs (participants of SATH-CAP study)	Age at first drink affects multiple sex partners through age at sexual debut and injection drug use, but no effect on unprotected sex; age at first drug use not related to sexual risk behaviors.
Buttmann et al., 2011 [22]	Denmark	$N = 23{,}080$ (M; 18–45)	Cross-sectional	Male residents of Denmark	Men who had sex with a commercial sex worker and those who reported >8 lifetime partners or ≥2 recent sex partners were more likely to have other risk taking behaviors. Men who started sexual activity at a young age, defined as ≤14 years, were also more likely to report >8 sexual partners.
Cavazos-Rehg et al., 2011 [59]	USA	$N = 13{,}580$ (M,F; 17 years and older)	Cross-sectional	High school seniors (participants in the 1999–2007 YRBS survey)	Severity of substance use was more closely related to higher number of sexual partners than age of substance use onset.
Cavazos-Rehg et al., 2012 [66]	USA	$N = 8{,}219$ (F; 15 years and younger)	Cross-sectional	Adolescent girls (participants in the 1999–2003 YRBS survey)	Pregnancy linked with substance use onset; of girls pregnant by age 15 years 16% had smoked marijuana by age 10 years and >20% had smoked cigarettes and initiated alcohol use by age 10 years and marijuana use by age 14 years.
Celentano et al., 2008 [67]	Chiang Mai, Thailand	$N = 658$ (M,F; 18–25)	Cross-sectional	Sexually active young adults	Men reported greater number of sexual partners than women, infrequent condom use at last sex; women ≥20 years of age, with ≥2 heterosexual partners in the past year and a younger age at sexual debut, were significantly more likely to have a prevalent STI.
Cheng et al., 2006 [45]	Chiang Mai Province, Thailand	2,231 (M,F; 12 years and older)	Cross-sectional	Opiate- or methamphetamine-dependent individuals receiving inpatient treatment	Age of drug initiation and having multiple sex partners were both associated with increased risk of injection initiation.
Cooper et al., 2007 [24]	Cape Town, South Africa	$N = 2{,}065$ (F; <60 years)	Case-control	Women (resident of Cape Town)	Early sexual debut associated with increased number of lifetime partners and alcohol use; number of sexual partners associated with sexual debut.
Cornelius et al., 2007 [60]	Pittsburgh, USA	$N = 136$ (M; 10–12)	Cohort	Adolescents (from high risk families based on fathers' SUD)	Earlier age at first intercourse and deviant activities of peers each predicted a significantly higher risk of subsequently developing substance use disorders (SUD).
de Carvalho et al., 2006 [68]	Porto Alegre, Brazil	$N = 176$ (M,F; 10–18)	Cross-sectional	Children and youth in street circumstances	Correlates of unsafe sex included younger age of sexual debut and having a steady sex partner; correlates of illicit drug use included lack of family contact, increased hours in the street daily, having had an HIV test, and older age.
Dillon et al., 2010 [25]	Florida, USA	$N = 316$ (F)	Cross-sectional	Latina mother-daughter dyads (living in urban area)	Having a mother who used drugs during the participants' childhood or adolescence was significantly related to age of sexual debut; younger ages of sexual debut were associated with drug abuse and more sexual risk behaviors.
Dorjgochoo et al., 2009 [69]	Port-au-Prince, Haiti	3,391 (M,F; 13–25)	Cross-sectional	Young adults and adolescents receiving voluntary HIV testing	HIV was associated with drug use and sexual debut with a casual/unknown person among males and suspected/confirmed STI and years of sexual activity among females. Among males, sexual debut >16 years old was positively associated with HIV-infection. Later sexual debut was not protective from HIV in women or men.

Table 2: Continued.

Study	Study location	Sample size (N) (sex; age)	Study design	Study population	Summary of findings
Drain et al., 2004 [70]	122 developing countries	(M,F)	Cross-sectional (ecologic/population-level analysis)	HIV seroprevalences per 100 adults 15–49 years old and number of children (younger than 15 years of age) living with HIV infection for the beginning of the year 2000 from the Joint United Nations Programme on HIV	Countries with earlier ages at first sex, higher teenage birth rates, and higher fertility rates had higher HIV seroprevalence.
Duong et al., 2008 [71]	Hai Phong, Vietnam	$N = 643$ (M,F; 18–29)	Cross-sectional	Young men and women	Early age at first intercourse was associated with having sex with a sex worker.
Fatusi and Wang, 2009 [26]	Nigeria	$N = 1{,}278$ (M; 15–24)	Cross-sectional	Sexually experienced never-married young males	Early sexual debut was associated with STIs; multiple sexual partnership is a mediator of the association between early debut and STI.
Fuller et al., 2001 [72]	Maryland, USA	$N = 226$ (M,F; 15–30)	Cross-sectional	Street IDUs (adolescence versus young adulthood)	Factors significantly associated with adolescent initiation of IDU included race other than African American and practices prior to initiating injection including condom use, lack of cocaine use, exclusive crack smoking just prior to initiation, and smoking marijuana.
Fuller et al., 2005 [61]	Maryland, USA	$N = 144$ (M,F; 15–30)	Cross-sectional	Street IDUs with ≤5 years of injection use	Adolescent-initiating IDUs were less likely than adult-initiating IDUs to report high-risk sex and injection behaviors and more likely to report high-risk networks. African American IDUs from neighborhoods with large percentages of minority residents and low adult educational levels were more likely to initiate injection during adolescence than White IDUs from neighborhoods with low percentages of minority residents and high adult education levels.
Gore-Felton et al., 2003 [73]	St. Petersburg, Russia	$N = 188$ (M,F; 14–25)	Cross-sectional	Young adult IDUs	Males who initiate sex at a younger age are more likely to report multiple sex partners.
Hadland et al., 2010 [74]	Vancouver, Canada	$N = 560$ (M,F; 14–26)	Cross-sectional	Street youth (participants of At Risk Youth Study)	Youth previously injected were more likely to have engaged in noninjection use of heroin or of crystal methamphetamine.
Hallett et al., 2007 [75]	Rural Zimbabwe	$N = 9{,}086$ (M,F; 17–54, 15–44; resp.)	Cross-sectional	Household couple (Zimbabwe household census)	Age at first sex declined among males over the past 30 years but increased recently among females; early sexual debut before marriage precedes a lifetime of greater sexual activity but with more consistent condom use; women who begin to have sex earlier than others of their age are more likely to be infected with HIV.
Hansen et al., 2010 [27]	Denmark, Iceland, Norway, and Sweden	$N = 69{,}486$ (F; 18–45)	Cross-sectional	Women who initiated smoking early (before age 15) and later (at 15 or later) and never smokers	Adult women who initiated smoking early reported more lifetime and recent sexual partners and less condom use and had lower debut ages for coitus, pregnancy, and alcohol consumption.
Harrison et al., 2005 [28]	Rural South KwaZulu/Natal South Africa	$N = 314$ (M; 15–24)	Cross-sectional	Adults (household census)	Men with sexual debut at less age than 15 were more likely to report risk behaviors at first sexual experience: no condom use (19%), a casual partner (26.8%), and not feeling they had been "ready and wanted to have sex" (19.5%); early sexual debut was strongly associated with >3 partners in the past 3 years.

Table 2: Continued.

Study	Study location	Sample size (N) (sex; age)	Study design	Study population	Summary of findings
Jackson et al., 2012 [76]	Glasgow City, UK	N = 3,104 (M,F; 15 and 18-19)	Cohort	Adolescents and Young Adults (participants in two cohorts, born 12 years apart)	Strong association between substance use and sexual risk behavior during early and late adolescence; significant between-cohort difference was a stronger association between female early adolescent smoking and early sexual initiation in the later cohort. Also, relationships between illicit drug use and both early sexual initiation and multiple sexual partners in late adolescence were significantly stronger among girls.
Kaestle et al., 2005 [77]	USA	9,844 (M,F; 18–26)	Longitudinal	Adolescents and young adults with STIs in wave 3 of National Longitudinal Study of Adolescent Health	Younger ages at first intercourse were associated with higher odds of STI in comparison with older ages, but the effect diminished with increasing current age. The association between timing of first intercourse and STIs did not vary by gender, race, ethnicity, or parental education.
Langille et al., 2010 [78]	Cape Breton, Nova Scotia, Canada	N = 797 (F; 15–19)	Cross-sectional	High school girls	Early vaginal intercourse was associated with not using a condom at last intercourse, unplanned intercourse in the previous year due to substance use, having a casual partner at last intercourse, and having three or more partners for vaginal intercourse in the previous year.
Liu et al., 2006 [79]	Northern Thailand	N = 1,725 (M,F; 15–21)	Cross-sectional	Vocational school students	Sexual initiation was associated with using alcohol or methamphetamine; for males, initiation was associated with friend as a confidant, tobacco use, high perceived risk for HIV, and high STI knowledge; for females, other factors associated with earlier initiation were younger age at interview, living away from family, lacking a family member as a confidant, high-perceived risk for STIs, and ever having smoked marijuana.
Lyons et al., 2012 [29]	Australia	N = 845 (M; 16–65)	Cross-sectional	Gay men born between 1994 and 1993	HIV-positive men were found to be significantly younger on average when they first had anal intercourse compared with HIV-negative men; men with a history of other STIs were significantly younger; engaging in higher risk sexual behavior was a likely factor, with AFAI generally younger among men who reported >10 sexual partners in the past year and who engaged in group sex and receptive anal intercourse or were drug or alcohol affected during their most recent sexual encounter.
Magnusson et al., 2011 [14]	USA	N = 3,588 (F; 15–44)	Cross-sectional	Fertile women (participants of the 2006–2008 National Survey of Family Growth)	Compared with women who were 18 or older at first intercourse, women who were <15 years of age at the time of first intercourse were nearly two times as likely to report a gap in contraceptive use.
McGuire et al., 2012 [37]	Mississippi, USA	(M,F)	Cross-sectional	High school students (participants of the 2009 Mississippi Youth Risk Behavior Survey)	Older age, being a black, drinking alcohol, or using marijuana or other drugs were associated with early sexual initiation and having multiple sexual partners; heavy smoking was associated with early sexual initiation.
Medhi et al., 2012 [80]	Nagaland, India	N = 426 (F; ≥18 years)	Cross-sectional	FSWs (participants in Integrated Biological Behavioural Assessment study)	Initiating sexual intercourse before the age of 15, more than 2 years of sex work, testing positive for more than 1 STIs, lifetime IDU history, exchange sex for drugs, and having IDU sexual partners were all associated with HIV seropositivity. Sexual debut <15 was independently associated with HIV.

Table 2: Continued.

Study	Study location	Sample size (N) (sex; age)	Study design	Study population	Summary of findings
Miller et al., 2006 [81]	Vancouver, Canada	$N = 542$ (M,F; ≤16 years and ≤ 25 years)	Cohort	IDUs (participants of the Vancouver Injection Drug Users Study)	Proportion of young initiators was greater among, females, sex workers, binge drug users, and those who have been in juvenile detention or jail; early initiates were more likely to be infected with HIV and hepatitis C virus.
Mitchell et al., 2007 [82]	South Dakota, USA	$N = 474$ (M,F; 14–18)	Cross-sectional	Cohorts of American Indian youths (participants of The Voices of Indian Teens (VOICES, 1993–1995; Waves 1–3) and Pathways of Choices (CHOICES, 1996–1999; Waves 4–7)	For young men, younger initiation of sex was predicted by a greater likelihood of having used alcohol or drugs at first sex; for young women, earlier initiation was related to having mothers who had their first child at an early age and using alcohol/drugs at first sex; higher cumulative risk was associated with elevated risk of sexual initiation.
Mohammad et al., 2007 [83]	Tehran, Iran	$N = 1,385$ (M; 15–18)	Cross-sectional	Unmarried adolescent males	Having no access to Internet, feeling regretful at sexual debut, having one sexual partner in lifetime, and lower knowledge of condoms predictors of condom nonuse; older age, using alcoholic drinks, early sexual debut, and poor knowledge of reproductive physiology are predictors of multiple sexual partners.
Muga et al., 2003 [84]	Barcelona, Spain	1,111 (M,F)	Cross-sectional	IDUs admitted to hospital detoxification unit	Age at start of and duration of injection drug use were associated with HIV infection ($P < .001$).
Nkansah-Amankra et al., 2011 [85]	Colorado, USA	1,498 (M,F)	Cross-sectional	Public high school students	Female teens using 2 illicit substances were 12 times more likely to report early debuts than abstinent teens; females using 3 illicit substances were 44 times more likely to report early debuts.
Novelli et al., 2005 [86]	Maryland, USA	$N = 420$ (M,F; 15–30)	Cross-sectional	Young urban IDUs (participants of the REACH III study)	Adjusting for race, gender, and homelessness, following variables independently associated with recent receptive syringe sharing: age at first hit, self-injection at initiation, and using a syringe that had previously been used by someone else at first hit.
O'Donnell et al., 2001 [30]	New York, USA	$N = 1,287$ (M,F)	Cross-sectional	Urban minority adolescents in 7th and 8th grade.	Early initiators had an increased likelihood of having had multiple sex partners, forced a partner to have sex, had frequent intercourse, and had sex while drunk or high.
Olesen et al., 2012 [31]	Denmark, Iceland, Norway, and Sweden	$N = 64,659$ (F; 18–45)	Cross-sectional	Women in four Nordic countries	OR of reporting >10 lifetime sexual partners was almost four times higher among women who reported a young age at first intercourse; women who were young at first intercourse were more likely to report two or more recent partners and to have a history of STIs; young age at first intercourse was associated with current smoking and binge drinking.
Outlaw et al., 2011 [87]	USA: New York, North Carolina, Michigan, Texas, and California	$N = 363$ (M; 13–24)	Cross-sectional	Non-White MSM	Participants having a MSM sexual debut before the age of 16 reported more exchange sex, drug use, and emotional/psychological problems related to substance use.
Parviz et al., 2006 [88]	Karachi, Pakistan	242 (M)	Cross-sectional	IDUs	Younger age of first injection was associated with subsequent receptive needle sharing. 47% of respondents shared needles and 22% had sexual intercourse—of whom 7% used condoms. No respondents cleaned needles with bleach.
Pechansky et al., 2011 [89]	Porto Alegre, Brazil	$N = 200$ (M,F)	Cross-sectional	Ecstasy and LSD users	Participants with early sexual debut (<14) more likely to report lifetime use of marijuana and powder and crack cocaine; early sexual debut was associated with past year sexual risk behaviors, including having sex while high and having two or more sex partners.

Table 2: Continued.

Study	Study location	Sample size (N) (sex; age)	Study design	Study population	Summary of findings
Perngmark et al., 2003 [90]	Southern Thailand	$N = 272$ (M,F)	Cross-sectional	Active IDU	HIV seropositivity among ethnic Thai was independently correlated with past history of needle sharing, injecting immediately at drug onset, and starting first injection at younger age.
Pettifor et al., 2004 [32]	In and around Harare, Zimbabwe	$N = 4,393$ (F; 18–35)	Cross-sectional	Sexually active women (from public sector family planning clinic)	Women with early coital debut had a significantly higher risk profile, including multiple lifetime partners; HIV risk was increased for women reporting early age of coital debut.
Pettifor et al., 2009 [91]	South Africa	$N = 7,692$ (M,F; 15–24)	Cross-sectional	Sexually active youth	Lack of condom use at first sex associated with early coital debut and forced sex for males; among females, the likelihood of nonuse elevated for respondents who had an early debut but had not had forced sex, and among those who had had both a later debut and forced sex.
Prado et al., 2009 [92]	Florida, USA	$N = 254$ (M,F)	Cross-sectional	Hispanic Adolescents of seventh grade year	Larger proportion with high intrapersonal risk for unsafe sex (irrespective of ecodevelopmental risk) report early sex initiation and sexually transmitted disease incidence.
Rothman et al., 2009 [62]	Massachusetts, USA	$N = 11,110$ (M,F; 14–21)	Cross-sectional	Black, Hispanic, and White adolescents	Age at first sex decreased linearly with decreasing age at first drink for all adolescents; significant positive trends between age at first drink and age at first sex were observed for all race and ethnic subgroups.
Sandfort et al., 2008 [33]	San Francisco, USA	$N = 8,466$ (M,F; 18 years and older)	Cross-sectional	US adult population (participants of the 1996 National Sexual Health Survey)	Early initiation of sexual intercourse was associated with various sexual risk factors, whereas late initiation was associated with fewer risk factors.
Santelli et al., 2001 [34]	USA	$N = 7,441$ (M,F; 14–22)	Cross-sectional	Unmarried young people (participants of the 1992 YRBS survey)	Failure to use a condom was strongly associated with the lifetime substance-use scale or, alliteratively, with age at initiation of alcohol.
Stanton et al., 2001 [63]	Maryland, USA	$N = 383$ (M,F; 9–15)	Cohort	African-American adolescents	Early initiators of sex were significantly more likely to report involvement in substance use and drug-delivery/sales.
Stueve and O'Donnell, 2005 [64]	New York, USA	$N = 1,034$ (M,F; 11–14)	Cross-sectional	African American and Hispanic youths at 7th and 8th grade	Early drinking was associated with alcohol and sexual risks through midadolescence; more likely to report subsequent alcohol problems, unprotected sexual intercourse, multiple partners, being drunk or high during sexual intercourse.
Subramaniam and Stitzer, 2009 [93]	Baltimore, Maryland	$N = 94$ (M,F; 14–18)	Cross-sectional	Treatment-seeking OUD adolescents	Roughly 50% injection heroin users reported sharing injection equipment/paraphernalia and 40% of total sample (opioid and heroin users) engaged in HIV-sexual risk behaviors.
Trenz et al., 2012 [94]	Maryland, USA	$N = 651$ (M,F)	Cross-sectional	Adult IDUs and non-IDUs (participants of the NEURO-HIV Epidemiologic Study)	IDUs differed from non-IDUs in age of initiation for cigarettes, marijuana, and alcohol.
Uusküla et al., 2010 [95]	Tallinn, Estonia	$N = 350$ (M,F; 18 years or older)	Cross-sectional	IDUs	Individual with earlier IDU initiation, injecting opioids, and receptive syringe sharing as significant predictors of individual HIV-positive status.
Vicknasingam et al., 2009 [96]	Malaysia	$N = 526$ (M,F)	Cross-sectional	IDUs in nontreatment settings	Being 44 years or younger; not holding regular job; initiating drug use at age 23 or younger; being a morphine user; sharing injecting equipment and having multiple-sex partners were all risk factors associated with HIV seropositivity, though only last 2 remained significant in multivariate analysis.

Table 2: Continued.

Study	Study location	Sample size (N) (sex; age)	Study design	Study population	Summary of findings
Wand and Ramjee, 2012 [97]	Durban, South Africa	$N = 3{,}492$ (F; 18–49)	Cross-sectional	Sexually active women (participants of MIRA study)	Lowest quintiles of age at sexual debut, a higher number of lifetime sexual partners, and being diagnosed as having STIs were significantly associated with prevalent HIV infection.
Wang et al., 2011 [98]	Southern, Midwestern, and Eastern regions of USA	$N = 7{,}372$ (M,F; 14 years and older)	Cross-sectional	Entering freshmen on HBCU campuses (participants of HBCU Substance Use Survey)	Early sex was modestly associated with subsequent illegal drug initiation, particularly among females.
Yode and LeGrand, 2012 [99]	Burkina Faso, Malawi, and Uganda	$N = 2{,}842$ (M,F; 14–19)	Cross-sectional	Adolescents (participants of the 2004 National Surveys of Adolescents)	Initiation of sexual activity <14 years of age was more likely to be associated with having a casual sex partner and less likely to be associated with condom use at first sexual relation or with systematic condom use in the past 12 months.
Zuma et al., 2010 [35]	South Africa	$N = 2{,}875$ (M,F; 15–24)	Cross-sectional	Sexually active youth	Having multiple sexual partners was significantly more common among those that had early sexual debut.

A similar rationale has been proffered to explain the link between early substance initiation and IDU behavior later in life. Earlier exposure and access to substances during a period of psychosocial development, marked by relatively rapid cognitive changes and strong peer influence, create a greater window of potential risk [94]. Additionally, poorer performance on executive functioning tasks among adolescent substance users suggest a reduced ability to control behavior, make healthy long-term decisions, and attend to environmental stimuli which may put individuals at greater risk for substance use later in life [58, 94]. Thus, considered as a whole, studies to date indicate that early initiation of sex- and drug-related behaviors may exert substantial influence on youth from diverse backgrounds and geographical regions and may set them on a different HIV risk trajectory relative to their counterparts who do not have an early debut of such behaviors.

4.1. Study Limitations. Some of the limitations of this systematic review should be acknowledged. First, the review was restricted to peer-reviewed journal articles published in English, which likely biased our collection toward primarily English-speaking countries. The search itself was restricted to one database, although this is unlikely to have been a major limitation as PubMed Central (PMC), with nearly 2.4 million biomedical articles, is the largest repository of full-text open-access biomedical articles in the world. In addition, only abstracts were screened for this review to determine whether the study investigated the impact of early sexual and substance use debuts on HIV risk behavior outcomes. Thus, any secondary findings and analyses relevant to our topics of interest not mentioned within the abstracts may have been excluded from this review. Many behaviors were self-reported, often at much later time points, making response bias and social desirability potential limiting factors.

We should also add that, due to a reliance on cross-sectional designs in many of the studies included, it is not possible to establish causal inferences and, hence, precludes any definitive interpretations regarding the processes by which sexual and substance use debuts independently lead to later risky behaviors or the precise sequence of their trajectories. Since certain antecedents and common underlying factors, such as PTSD and CSA (childhood sexual abuse), parental substance use history, peer influence, and the role of genetic predispositions to substance dependence were not the foci of most of the studies included in this literature review, disentangling these potential confounders was well beyond the scope of our review.

4.2. Future Directions. Despite the noted limitations, the findings of this study have implications for future interventions and HIV risk prevention programs. Of the Centers for Disease Control and Prevention's (CDC) 18 evidence-based HIV Risk Prevention Interventions targeting "high-risk youth," eight address both drug and sexual risk behaviors. Of those, however, five are designed for either nonsubstance dependent or precoital adolescents, and only two of which meet the CDC's best evidence criteria of showing empirical evidence that demonstrates a reduction in HIV/STD incidence, reduced HIV-related risk behaviors, reduction in HIV viral load, or improvement in HIV medication adherence behaviors. Thus, a need exists for innovative EBIs that optimally target high risk youth in a manner that prevents or disrupts the linkage between the initiation of sex- and drug-related behaviors and subsequent HIV risk. Screening adolescents for risk factors may also prove a potent preventative measure given the established association between early debuts of substance use, sexual intercourse, or both, as it could potentially obviate later secondary and tertiary prevention efforts.

Interventions that cross multiple domains of risk (i.e., focus on delaying the initiations of sexual behaviors and substance use and reducing harm following initiation) may have a larger impact than addressing either one by itself in reducing the risk for STD transmission, pregnancy, initiation of IDU, and HIV infection. Interventions are needed that focus on the associations between substance use, multiple sexual partners, failure to use condoms, and HIV infection and that stress the potential harms of alcohol and other substances on judgment and risk taking. Secondly, interventions should confront attitudes about condom use and sexual norms in a culturally competent and relevant manner—tailoring messages to fit within the target audience's larger religious, social, and cultural contexts [31, 62, 83]. A "one size fits all" approach would overlook the diverse findings of the studies reviewed that vary among different ethnic groups and communities of disparate socioeconomic statuses. Environmental context, race, sexual orientation [29, 87], and gender must all be considered when designing behavioral interventions targeting adolescents [61].

Lastly, future prevention interventions should target younger, precoital adolescents in late elementary and early middle school who are cognitively susceptible to experimenting with a range of risk-taking behaviors. Early screening to assess for behaviors such as drinking and cigarette smoking might help to quickly identify those beginning to experiment and assist them in averting a trajectory with potentially deleterious health outcomes. Similarly, an efficacious assessment tool could provide an early warning sign to parents, school counselors, medical professionals, and other professionals in positions to provide proper education and counseling regarding the short- and long-term health consequences of initiating risky behaviors during adolescence.

Appendix

For more details see Table 2.

References

[1] B. M. Mathers, L. Degenhardt, B. Phillips et al., "Global epidemiology of injecting drug use and HIV among people who inject drugs: a systematic review," *The Lancet*, vol. 372, no. 9651, pp. 1733–1745, 2008.

[2] Centers for Disease Control and Prevention, *Diagnoses of HIV Infection and AIDS in the United States and Dependent*

Areas, 2011, vol. 23 of *HIV Surveillance Report*, 2013, http://www.cdc.gov/hiv/pdf/statistics_2011_HIV_Surveillance_Report_vol_23.pdf.

[3] B. J. Lohman and A. Billings, "Protective and risk factors associated with adolescent boys' early sexual debut and risky sexual behaviors," *Journal of Youth and Adolescence*, vol. 37, no. 6, pp. 723–735, 2008.

[4] D. K. Eaton, L. Kann, S. Kinchen et al., "Youth risk behavior surveillance—United States, 2011," *Morbidity and Mortality Weekly Report*, vol. 61, no. 4, pp. 1–162, 2012.

[5] P. A. Cavazos-Rehg, M. J. Krauss, E. L. Spitznagel et al., "Age of sexual debut among US adolescents," *Contraception*, vol. 80, no. 2, pp. 158–162, 2009.

[6] N. Abdala, N. B. Hansen, O. V. Toussova, T. V. Krasnoselskikh, A. P. Kozlov, and R. Heimer, "Age at first alcoholic drink as predictor of current HIV sexual risk behaviors among a sample of Injection Drug Users (IDUs) and non-IDUs who are sexual partners of IDUs, in St. Petersburg, Russia," *AIDS and Behavior*, vol. 16, no. 6, pp. 1597–1604, 2012.

[7] J. C. Anthony and K. R. Petronis, "Early-onset drug use and risk of later drug problems," *Drug and Alcohol Dependence*, vol. 40, no. 1, pp. 9–15, 1995.

[8] D. W. Brook, J. S. Brook, C. Zhang, P. Cohen, and M. Whiteman, "Drug use and the risk of major depressive disorder, alcohol dependence, and substance use disorders," *Archives of General Psychiatry*, vol. 59, no. 11, pp. 1039–1044, 2002.

[9] B. T. Conner, G. S. Hellemann, T. L. Ritchie, and E. P. Noble, "Genetic, personality, and environmental predictors of drug use in adolescents," *Journal of Substance Abuse Treatment*, vol. 38, no. 2, pp. 178–190, 2010.

[10] S. Hansell and H. R. White, "Adolescent drug use, psychological distress, and physical symptoms," *Journal of Health and Social Behavior*, vol. 32, no. 3, pp. 288–301, 1991.

[11] R. W. Hingson, J.-P. Assailly, and A. F. Williams, "Underage drinking: frequency, consequences, and interventions," *Traffic Injury Prevention*, vol. 5, no. 3, pp. 228–236, 2004.

[12] R. W. Hingson, T. Heeren, and M. R. Winter, "Age at drinking onset and alcohol dependence: age at onset, duration, and severity," *Archives of Pediatrics and Adolescent Medicine*, vol. 160, no. 7, pp. 739–746, 2006.

[13] K. M. King and L. Chassin, "A prospective study of the effects of age of initiation of alcohol and drug use on young adult substance dependence," *Journal of Studies on Alcohol and Drugs*, vol. 68, no. 2, pp. 256–265, 2007.

[14] B. M. Magnusson, S. W. Masho, and K. L. Lapane, "Adolescent and sexual history factors influencing reproductive control among women aged 18–44," *Sexual Health*, vol. 8, no. 1, pp. 95–101, 2011.

[15] D. W. Zeigler, C. C. Wang, R. A. Yoast et al., "The neurocognitive effects of alcohol on adolescents and college students," *Preventive Medicine*, vol. 40, no. 1, pp. 23–32, 2005.

[16] A. L. Spriggs and C. T. Halpern, "Sexual debut timing and depressive symptoms in emerging adulthood," *Journal of Youth and Adolescence*, vol. 37, no. 9, pp. 1085–1096, 2008.

[17] S. Armour and D. L. Haynie, "Adolescent sexual debut and later delinquency," *Journal of Youth and Adolescence*, vol. 36, no. 2, pp. 141–152, 2007.

[18] A. Parkes, D. Wight, M. Henderson, and P. West, "Does early sexual debut reduce teenagers' participation in tertiary education? Evidence from the SHARE longitudinal study," *Journal of Adolescence*, vol. 33, no. 5, pp. 741–754, 2010.

[19] A.-K. Valle, E. Røysamb, J. Sundby, and K. I. Klepp, "Parental social position, body image, and other psychosocial determinants and first sexual intercourse among 15- and 16-year olds," *Adolescence*, vol. 44, no. 174, pp. 479–498, 2009.

[20] T. R. Raine, R. Jenkins, S. J. Aarons et al., "Sociodemographic correlates of virginity in seventh-grade black and Latino students," *Journal of Adolescent Health*, vol. 24, no. 5, pp. 304–312, 1999.

[21] B. M. Magnusson, S. W. Masho, and K. L. Lapane, "Early age at first intercourse and subsequent gaps in contraceptive use," *Journal of Women's Health*, vol. 21, no. 1, pp. 73–79, 2012.

[22] N. Buttmann, A. Nielsen, C. Munk, K. L. Liaw, and S. K. Kjaer, "Sexual risk taking behaviour: prevalence and associated factors. A population-based study of 22,000 Danish men," *BMC Public Health*, vol. 11, article 764, 2011.

[23] P. A. Cavazos-Rehg, M. J. Krauss, E. L. Spitznagel et al., "Type of contraception method used at last intercourse and associations with health risk behaviors among US adolescents," *Contraception*, vol. 82, no. 6, pp. 549–555, 2010.

[24] D. Cooper, M. Hoffman, H. Carrara et al., "Determinants of sexual activity and its relation to cervical cancer risk among South African women," *BMC Public Health*, vol. 7, article 341, 2007.

[25] F. R. Dillon, M. de La Rosa, S. J. Schwartz, P. Rojas, R. Duan, and R. M. Malow, "US Latina age of sexual debut: long-term associations and implications for HIV and drug abuse prevention," *AIDS Care*, vol. 22, no. 4, pp. 431–440, 2010.

[26] A. Fatusi and W. Wang, "Multiple sexual partnership mediates the association between early sexual debut and sexually transmitted infection among adolescent and young adult males in Nigeria," *The European Journal of Contraception and Reproductive Health Care*, vol. 14, no. 2, pp. 134–143, 2009.

[27] B. T. Hansen, S. K. Kjær, C. Munk et al., "Early smoking initiation, sexual behavior and reproductive health—a large population-based study of Nordic women," *Preventive Medicine*, vol. 51, no. 1, pp. 68–72, 2010.

[28] A. Harrison, J. Cleland, E. Gouws, and J. Frohlich, "Early sexual debut among young men in rural South Africa: heightened vulnerability to sexual risk?" *Sexually Transmitted Infections*, vol. 81, no. 3, pp. 259–261, 2005.

[29] A. Lyons, M. Pitts, J. Grierson, A. Smith, S. McNally, and M. Couch, "Age at first anal sex and HIV/STI vulnerability among gay men in Australia," *Sexually Transmitted Infections*, vol. 88, no. 4, pp. 252–257, 2012.

[30] L. O'Donnell, C. R. O'Donnell, and A. Stueve, "Early sexual initiation and subsequent sex-related risks among urban minority youth: the reach for health study," *Family Planning Perspectives*, vol. 33, no. 6, pp. 268–275, 2001.

[31] T. B. Olesen, K. E. Jensen, M. Nygård et al., "Young age at first intercourse and risk-taking behaviours—a study of nearly 65000 women in four Nordic countries," *European Journal of Public Health*, vol. 22, no. 2, pp. 220–224, 2012.

[32] A. E. Pettifor, A. van der Straten, M. S. Dunbar, S. C. Shiboski, and N. S. Padian, "Early age of first sex: a risk factor for HIV infection among women in Zimbabwe," *AIDS*, vol. 18, no. 10, pp. 1435–1442, 2004.

[33] T. G. M. Sandfort, M. Orr, J. S. Hirsch, and J. Santelli, "Long-term health correlates of timing of sexual debut: results from a national US study," *American Journal of Public Health*, vol. 98, no. 1, pp. 155–161, 2008.

[34] J. S. Santelli, L. Robin, N. D. Brener, and R. Lowry, "Timing of alcohol and other drug use and sexual risk behaviors among

unmarried adolescents and young adults," *Family Planning Perspectives*, vol. 33, no. 5, pp. 200–205, 2001.

[35] K. Zuma, G. Setswe, T. Ketye, T. Mzolo, T. Rehle, and N. Mbelle, "Age at sexual debut: a determinant of multiple partnership among South African youth," *African Journal of Reproductive Health*, vol. 14, no. 2, pp. 47–54, 2010.

[36] M. Durbin, R. J. DiClemente, D. Siegel, F. Krasnovsky, N. Lazarus, and T. Camacho, "Factors associated with multiple sex partners among junior high school students," *Journal of Adolescent Health*, vol. 14, no. 3, pp. 202–207, 1993.

[37] J. McGuire, B. Wang, and L. Zhang, "Substance use and sexual risk behaviors among Mississippi public high school students," *Journal of the Mississippi State Medical Association*, vol. 53, no. 10, pp. 323–328, 2012.

[38] S. N. Seidman, W. D. Mosher, and S. O. Aral, "Predictors of high-risk behavior in unmarried American women: adolescent environment as risk factor," *Journal of Adolescent Health*, vol. 15, no. 2, pp. 126–132, 1994.

[39] S. A. Burgard and S. M. Lee-Rife, "Community characteristics, sexual initiation, and condom use among young black South Africans," *Journal of Health and Social Behavior*, vol. 50, no. 3, pp. 293–309, 2009.

[40] A. Agrawal, J. D. Grant, M. Waldron et al., "Risk for initiation of substance use as a function of age of onset of cigarette, alcohol and cannabis use: findings in a Midwestern female twin cohort," *Preventive Medicine*, vol. 43, no. 2, pp. 125–128, 2006.

[41] S. Behrendt, H.-U. Wittchen, M. Höfler, R. Lieb, and K. Beesdo, "Transitions from first substance use to substance use disorders in adolescence: is early onset associated with a rapid escalation?" *Drug and Alcohol Dependence*, vol. 99, no. 1–3, pp. 68–78, 2009.

[42] S. Behrendt, K. Beesdo-Baum, M. Höfler et al., "The relevance of age at first alcohol and nicotine use for initiation of cannabis use and progression to cannabis use disorders," *Drug and Alcohol Dependence*, vol. 123, no. 1–3, pp. 48–56, 2011.

[43] N. Breslau, N. Fenn, and E. L. Peterson, "Early smoking initiation and nicotine dependence in a cohort young adults," *Drug and Alcohol Dependence*, vol. 33, no. 2, pp. 129–137, 1993.

[44] A. F. Buchmann, B. Schmid, D. Blomeyer et al., "Drinking against unpleasant emotions: possible outcome of early onset of alcohol use?" *Alcoholism*, vol. 34, no. 6, pp. 1052–1057, 2010.

[45] Y. Cheng, S. G. Sherman, N. Srirat et al., "Risk factors associated with injection initiation among drug users in Northern Thailand," *Harm Reduction Journal*, vol. 3, article 10, 2006.

[46] D. A. Dawson, R. B. Goldstein, S. Patricia Chou, W. June Ruan, and B. F. Grant, "Age at first drink and the first incidence of adult-onset DSM-IV alcohol use disorders," *Alcoholism*, vol. 32, no. 12, pp. 2149–2160, 2008.

[47] D. J. DeWit, E. M. Adlaf, D. R. Offord, and A. C. Ogborne, "Age at first alcohol use: a risk factor for the development of alcohol disorders," *The American Journal of Psychiatry*, vol. 157, no. 5, pp. 745–750, 2000.

[48] P. L. Ellickson, J. S. Tucker, D. J. Klein, and H. Saner, "Antecedents and outcomes of marijuana use initiation during adolescence," *Preventive Medicine*, vol. 39, no. 5, pp. 976–984, 2004.

[49] K. Poikolainen, A. Tuulio-Henriksson, T. Aalto-Setälä, M. Marttunen, T. Anttila, and J. Lönnqvist, "Correlates of initiation to cannabis use: a 5-year follow-up of 15–19-year-old adolescents," *Drug and Alcohol Dependence*, vol. 62, no. 3, pp. 175–180, 2001.

[50] J. Abelson, C. Treloar, J. Crawford, S. Kippax, I. van Beek, and J. Howard, "Some characteristics of early-onset injection drug users prior to and at the time of their first injection," *Addiction*, vol. 101, no. 4, pp. 548–555, 2006.

[51] B. Brands, J. Blake, B. Sproule, D. Gourlay, and U. Busto, "Prescription opioid abuse in patients presenting for methadone maintenance treatment," *Drug and Alcohol Dependence*, vol. 73, no. 2, pp. 199–207, 2004.

[52] Y.-I. Hser, C. E. Grella, C. Collins, and C. Teruya, "Drug-use initiation and conduct disorder among adolescents in drug treatment," *Journal of Adolescence*, vol. 26, no. 3, pp. 331–345, 2003.

[53] C. S. Meade, L. J. McDonald, and R. D. Weiss, "HIV risk behavior in opioid dependent adults seeking detoxification treatment: an exploratory comparison of heroin and oxycodone users," *The American Journal on Addictions*, vol. 18, no. 4, pp. 289–293, 2009.

[54] M. L. Schoeneberger, T. K. Logan, and C. G. Leukefeld, "Age differences in HIV risk behaviors and drug treatment utilization among drug users in Kentucky," *Substance Use and Misuse*, vol. 36, no. 6-7, pp. 867–925, 2001.

[55] B. Sproule, B. Brands, S. Li, and L. Catz-Biro, "Changing patterns in opioid addiction: characterizing users of oxycodone and other opioids," *Canadian Family Physician*, vol. 55, no. 1, pp. 68.e5–69.e5, 2009.

[56] C. Guerri and M. Pascual, "Mechanisms involved in the neurotoxic, cognitive, and neurobehavioral effects of alcohol consumption during adolescence," *Alcohol*, vol. 44, no. 1, pp. 15–26, 2010.

[57] J. D. Grant, J. F. Scherrer, M. T. Lynskey et al., "Adolescent alcohol use is a risk factor for adult alcohol and drug dependence: evidence from a twin design," *Psychological Medicine*, vol. 36, no. 1, pp. 109–118, 2006.

[58] L. M. Squeglia, J. Jacobus, and S. F. Tapert, "The influence of substance use on adolescent brain development," *Clinical EEG and Neuroscience*, vol. 40, no. 1, pp. 31–38, 2009.

[59] P. A. Cavazos-Rehg, M. J. Krauss, E. L. Spitznagel, M. Schootman, L. B. Cottler, and L. J. Bierut, "Number of sexual partners and associations with initiation and intensity of substance use," *AIDS and Behavior*, vol. 15, no. 4, pp. 869–874, 2011.

[60] J. R. Cornelius, D. B. Clark, M. Reynolds, L. Kirisci, and R. Tarter, "Early age of first sexual intercourse and affiliation with deviant peers predict development of SUD: a prospective longitudinal study," *Addictive Behaviors*, vol. 32, no. 4, pp. 850–854, 2007.

[61] C. M. Fuller, L. N. Borrell, C. A. Latkin et al., "Effects of race, neighborhood, and social network on age at initiation of injection drug use," *American Journal of Public Health*, vol. 95, no. 4, pp. 689–695, 2005.

[62] E. F. Rothman, L. A. Wise, E. Bernstein, and J. Bernstein, "The timing of alcohol use and sexual initiation among a sample of black, hispanic, and white adolescents," *Journal of Ethnicity in Substance Abuse*, vol. 8, no. 2, pp. 129–145, 2009.

[63] B. Stanton, X. Li, L. Cottrell, and L. Kaljee, "Early initiation of sex, drug-related risk behaviors, and sensation-seeking among urban, low-income African-American adolescents," *Journal of the National Medical Association*, vol. 93, no. 4, pp. 129–138, 2001.

[64] A. Stueve and L. N. O'Donnell, "Early alcohol initiation and subsequent sexual and alcohol risk behaviors among urban youths," *American Journal of Public Health*, vol. 95, no. 5, pp. 887–893, 2005.

[65] M. Makenzius and M. Larsson, "Early onset of sexual intercourse is an indicator for hazardous lifestyle and problematic life situation," *Scandinavian Journal of Caring Sciences*, vol. 27, no. 1, pp. 20–26, 2013.

[66] P. A. Cavazos-Rehg, M. J. Krauss, E. L. Spitznagel, M. Schootman, L. B. Cottler, and L. J. Bierut, "Brief report: pregnant by age 15 years and substance use initiation among US adolescent girls," *Journal of Adolescence*, vol. 35, no. 5, pp. 1393–1397, 2012.

[67] D. D. Celentano, B. Sirirojn, C. G. Sutcliffe et al., "Sexually transmitted infections and sexual and substance use correlates among young adults in Chiang Mai, Thailand," *Sexually Transmitted Diseases*, vol. 35, no. 4, pp. 400–405, 2008.

[68] F. T. de Carvalho, L. Neiva-Silva, M. C. Ramos et al., "Sexual and drug use risk behaviors among children and youth in street circumstances in Porto Alegre, Brazil," *AIDS and Behavior*, vol. 10, supplement 1, pp. S57–S66, 2006.

[69] T. Dorjgochoo, F. Noel, M. M. Deschamps et al., "Risk factors for HIV infection among haitian adolescents and young adults seeking counseling and testing in port-au-prince," *Journal of Acquired Immune Deficiency Syndromes*, vol. 52, no. 4, pp. 498–508, 2009.

[70] P. K. Drain, J. S. Smith, J. P. Hughes, D. T. Halperin, and K. K. Holmes, "Correlates of national HIV seroprevalence: an ecologic analysis of 122 developing countries," *Journal of Acquired Immune Deficiency Syndromes*, vol. 35, no. 4, pp. 407–420, 2004.

[71] C. T. Duong, T. H. Nguyen, T. T. H. Hoang et al., "Sexual risk and bridging behaviors among young people in Hai Phong, Vietnam," *AIDS and Behavior*, vol. 12, no. 4, pp. 643–651, 2008.

[72] C. M. Fuller, D. Vlahov, A. M. Arria, D. C. Ompad, R. Garfein, and S. A. Strathdee, "Factors associated with adolescent initiation of injection drug use," *Public Health Reports*, vol. 116, supplement 1, pp. 136–145, 2001.

[73] C. Gore-Felton, A. M. Somlai, E. G. Benotsch, J. A. Kelly, D. Ostrovski, and A. Kozlov, "The influence of gender on factors associated with HIV transmission risk among young Russian injection drug users," *The American Journal of Drug and Alcohol Abuse*, vol. 29, no. 4, pp. 881–894, 2003.

[74] S. E. Hadland, T. Kerr, B. D. L. Marshall et al., "Non-Injection drug use patterns and history of injection among street youth," *European Addiction Research*, vol. 16, no. 2, pp. 91–98, 2010.

[75] T. B. Hallett, J. J. C. Lewis, B. A. Lopman et al., "Age at first sex and HIV infection in rural Zimbabwe," *Studies in Family Planning*, vol. 38, no. 1, pp. 1–10, 2007.

[76] C. Jackson, H. Sweeting, and S. Haw, "Clustering of substance use and sexual risk behaviour in adolescence: analysis of two cohort studies," *BMJ Open*, vol. 2, no. 1, Article ID e000661, 2012.

[77] C. E. Kaestle, C. T. Halpern, W. C. Miller, and C. A. Ford, "Young age at first sexual intercourse and sexually transmitted infections in adolescents and young adults," *American Journal of Epidemiology*, vol. 161, no. 8, pp. 774–780, 2005.

[78] D. B. Langille, M. Asbridge, G. Flowerdew, and M. Allen, "Associations of sexual risk-taking with having intercourse before 15 years in adolescent females in Cape Breton, Nova Scotia, Canada," *Sexual Health*, vol. 7, no. 2, pp. 199–204, 2010.

[79] A. Liu, P. Kilmarx, R. A. Jenkins et al., "Sexual initiation, substance use, and sexual behavior and knowledge among vocational students in Northern Thailand," *International Family Planning Perspectives*, vol. 32, no. 3, pp. 126–135, 2006.

[80] G. K. Medhi, J. Mahanta, R. S. Paranjape, R. Adhikary, N. Laskar, and P. Nqully, "Factors associated with HIV among female sex workers in a high HIV prevalent state of India," *AIDS Care*, vol. 24, no. 3, pp. 369–376, 2012.

[81] C. L. Miller, S. A. Strathdee, T. Kerr, K. Li, and E. Wood, "Factors associated with early adolescent initiation into injection drug use: implications for intervention programs," *The Journal of Adolescent Health*, vol. 38, no. 4, pp. 462–464, 2006.

[82] C. M. Mitchell, N. R. Whitesell, P. Spicer, J. Beals, and C. E. Kaufman, "Cumulative risk for early sexual initiation among American Indian youth: a discrete-time survival analysis," *Journal of Research on Adolescence*, vol. 17, no. 2, pp. 387–412, 2007.

[83] K. Mohammad, F. K. A. Farahani, M. R. Mohammadi et al., "Sexual risk-taking behaviors among boys aged 15–18 years in Tehran," *Journal of Adolescent Health*, vol. 41, no. 4, pp. 407–414, 2007.

[84] R. Muga, A. Sanvisens, J. M. Egea, J. Tor, and C. Rey-Joly, "Trends in human immunodeficiency virus infection among drug users in a detoxification unit," *Clinical Infectious Diseases*, vol. 37, supplement 5, pp. S404–S409, 2003.

[85] S. Nkansah-Amankra, A. Diedhiou, H. L. K. Agbanu, C. Harrod, and A. Dhawan, "Correlates of sexual risk behaviors among high school students in Colorado: analysis and implications for school-based HIV/AIDS programs," *Maternal and Child Health Journal*, vol. 15, no. 6, pp. 730–741, 2011.

[86] L. A. Novelli, S. G. Sherman, J. R. Havens, S. A. Strathdee, and M. Sapun, "Circumstances surrounding the first injection experience and their association with future syringe sharing behaviors in young urban injection drug users," *Drug and Alcohol Dependence*, vol. 77, no. 3, pp. 303–309, 2005.

[87] A. Y. Outlaw, G. Phillips, L. B. Hightow-Weidman et al., "Age of MSM sexual debut and risk factors: results from a multisite study of racial/ethnic minority YMSM living with HIV," *AIDS Patient Care and STDs*, vol. 25, no. 1, pp. S23–S29, 2011.

[88] S. Parviz, Z. Fatmi, A. Altaf et al., "Background demographics and risk behaviors of injecting drug users in Karachi, Pakistan," *International Journal of Infectious Diseases*, vol. 10, no. 5, pp. 364–371, 2006.

[89] F. Pechansky, L. Remy, H. L. Surratt et al., "Age of sexual initiation, psychiatric symptoms, and sexual risk behavior among ecstasy and LSD users in Porto Alegre, Brazil: a preliminary analysis," *Journal of Drug Issues*, vol. 41, no. 2, pp. 217–232, 2011.

[90] P. Perngmark, D. D. Celentano, and S. Kawichai, "Risk factors for HIV infection among drug injectors in southern Thailand," *Drug and Alcohol Dependence*, vol. 71, no. 3, pp. 229–238, 2003.

[91] A. Pettifor, K. O'Brien, C. MacPhail, W. C. Miller, and H. Rees, "Early coital debut and associated HIV risk factors among young women and men in South Africa," *International Perspectives on Sexual and Reproductive Health*, vol. 35, no. 2, pp. 82–90, 2009.

[92] G. J. Prado, S. J. Schwartz, M. Maldonado-Molina et al., "Ecodevelopmental x intrapersonal risk: substance use and sexual behavior in Hispanic adolescents," *Health Education and Behavior*, vol. 36, no. 1, pp. 45–61, 2009.

[93] G. A. Subramaniam and M. A. Stitzer, "Clinical characteristics of treatment-seeking prescription opioid vs. heroin-using adolescents with opioid use disorder," *Drug and Alcohol Dependence*, vol. 101, no. 1-2, pp. 13–19, 2009.

[94] R. C. Trenz, M. Scherer, P. Harrell, J. Zur, A. Sinha, and W. Latimer, "Early onset of drug and polysubstance use as predictors of injection drug use among adult drug users," *Addictive Behaviors*, vol. 37, no. 4, pp. 367–372, 2012.

[95] A. Uusküla, J. M. McMahon, M. Raag et al., "Emergent properties of HIV risk among injection drug users in Tallinn, Estonia: synthesis of individual and neighbourhood-level factors," *Sexually Transmitted Infections*, vol. 86, pp. iii79–iii84, 2010.

[96] B. Vicknasingam, S. Narayanan, and V. Navaratnam, "The relative risk of HIV among IDUs not in treatment in Malaysia," *AIDS Care*, vol. 21, no. 8, pp. 984–991, 2009.

[97] H. Wand and G. Ramjee, "The relationship between age of coital debut and HIV seroprevalence among women in Durban, South Africa: a cohort study," *BMJ Open*, vol. 2, no. 1, Article ID e000285, 2012.

[98] Y. Wang, C. Storr, D. C. Browne, and F. A. Wagner, "Early sexual experience and later onset of illegal drug use among African American students on HBCU campuses," *Substance Use and Misuse*, vol. 46, no. 4, pp. 543–551, 2011.

[99] M. Yode and T. LeGrand, "Association between age at first sexual relation and some indicators of sexual behaviour among adolescents," *African Journal of Reproductive Health*, vol. 16, no. 2, pp. 173–188, 2012.

[100] J. R. Busza, O. M. Balakireva, A. Teltschik et al., "Street-based adolescents at high risk of HIV in Ukraine," *Journal of Epidemiology and Community Health*, vol. 65, no. 12, pp. 1166–1170, 2011.

[101] B. Albert, S. Brown, and C. M. Flanigan, *14 and Younger: The Sexual Behaviors of Young Adolescents*, National Campaign to Prevent Teen Pregnancy, Washington, DC, USA, 2003.

[102] L. Degenhardt, W. T. Chiu, K. Conway et al., "Does the gateway matter? Associations between the order of drug use initiation and the development of drug dependence in the national comorbidity study replication," *Psychological Medicine*, vol. 39, no. 1, pp. 157–167, 2009.

[103] K. Peltzer, "Early sexual debut and associated factors among in-school adolescents in eight African countries," *Acta Paediatrica*, vol. 99, no. 8, pp. 1242–1247, 2010.

[104] A. K. Turner, C. Latkin, F. Sonenstein, and S. D. Tandon, "Psychiatric disorder symptoms, substance use, and sexual risk behavior among African-American out of school youth," *Drug and Alcohol Dependence*, vol. 115, no. 1-2, pp. 67–73, 2011.

[105] S. F. Tapert, G. A. Aarons, G. R. Sedlar, and S. A. Brown, "Adolescent substance use and sexual risk-taking behavior," *Journal of Adolescent Health*, vol. 28, no. 3, pp. 181–189, 2001.

[106] C. J. Sullivan, K. K. Childs, and D. O'Connell, "Adolescent risk behavior subgroups: an empirical assessment," *Journal of Youth and Adolescence*, vol. 39, no. 5, pp. 541–562, 2010.

[107] W. Udell, T. Sandfort, E. Reitz, H. Bos, and M. Dekovic, "The relationship between early sexual debut and psychosocial outcomes: a longitudinal study of dutch adolescents," *Archives of Sexual Behavior*, vol. 39, no. 5, pp. 1133–1145, 2010.

[108] K. Edgardh, "Sexual behaviour and early coitarche in a national sample of 17 year old Swedish girls," *Sexually Transmitted Infections*, vol. 76, no. 2, pp. 98–102, 2000.

Predictors of Adherence to Antiretroviral Therapy among HIV/AIDS Patients in the Upper West Region of Ghana

Christian Obirikorang,[1] Peter Kuugemah Selleh,[2] Jubilant Kwame Abledu,[3] and Chris Opoku Fofie[4]

[1] *Department of Molecular Medicine, School of Medical Sciences, College of Health Sciences, Kwame Nkrumah University of Science and Technology (KNUST), Kumasi, Ghana*
[2] *Department of Medical Laboratory Technology, Faculty of Allied Health, College of Health Sciences, Kwame Nkrumah University of Science and Technology (KNUST), Kumasi, Ghana*
[3] *School of Veterinary Medicine, University of Ghana, Legon, Ghana*
[4] *Ghana Health Service, Upper West Regional Hospital, Wa, Upper West Region, Ghana*

Correspondence should be addressed to Christian Obirikorang; krisobiri@yahoo.com

Academic Editors: R. Ansari and V. C. Bond

Background. The effectiveness of ART interventions is only realized in maximal levels of adherence. A near perfect adherence level of >95% is required for the effective suppression of HIV/AIDS virus. The main objective of this study was to identify the sociodemographic and socioeconomic factors that facilitate adherence to antiretroviral therapy among HIV/AIDS patients. *Methods.* This descriptive cross-sectional study was conducted between March and May 2013 at the Upper West Regional Hospital, Wa. A total of 201 confirmed HIV 1 seropositive subjects (mean age 36.6±9.9 years) receiving antiretroviral therapy were interviewed using a structured questionnaire. The collected data was analyzed using GraphPad Prism version 5. A P value of <0.05 was considered statistically significant for all statistical analyses. *Results.* Overall lifetime adherence was found to be 62.2% while medication adherence in the last six months, last three months, last month, and last week were 73.6%, 87.1%, 91.0%, and 86.0%, respectively. The study revealed a positive association between adherence to ART and immunological success, with nonadherence increasing the risk (OR (95% CI): 9.2 (3.2–26.9)) of immunological failure. Univariate logistic regression analysis of the data showed that other ailments and side effects of drug were negatively associated with adherence to ART whereas self-perceived wellness, family support, and regular followup were positively associated with adherence to ART. *Conclusion.* Regular attendance at followup and family support are vital factors for 100% lifetime medication adherence. Effective counseling sessions on adherence for patients on antiretroviral therapy are paramount for the realization of the purpose of antiretroviral therapy programmes in Ghana.

1. Introduction

The effect of HIV infection at the individual level is the continued breakdown of the immune system of the host which ultimately results in the onset of AIDS. All infected persons are at risk of illness and death from opportunistic infections and neoplastic complications [1]. Infection to noninfected individuals with HIV occurs mainly through the exposure to biological fluids, especially semen and blood, of the infected individuals. Globally, the principal route of transmission is unprotected heterosexual intercourse (>75%). This accounts for the increasing number of women being affected worldwide. Homosexual intercourse is the second commonest route of transmission [2].

Sub-Saharan Africa bears the greatest burden with more than two-thirds (68%) of all persons infected with HIV. An estimated 1.8 million adults and children became infected with the disease in Sub-Saharan Africa. It is recorded that out of 260,000 child deaths that occurred globally from HIV/AIDS in 2009, 88% occurred in Sub-Saharan Africa [3].

The HIV/AIDS epidemic in Ghana continues to be a generalized epidemic with a prevalence of more than 1% in the general population. Promising developments have been seen in recent years in global efforts to address the AIDS epidemic, including increased access to effective treatment and prevention programmes [4].

The number of HIV patients receiving ART in Ghana increased more than 200-fold from 197 in 2003 to over 45,000 in 2010. Some regions report ART enrollment lower than their percent share of number of HIV infected persons in the country [5]. The world Health Organization recommendations on the use of ART in resource-limited settings recognize the critical role of adherence in order to achieve clinical and pragmatic success. Good adherence to ART is necessary to achieve the best antivirological response, lower the risk that drug resistance will develop, and reduce morbidity [6].

Combination therapies of ARV drugs are the treatment of choice in HIV, and nonadherence is a major, if not the most important, factor in treatment failure and the development of resistance. 100% medication adherence is paramount for the effective management of HIV [2] and provision of free treatment without adequate patient preparation and adherence support may compromise the success of ART scale-up programmes [7]. A major concern with scaling up of antiretroviral therapy (ART) in resource-limited settings is the emergence of drug resistant viral strains due to suboptimal adherence and the transmission of these resistant viral strains in the population [7].

In view of the changing trend in prevalence of HIV in Ghana and the lack of data surrounding medication adherence in this population, this study therefore proposed to assess the level of and validate (using CD4 results) self-reported adherence and its predictors among patients attending the HIV Clinic of Upper West Regional Hospital, Wa.

2. Materials and Methods

This descriptive cross-sectional study was conducted at the Upper West Regional Hospital situated in the southern part of the capital Wa. It is the only specialized referral hospital in the region and the HIV unit currently provides service to over 1600 registered HIV/AIDS patients on antiretroviral drugs. The study was conducted between the months of March and May 2013. A total of two hundred and one (201) confirmed HIV 1 seropositive subjects receiving antiretroviral therapy were interviewed using a structured questionnaire with both open and close ended questions. Primary data was also obtained from their medical records after obtaining permission from the health facility administrators and consent from patients. The Committee on Human Research, Publications and Ethics, School of Medical Sciences, Kwame Nkrumah University of Science and Technology, gave ethical approval for the study to be conducted. Confidentiality, anonymity, and privacy were guaranteed.

2.1. Data Collection. A structured questionnaire which was developed from different literatures was used for the data collection. The dependent variable was adherence to highly active antiretroviral therapy (HAART) among PLWHA. The independent variables were sociodemographic (age, sex, weight, level of education, occupation, marital status, and family type), socioeconomic variables (income), psychosocial (social support, active substance and alcohol use, disclosure of HIV serostatus, and perception of well-being), disease characteristics (duration of HIV infection), regimen related variables (types of ART, dietary related demands/restriction, and side effect), CD4 at diagnosis and current value, followups, adherence to treatment information and symptoms associated with treatment.

Many researchers who have conducted studies in this area found that there is no existing gold standard by which adherence can be quantified and many predictors have been reported to influence it. The study therefore chose five measurement tools to quantify adherence from self-recalled report data collected from participants at exit face-to-face interviews:

(A) lifetime self-recall adherence,

(B) last 6 months' self-recall adherence,

(C) last 3 months' self-recall adherence,

(D) last month's self-recall adherence,

(E) last week's self-recall adherence.

Participants were asked if they had ever missed medication in their lifetime beginning from the time s/he was put on antiretroviral therapy. Self-reported adherence was classified as "adherent" when not a single dose was missed or non-adherent if the patient admitted having missed at least one dose. They were asked about adherence to medication since initiation of ART as listed above. This means that patients' memory of medicine intake was likely to be good.

However, in such face-to-face interviews patients might feel ashamed to report missed medications. Hence participants were assured of confidentiality for their response and they were made aware that, even though medically precarious, every individual could miss medication for one reason or the other.

2.2. Data Management and Analysis. Data collected was sorted, coded, and entered into an Excel spreadsheet for analysis using GraphPad Prism for Windows version 5.0 (GraphPad Software, San Diego, CA, USA). Descriptive statistics such as mean, frequencies, and percentages were used to summarize the data. Overall lifetime adherence to medication was determined from the data and predictors determined. Analysis of contingency tables was done and Fisher's exact test and the chi-square test were used where necessary to compare proportions. Logistic regression analysis was used to determine the relationships between adherence and other variables (level of significance, $P < 0.05$).

3. Results

The cross-sectional study included 201 individuals diagnosed with HIV, who had since been receiving ART at the Regional Hospital at Wa in the Upper West Region of Ghana between 2003 and 2012. The patients' demographic and clinical data are presented in Tables 1 and 2. The age range of patients was 20–74 years with the mean ± standard deviation of the age

TABLE 1: Patient demographics relative to medication adherence.

Parameter	Total (%)	No (%)	Yes (%)	P value
Missed medications in lifetime				
Ever missed medications since starting ART	201 (100)	125 (62.2)	76 (37.8)	
Missed medications in the last 6 months	201 (100)	148 (73.6)	53 (26.4)	
Missed medications in the last 3 months	201 (100)	175 (87.1)	26 (12.9)	
Missed medications in the last month	201 (100)	183 (91.0)	18 (9.0)	
Missed medications in the last week	201 (100)	172 (86.0)	28 (14.0)	
Age				
20–30	64 (32.5)	38 (59.4)	26 (40.6)	
31–40	83 (42.1)	53 (63.9)	30 (36.1)	0.3401
>40	50 (25.4)	34 (68.0)	16 (32.0)	
Sex				
Male	42 (20.9)	24 (57.1)	18 (42.9)	0.4774
Female	159 (79.1)	101 (63.5)	58 (36.5)	
Marital status				
Married	105 (52.2)	62 (59.0)	43 (41.0)	
Widowed	45 (22.4)	28 (62.2)	17 (37.8)	0.7060
Divorced	30 (14.9)	21 (70.0)	9 (30.0)	
Single	21 (10.4)	14 (66.7)	7 (33.3)	
Education				
No education	102 (50.7)	62 (60.8)	40 (39.2)	
Primary	31 (15.4)	21 (67.4)	10 (32.3)	
JHS/middle school	49 (24.4)	30 (61.2)	19 (38.8)	0.7223
SHS	10 (5.0)	5 (50.0)	5 (50.0)	
Tertiary	9 (4.5)	7 (77.8)	2 (22.2)	
Family type				
Nuclear	106 (52.7)	59 (55.7)	47 (44.3)	
Extended	67 (33.3)	46 (68.7)	21 (31.3)	0.1268
Living alone	28 (13.9)	20 (71.4)	8 (28.6)	
Monthly income				
≤100	104 (92.0)	71 (68.3)	33 (31.7)	
101–500	7 (6.2)	5 (71.4)	2 (28.6)	0.6238
>500	2 (1.8)	2 (100.0)	0 (0.0)	
Time since ART (years)				
<1	7 (3.5)	1 (14.3)	6 (85.7)	
1–4	163 (81.1)	66 (40.5)	97 (58.4)	0.2058
5+	31 (15.4)	9 (29.0)	22 (71.0)	
Time since diagnosis (years)				
<1	3 (1.5)	0 (0.0)	3 (100.0)	
1–4	158 (78.6)	62 (39.2)	96 (60.8)	0.3507
5+	40 (19.9)	14 (35.0)	26 (65.0)	
Immunological success				
Yes	96 (78.7)	66 (68.8)	30 (31.3)	**0.001***
No*	26 (21.3)	5 (19.2)	21 (80.8)	

Data are presented as proportions. Proportions are compared using Fisher's exact test and the chi-square test where applicable. *(OR: 9.2; 95% CI: 3.2–26.9).

being 36.6 ± 9.9 years. The males (42.3 ± 11.0 years) were significantly older ($P < 0.0001$) than the females (35.1 ± 9.0 years) although the latter constituted the majority (79.1%) of the population. Whereas only 4.5% had attained higher (tertiary) education, 52.2% were married and as many as 52.7% were living with their nuclear family. Monthly income not exceeding GH¢ 100.00 was earned by as many as 92.0% of the patients.

Most patients (80.1%) were diagnosed during the last four years (i.e., 2008–2012), with 158 patients attending regular followup, that is, attending greater than 90% of 3 monthly appointments. The overall lifetime medication adherence

TABLE 2: Patient antiretroviral therapy and disease characteristics.

Parameter	Frequency/percentage
CD4 at diagnosis (cells/mm^3)	
<100	26 (15.1)
101–200	35 (20.3)
201–300	56 (32.6)
>300	55 (32.0)
Current ART regimen	
Nevirapine based	84 (41.8)
Efavirenz based	66 (32.8)
Nevirapine based + septrin	30 (14.9)
Efavirenz based + septrin	17 (8.5)
Septrin	4 (2.0)
Current CD4 (cells/mm^3)	
<100	1 (0.6)
101–200	4 (2.4)
201–300	21 (12.5)
>300	142 (84.5)
Reason for missing ART	
Forgetfulness	35 (46.1)
No food to take with	7 (9.2)
Away from home	12 (15.8)
Felt sick	2 (2.6)
Busy	3 (3.9)
Run out of drugs	32 (42.1)

Data are presented as frequency and percentage. Data may not add up to 201 due to missing data.

(i.e., taking all medications everyday as prescribed) since initiating ART was found to be 62.2% (n = 125). Of the respondents who had participated in the study, as many as 73.6%, 87.1%, 91.0%, and 86.0% had adhered to medication in the last six months, last three months, last month, and last week, respectively (Table 1).

Of those who enumerated reasons for missing ART, 46.1% attributed it to forgetfulness and 7.2% said they had no food, among other reasons as shown in Table 2. The median rise in CD4 cell count from baseline to now was 119 cells/mm^3, with a proportion of 21.3% meeting the criteria for immunological failure (i.e., a drop in CD4 cell count to pretreatment levels or <100 cells/mm^3) (Table 1). Besides that, about 15.1% of subjects had a CD4 count of <100 cells/mm^3 at diagnosis and 0.6% had a current CD4 count of <100 cells/mm^3.

All except four subjects were on NNRTI and NRTI or in combination with septrin prophylaxis. The four exceptional subjects were on septrin prophylaxis only. As many as 41.8% were on nevirapine-based combination therapy and 32.8% on efavirenz-based combination therapy as shown in Table 2.

Univariate analysis of individual patient factors associated with medication adherence is recorded in Table 3. Gender, education, marital status, type of family, disclosure of status to other persons, time since diagnosis was made, time since ART was initiated, perceived difficulty of drug regimen, and food restrictions were not associated ($P > 0.05$) with medication adherence. Although not statistically significant, positive trends for medication adherence were seen for increasing age ($P = 0.3401$) and monthly income ($P = 0.6238$). However, as shown in the univariate analysis (Table 3), regular followup (OR: 10.4; CI: 4.6–23.6; $P < 0.0001$), perceiving oneself as very healthy (OR: 9.0; CI: 3.4–23.9; $P < 0.0001$), and family support (OR: 1.9; CI: 1.1–3.5; $P = 0.0401$) were the most significant positive factors associated with increased medication adherence. On the other hand, adherence to medication was significantly reduced in patients who suffered other ailments (OR: 0.2; CI: 0.1–0.5; $P = 0.0004$) and those who suffered side effects of drug (OR: 0.2; CI: 0.1–0.4; $P < 0.0001$). Some of the patients perceived their ART regimen as simple (n = 94) and moderate (n = 100). Although self-perceived well-being was generally high (normal (n = 143) and very healthy (n = 54)), 17.4% of patients reported having side effects of the drugs, 14.4% presented with some other ailments, whilst about 91.5% were currently placed on food/substance restriction. Also, some participants (79.0%) reported having disclosed their HIV status to at least one person and 69.2% were satisfied by their family support.

To construct a predictive model of the determinants of adherence, the significant independent factors were entered simultaneously into a multivariate logistic regression model. The results are presented in Table 3. All other factors but family support (OR: 0.9; CI: 0.40–1.97; $P = 0.7683$) retained their significance. In this adjusted model, patients who suffered other ailments (OR: 0.3; CI: 0.10–0.81; $P = 0.0178$) improved slightly on adherence to medication although the association maintained its negativity; side effects of drug (OR: 0.2; CI: 0.1–0.6; $P = 0.0016$) maintained a constant negative association with adherence as was in the univariate analysis, while regular followups (OR: 6.9; CI: 2.8–17.0; $P < 0.0001$) and perceiving oneself as very healthy (OR: 4.2; CI: 1.5–12.1; $P = 0.0078$) slightly decrease adherence (as compared to the univariate analysis) albeit maintaining their positive association with medication adherence.

Figure 1 shows the adherence levels based on patient's ART combinations. With the exception of few respondents who were taking septrin alone (2.0%), all other participants were taking the three combinations of ART from the nucleotide and nucleoside reverse transcriptase inhibitors and the nonnucleoside reverse transcriptase inhibitors classes. The majority of the respondents (25.9%) were taking stavudine (d4t)/lamivudine (3TC)/nevirapine (NVP) combination. Figure 1 presents the adherence pattern based on the different combinations of ART the respondents were taking. The majority of nonadherent participants were on efavirenz based combination therapy and most adhering respondents were on nevirapine-based combination therapy. Patients taking a combination of efavirenz and septrin had comparatively reduced adherence as compare to those on efavirenz only.

4. Discussion

Antiretroviral therapy adherence levels of ≥95% optimize outcomes and minimize viral resistance [6]. The overall lifetime adherence (i.e., taking all medications everyday as prescribed and abiding by the food/substance restrictions) since

TABLE 3: Logistic regression of patient characteristics associated with medication adherence.

Characteristic	Total	Nonadherent	Adherent	OR (95% CI)	P value	aOR (95% CI)	P value
Food restriction							
Yes	183 (91.5)	71 (38.8)	112 (61.2)	0.7 (0.2–1.9)	0.3896		
Other ailments							
Yes	29 (14.4)	20 (69.0)	9 (31.0)	0.2 (0.1–0.5)	**0.0004**	0.3 (0.1–0.8)	**0.0178**
No*	167 (85.2)	54 (32.3)	113 (67.7)	1		1	
Side effects							
Yes	35 (17.4)	26 (74.2)	9 (25.7)	0.2 (0.1–0.4)	**<0.0001**	0.2 (0.1–0.6)	**0.0016**
No*	166 (82.6)	50 (30.1)	116 (69.9)	1		1	
Perceived difficulty of drug regimen							
Simple*	94 (46.8)	41 (43.6)	53 (56.4)	1			
Moderate	100 (49.8)	31 (31.0)	69 (69.0)	1.7 (1.0–3.1)	0.0701		
Difficult	7 (3.4)	4 (57.1)	3 (42.9)	0.6 (0.1–2.7)	0.4916		
Perceived well-being							
Normal*	143 (71.5)	69 (48.3)	74 (51.7)	1		1	
Very healthy	54 (27.0)	5 (9.3)	49 (90.7)	9.0 (3.4–23.9)	**<0.0001**	4.2 (1.5–12.1)	**0.0078**
Sick	3 (1.5)	2 (66.7)	1 (33.3)	0.5 (0.1–5.2)	0.5299		
Disclosure							
Yes	158 (79.0)	63 (39.9)	95 (60.1)	1.5 (0.7–3.1)	0.2915		
No*	42 (21.0)	13 (31.0)	29 (69.0)	1			
Family support							
Yes	139 (69.2)	46 (33.1)	93 (66.9)	1.9 (1.1–3.5)	**0.0401**	0.9 (0.4–2.0)	**0.7683**
No*	62 (30.8)	30 (48.4)	32 (51.6)	1		1	
Followup							
Regular	158 (78.6)	42 (26.6)	116 (73.4)	10.4 (4.6–23.6)	**<0.0001**	6.9 (2.8–17.0)	**<0.0001**
Irregular*	43 (21.4)	34 (79.1)	9 (20.9)	1		1	

*Reference. Data are presented as proportions. Regular followup implies more than 90% attendance at 3 monthly appointments. OR: odds ratio, aOR: adjusted odds ratio, CI: confidence interval. Data may not add up to 201 due to missing data. Other ailments (0: no; 1: yes); perception of well-being (1: normal; 2: very healthy; 3: sick); side effects (0: no; 1: yes); support from family (0: no; 1: yes); followup (0: irregular; 1: regular-0) Perceived difficulty of drug regimen (simple: 1; moderate: 2; difficult: 3) Disclosure (yes: 1; no: 0).

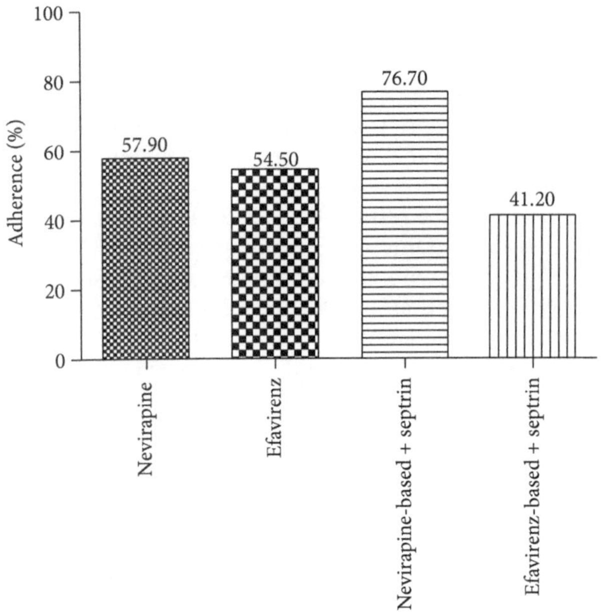

FIGURE 1: Adherence levels based on patient's antiretroviral therapy combinations.

initiating ART therapy was found to be suboptimal (62.2%). This adherence level is similar to a study report in Bangalore, India [2], where overall lifetime adherence was 60.4%. On the other hand, high proportions of the study respondents had not missed medication in the last three months, last month and last week (87.1%, 91.0%, and 86%, resp.). The overall lifetime adherence level of the present study is higher than the adherence level in the developed countries (55%), as shown in a meta-analysis of adherence to ART in both developed and developing countries [8]. The many study reviews conducted in this field in Africa revealed an adherence level similar or higher than the adherence level in the developed countries. This review finding is against the initial fears raised prior to ART initiation in the African continent and has shown that a higher adherence level can be achieved in Africa despite limited resources.

There are concerns that patients on ART have the tendency to be nonadherent once they feel physically better [9]. The current study however revealed, on the contrary, that respondents with high perception of well being were more adherent to ART therapy. This could be due to respondents' realization of the usefulness of the medication and the fact that they were heeding the counseling instructions offered prior to ART initiation. This deduction is buttressed by a study conducted by Mills et al. [8] on "Meta-analysis of ART adherence in both developed and developing countries." There was no significant relationship ($P > 0.05$) in levels of adherence in relation to the duration a patient had been taking ART as well as food/substance restriction as shown in Tables 1 and 3, respectively.

In univariate analysis, regular followup, family support, and perception of well being were positively associated with adherence to medication as shown in Table 3. Traditionally, before the infiltration of Western culture, Africans were identified by the extended family system which has its own benefits and demerits. The results of our study show no statistically significant relationship between family type and adherence to antiretroviral therapy. However patients who had family support adhered to the antiretroviral therapy ($P = 0.0401$). This is consistent with a study report from Southwest Ethiopia where participants who had family support were two times more likely to adhere than respondents on the other side of the coin [10]. This study finding is also in support of study review findings in Kenya where family support was characteristic of patients who achieved optimal adherence [6].

The majority of patients (79%) in our study had disclosed their status to at least one relative, a reflection that the study site is complying with the national guidelines for managing HIV/AIDS patients on ART. Besides that, about 69.2% of study participants reported they had support from family members in the form of emotional/psychological, physical, and food provision. These could be the promoters of optimal adherence among these participants as family members could remind them to take the ART, give comfort, and provide food to take ART with. The findings of this study suggest that a poor psychological state could be associated with poor adherence. Other studies have also shown a significant association between poor psychological states and nonadherence [11].

Moreover, regular followup is another positive predictor of adherence to ART per the results of our study ($P < 0.0001$). This finding is consistent with the numerous studies from both developed and developing countries [2, 8]. Of those who reported regular followup, 73.4% were adherent. This could be due to constant counseling, patients being able to express concerns about medication and their health, and receiving medications thus avoiding running out of drugs.

The study results demonstrated positive correlation between adherence to ART and immunological success; nonadherent subjects were nine times (OR (95% CI): 9.2 (3.2–26.9)) at risk of progressing to immunological failure (that is, a drop in CD4 cell count to pretreatment value or <100 cells/mm^3 whilst on treatment for a period of time) compared to their adherent counterparts as depicted in Table 1. This immunological finding indicates that body systems of respondents in this category responded positively to the ARV. A greater proportion of these participants also had good perception of well-being. This finding is similar to a study report from the resource-limited setting of Southwest Ethiopia [10]. Our study revealed that about 21.3% of respondents met the criterion for immunological failure where most of these persons constituted the nonadherent group of this study. Our study found no statistically significant relationship between gender and adherence to ART. However, females constituted a greater proportion (79.1%) of the study participants; "this is a reflection of the gender distribution of HIV/AIDS" in Ghana as revealed by other studies [12]. It can be argued that females are more aware of their status and have access to ART therapy. This is consistent with study reports from most resource-limited settings like the neighboring Togo where out of 99 participants in a study, 76.8% were females [13].

The majority of the participants who did not adhere to ART provided varied motives for their defaults. A large proportion (46.1%) of people in this subset cited forgetfulness as reasons for missing therapy and 42.1% said they missed medication due to the fact that they ran out of drugs. Of those who did not adhere, 9.2% said they had no food to take with the drug and 15.8% said they were away from home as reasons for missing ART treatment. These findings were similar to works done in South West Ethiopia [10], India [7], Kenya [6], Zambia [14], and South Africa [11].

Some of the respondents (14.8%) suffered other ailments and adherence to ART was significantly reduced in this category of respondents. The most common ailments mentioned were coughing, hernia, diabetes, high blood pressure, chest pains, ulcer, rashes, general weakness, and skin itching. Our study found that adherence was negatively affected ($P < 0.001$) in respondents who suffered side effects of the drugs (17.4%). This finding is consistent with the study report by [13].

All study participants were on the standard first-line regimen proposed by WHO (2NRTI+1NNRTI) and all patients were managed on the three combinations as found in other study reports in Africa [12, 13]. The study found no significant relationship between type of ART combination and adherence although the majority of nonadherent participants were on efavirenz based combination therapy. Some of HIV/AIDS patients on ART experience side effects. However, side effects were cited by most respondents on efavirenz-based combination therapy. Almost all participants on efavirenz-based combination therapy in this class cited sleepiness and/or dizziness as side effects experienced. Other side effects mentioned by participants include headache, cold, general weakness, and excessive urination. Adherence to ART was negatively affected in these patients who experienced side effects. They skipped medication to avoid side effects and this could explain why the majority of nonadherent participants in this study are those on efavirenz-based combination therapy. This outcome is consistent with studies done in other African countries [6, 10].

5. Conclusion

The findings of the study show that the lifetime adherence was suboptimal. Factors such as regular followup and psychological and physical support were found to be positive promoters of ART adherence. However, other ailments and side effects of the drugs had a negative association with adherence to ART.

Conflict of Interests

The authors declare that they have no conflict of interests.

Authors' Contribution

Christian Obirikorang contributed to the conception of the research idea, designing, data analysis, and paper drafting, Chris Opoku Fofie designed the research and provided critical revision of the paper, and Peter Kuugemah Selleh contributed to collection of data, data analysis, interpretation, and paper drafting. Jubilant Kwame Abledu contributed to data analysis, interpretation and paper reviewing.

Acknowledgments

The authors wish to express their profound gratitude to all the staff and HIV clients at the HIV Clinic at the Upper West Regional Hospital who voluntarily participated in the research.

References

[1] A. R. Moss and P. Bacchetti, "Natural history of HIV infection," *AIDS*, vol. 3, no. 2, pp. 55–61, 1989.

[2] M. B. Cauldbeck, C. O'Connor, M. B. O'Connor et al., "Adherence to anti-retroviral therapy among HIV patients in Bangalore, India," *AIDS Research and Therapy*, vol. 6, article 7, 2009.

[3] UNAIDS, "Report on the Global AIDS Epidemic," Tech. Rep., UNAIDS, 2010.

[4] NACP, "HIV sentinel survey report," Tech. Rep., Ministry of Health, 2010.

[5] P. Dako-Gyeke, R. Snow, and A. E. Yawson, "Who is utilizing anti-retroviral therapy in Ghana: an analysis of ART service utilization," *International Journal for Equity in Health*, vol. 11, article 62, 2012.

[6] A. Nyambura, "Factors that influence adherence to ART among HIV/AIDS patients in central province, Kenya," 2009, http://ir-library.ku.ac.ke/handle/123456789/1725.

[7] A. Sarna, S. Pujari, A. K. Sengar, R. Garg, I. Gupta, and J. van Dam, "Adherence to antiretroviral therapy & its determinants amongst HIV patients in India," *Indian Journal of Medical Research*, vol. 127, no. 1, pp. 28–36, 2008.

[8] E. J. Mills, J. B. Nachega, D. R. Bangsberg et al., "Adherence to HAART: a systematic review of developed and developing nation patient-reported barriers and facilitators," *PLoS Medicine*, vol. 3, no. 11, article e438, 2006.

[9] B. Achappa, D. Madi, U. Bhaskaran, J. T. Ramapuram, S. Rao, and S. Mahalingam, "Adherence to antiretroviral therapy among people living with HIV," *North American Journal of Medical Sciences*, vol. 5, no. 3, pp. 220–223, 2013.

[10] A. Tiyou, T. Belachew, F. Alemseged, and S. Biadgilign, "Predictors of adherence to antiretroviral therapy among people living with HIV/AIDS in resource-limited setting of southwest ethiopia," *AIDS Research and Therapy*, vol. 7, article 39, 2010.

[11] N. O. Chabikuli, D. O. Datonye, J. Nachega, and D. Ansong, "Adherence to antiretroviral therapy, virologic failure and workload at the Rustenburg Provincial Hospital," *South African Family Practice*, vol. 52, no. 4, pp. 350–355, 2010.

[12] S. Ohene and E. Forson, "Care of patients on anti-retroviral therapy in kumasi metropolis," *Ghana Medical Journal*, vol. 43, no. 4, pp. 144–149, 2009.

[13] Y. Potchoo, K. Tchamdja, A. Balogou, V. P. Pitche, I. P. Guissou, and E. K. Kassang, "Knowledge and adherence to antiretroviral therapy among adult people living with HIV/AIDS treated in the health care centers of the association "Espoir Vie Togo" in Togo, West Africa," *BMC Clinical Pharmacology*, vol. 10, article 11, 2010.

[14] S. Chishimba and F. Zulu, "The 3×5 HIV and AIDS treatment plan, challenges for developing countries from zambian perspective," in *Proceedings of the International Conference of AIDS*, vol. 15, 2004.

Improvements in Immune Function and Activation with 48-Week Darunavir/Ritonavir-Based Therapy: GRACE Substudy

Christos Tsoukas,[1] Louise Gilbert,[2] Trevor Lewis,[1] George Hatzakis,[3] Ron Falcon,[4] and Joseph Mrus[4]

[1] *Department of Microbiology and Immunology, McGill University Health Centre, Room A5-140, 1650 Cedar Avenue, Montreal, QC, Canada H3G 1A4*
[2] *Montreal General Hospital, Flowcytometry Laboratory, 1650 Cedar Avenue, Room C10-166, Montreal, QC, Canada H3G 1A4*
[3] *LAC+USC Medical Center, 1200 N State Street, Room IPT-C4E100, Los Angeles, CA 90033, USA*
[4] *Janssen Services, LLC, Clinical Affairs, 1125 Trenton-Harbourton Road, Titusville, NJ 08560, USA*

Correspondence should be addressed to Christos Tsoukas; chris.tsoukas@muhc.mcgill.ca

Academic Editors: G. D'ettorre and C. Petrovas

Objective. During the course of HIV infection, progressive immune deficiency occurs. The aim of this prospective substudy was to evaluate the recovery of functional immunity in a subset of patients from the GRACE (Gender, Race, And Clinical Experience) study treated with a DRV/r-based regimen. *Methods*. The recovery of functional immunity with a darunavir/ritonavir-based regimen was assessed in a subset of treatment-experienced, HIV-1 infected patients from the GRACE study. *Results*. 19/32 patients (59%) enrolled in the substudy were virologically suppressed (<50 copies/mL). In these patients, median (range) CD4+ cell count increased from 222 (2, 398) cells/mm^3 at baseline to 398 (119, 812) cells/mm^3 at Week 48. CD8+% decreased significantly from baseline to Week 48 ($P = .03$). Proliferation of CD4+ lymphocytes in response to CD3+/CD28+, phytohemagglutinin, and pokeweed was significantly increased ($P < .01$) by Week 12. Proliferation in response to *Candida* and tetanus was significantly increased by Week 48 ($P < .01$ and $P = .014$, resp.). Staphylococcal enterotoxin B-stimulated tumor necrosis factor-alpha and interleukin-2 in CD4+ cells was significantly increased by Week 12 ($P = .046$) and Week 48 ($P < .01$), respectively. *Conclusions*. Darunavir/ritonavir-based therapy demonstrated improvements in CD4+ cell recovery and association with progressive functional immune recovery over 48 weeks. This trial is registered with NCT00381303.

1. Introduction

During the course of HIV-1 infection, multifactorial T-lymphocyte (T-cell)-mediated mechanisms contribute to the progressive loss of host immune function [1–5]. In infected individuals, immune dysregulation occurs early and is characterized by a decrease in CD4+ cell count, a concurrent rise in CD8+ cells, a progressive decline in the CD4+/CD8+ ratio, and defective thymocyte proliferation [6]. During late-stage disease, loss of T-cell homeostasis also occurs [7, 8].

T cells are chronically activated throughout the course of HIV infection, as indicated by an increase in the expression of the antigens Ki67, CD38, and human leukocyte antigen (HLA)-DR, with CD38 recognized as the most reliable marker of immune activation [1–3, 5, 9]. Immune activation provides the virus with a steady pool of target cells and has been linked with increased polyclonal T-cell proliferation and turnover, as well as increases in the apoptotic marker CD95 [10–13] and activation-induced cell death [12, 14–16].

Concomitant with the decline of CD4 cells in the peripheral blood, the frequency of the CD4+ CD28 null subset increases with disease progression and eventual progression to AIDS [10]. The presence of CD28 on T cells is critically important for the generation of T-cell responses. Interaction of this costimulatory molecule with its ligands increases the expression of antiapoptotic proteins and improves interleukin (IL)-2 production. The increase in circulation of T cells with a CD4+ CD28 null phenotype is consistent with a process known as replicative senescence [11, 13, 17–19]. T cells that lack CD28 surface expression are nonanergic, oligoclonally expanded, and terminally differentiated, with limited replicative capacity and increased sensitivity to apoptosis [20, 21]. These alterations in phenotype are accompanied by cytokine changes consistent with a chronic proinflammatory state. The failure to produce adequate amounts of IL-2 leads to a marked functional impairment of cellular and humoral immunity. Reduced IL-2 expression has been associated with a shift from Th1 cytokine responses to Th2 cytokine responses. It has been postulated that the Th1/Th2 imbalance may result in cellular immunity deficiency [4].

The dysregulation of cytokine secretion during the course of HIV infection has been examined using a wide range of methods, including enzyme-linked immunosorbent assay, reverse transcriptase-polymerase chain reaction, T-cell cloning, and, more recently, flow cytometric intracellular cytokine detection [4]. Of these methods, only flow cytometry allows quantitative and qualitative determination of cytokine expression patterns in individual T cells [4].

Successful antiretroviral (ARV) therapy results in improvements in circulating CD4+ T-cell levels with decreases in CD8+ counts and declines in immune activation and CD95 expression [1–5, 7, 9, 22–26]. Limited data on replicative senescence suggest a lack of significant improvement in the short term, despite adequate HIV suppression [10]. Some studies have suggested that protease inhibitor- (PI-) based regimens may have a greater effect on CD4+ count recovery than nonnucleoside reverse transcriptase inhibitor-based regimens [27, 28]. Some of the previous studies on immune recovery with ARV therapy have been cross-sectional in design, conducted primarily in white males, and focused on absolute CD4+ count or CD4+% recovery. Furthermore, most of these studies did not comprehensively assess the functional aspects of immune recovery [29]. Of the studies that did evaluate the influence of ARV therapy on functional immune parameters, most were drug class specific [30–32].

GRACE (Gender, Race, And Clinical Experience) is the largest ARV trial to focus on women with HIV-1 in North America and was designed to assess sex-based and race-based differences in efficacy, safety, and tolerability of the PI darunavir with low-dose ritonavir (DRV/r) plus an optimized background regimen over 48 weeks in a diverse, treatment-experienced patient population [33]. The aim of this prospective substudy was to quantitatively and qualitatively evaluate the recovery of functional immunity (T-cell function) with a DRV/r-based regimen in a subset of patients from the GRACE study.

2. Materials and Methods

2.1. Study Design and Patients. GRACE was a multicenter, open-label, single-arm, Phase IIIb study conducted at 65 sites across USA, Puerto Rico, and Canada that enrolled 429 treatment-experienced patients (viral load ≥ 1000 HIV-1 RNA copies/mL) aged at least 18 years with documented HIV-1 infection [33]. Full inclusion and exclusion criteria and the study flow diagram have been reported [33]. Patients received DRV/r 600/100 mg twice daily plus an investigator-selected background regimen that could include etravirine. Patients at participating GRACE study sites were eligible for the prospective immunology substudy, which aimed to enroll up to 100 subjects. A group of healthy, HIV seronegative volunteers were included for comparison.

2.2. Ethics Statement. The research has complied with all federal guidelines and institutional policies. All subjects were required to sign a separate, Independent Ethics Committee/Institutional Review Board (IRB) informed consent form specific to this substudy. The IRBs were Quorom Review Inc., Seattle, WA, Office of Human Research Ethics—UNC IRB, Chapel Hill, NC, and AIDS Research Consortium of Atlanta, Atlanta, GA. Each IRB approved of this study. The study was conducted in accordance with the principles of the Declaration of Helsinki and followed Good Clinical Practice guidelines.

2.3. Study Evaluations. Viral suppression in this analysis was defined as achieving HIV-1 RNA less than 50 copies/mL at Week 48. Immune function and phenotype were determined by flow cytometry at baseline and Weeks 12 and 48 in virologically suppressed and nonsuppressed patients. Changes in immune phenotype were determined from subsets of CD4+ and CD8+ T cells, with immune activation defined as increased expression of T-cell CD38 and HLA-DR surface markers, and immune replicative senescence by increased frequency of circulating CD28 null T cells. Changes in immune function were assessed by lymphocyte proliferation in response to *Candida* and tetanus (recall antigens), phytohemagglutinin (PHA) and pokeweed (mitogenic plant lectins), and CD3+/CD28+ and by intracellular cytokine expression of IL-2, interferon-gamma (IFN-γ), and tumor necrosis factor-alpha (TNF-α) in response to staphylococcal enterotoxin B.

2.4. Immunophenotyping. A whole blood lysing technique was used and subpopulations were assessed according to a standard protocol for 3-color and 4-color immunofluorescence flow cytometry using fluorochrome conjugated monoclonal antibodies and a fluorescence activated cell sorter. A panel of monoclonal antibodies was used to delineate total CD3+, total CD4+ and CD8+ T cells, CD4+/CD8+ ratio, activated T cells (CD38+/HLA-DR+), immune replicative senescence (CD4+/CD28+ or CD8+/CD28+), and apoptotic cells (CD95+).

2.5. Proliferation Assays. The Vybrant CFDA SE Cell Tracer Kit (Molecular Probes, Inc.) was used. Lymphocytes were labeled with carboxyfluorescein diacetate and succinimidyl ester CFDA SE and then incubated at 37°C with 5% carbon dioxide for 7 days. The label is inherited by daughter cells after division. Labeled lymphocytes with carboxyfluorescein diacetate and succinimidyl ester were detected by flow cytometry using CD45 markers for gating strategy. This method quantified mitogenic and recall antigen responses.

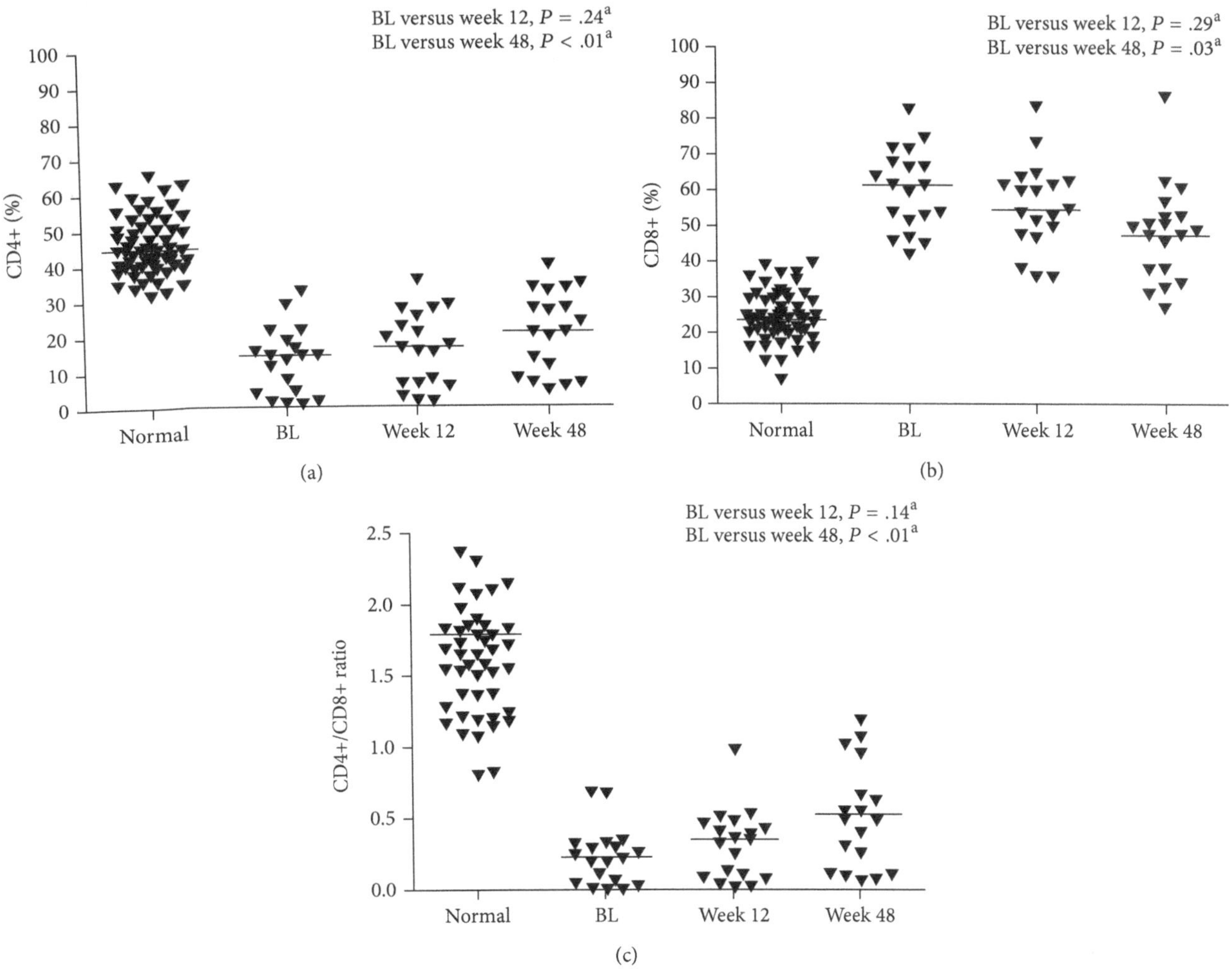

Figure 1: (a) Percent CD4+, (b) percent CD8+, and (c) CD4+/CD8+ ratio in virologically suppressed patients. Line represents median; [a]Wilcoxon rank-sum test; BL: baseline.

The reagents used were *Candida*, tetanus, CD3+/CD28+, PHA, and pokeweed.

2.6. Intracellular Cytokines. Flow cytometric intracellular cytokine detection of Th1 cytokines including IFN-γ, IL-2, and TNF-α was assessed using the BD Cytofix/Cytoperm Plus Fixation/Permeabilization (GolgiPlug protein transport inhibitor; BD Biosciences). Peripheral blood mononuclear cells were stimulated with staphylococcal enterotoxin B (Sigma) and a CEF control peptide pool (CMV, EBV, Influenza virus; NIH reagent 9808). This stimulation step was followed by the fixation and permeabilization of the cells. Then, surface and intracellular staining antibodies were added in a single staining step (Anti-Hu-IFN-γ/CD69/CD4/CD3, Anti-Hu-IL2/CD69/CD4/CD3, Anti-Hu-TNF-α/CD69/CD4/CD3; BD Biosciences). Cells were acquired and analyzed by flow cytometry.

2.7. Statistical Analysis. Immune recovery was evaluated in continuous and categorical outcome analyses. Wilcoxon rank-sum tests were used to assess immune parameter changes from baseline.

3. Results

3.1. Patient Population and Baseline Characteristics. A total of 32 patients with HIV-1 were enrolled in the substudy; 25 (78%) patients had Week 48 data and 19 (59%) were virologically suppressed at Week 48. The normal comparator group consisted of 34 healthy, HIV-seronegative individuals, 17 (50%) of whom were women and 25 (74%) of whom were white. Patient demographics and baseline characteristics for total and virologically suppressed patients are shown in Table 1.

3.2. Immune Phenotype. The median (range) CD4+ count at baseline for the total patient population was 191 (2, 463) and the median (range) CD4+ count in virologically suppressed patients at baseline was 222 (2, 398) cells/mm^3 (Table 1). At Week 48, the median (range) CD4+ count for the total population and virologically suppressed patients

TABLE 1: Demographics and baseline characteristics of patients enrolled into the immunology substudy of GRACE.

Parameter		All HIV+ patients ($N = 32$)	Virologically suppressed[a] patients at Wk 48 ($n = 19$)
Sex, n (%)	Men	19 (59.4)	13 (68.4)
	Women	13 (40.6)	6 (31.6)
Race, n (%)	Black	15 (46.9)	8 (42.1)
	Hispanic	10 (31.3)	6 (31.6)
	White	7 (21.9)	5 (26.3)
Mean (SD) viral load, $\log_{10}$ copies/mL		4.74 (0.84)	4.76 (0.82)
Median (range) CD4+ count, cells/mm^3		191 (2, 463)	222 (2, 398)

[a]HIV-1 RNA < 50 copies/mL at Wk 48 (or at Wks 36 and 52 if a Wk 48 sample was not available).

TABLE 2: Immune phenotype over the course of the GRACE immunology substudy.

Median (range)	Baseline		Wk 12		Wk 48	
	All[a]	Suppressed[b]	All[a]	Suppressed[b]	All[a]	Suppressed[b]
CD4+ (%)	15 (1, 33)	15 (1, 33)	16 (2, 36)	17 (2, 36)	21 (3, 40)	21 (5, 40)
CD8+ (%)	60.5 (39, 83)	62 (42, 83)	59 (35, 84)	55 (36, 84)	50 (27, 87)	49 (27, 87)
CD4+/CD8+ ratio (%)	0.22 (0.01, 0.70)	0.22 (0.01, 0.70)	0.30 (0.03, 1.00)	0.36 (0.03, 1.00)	0.41 (0.04, 1.21)	0.52 (0.08, 1.21)
CD4+/CD38+/DR+ (%)	22.5 (10, 88)	22 (10, 88)	19 (9, 76)	18 (9, 53)	13 (2, 36)	11 (2, 36)
CD8+/CD38+/DR+ (%)	48.5 (18, 76)	47 (18, 76)	36.5 (11, 71)	34 (11, 62)	25 (4, 68)	22 (4, 52)
CD4+/CD95+ (%)	15 (1, 35)	16 (1, 35)	21 (3, 38)	22 (3, 38)	23 (4, 41)	24 (6, 41)
CD8+/CD95+ (%)	71.5 (40, 87)	70 (40, 87)	69.5 (44, 88)	66 (44, 88)	55 (32, 80)	49 (32, 79)
CD3+/CD4+/CD28+ (%)	93 (46, 99)	95 (56, 99)	94 (67, 100)	94 (70, 100)	96 (67, 99)	96 (67, 99)
CD3+/CD8+/CD28+ (%)	59.5 (39, 86)	62 (39, 85)	50 (39, 79)	50.5 (39, 79)	56 (23, 82)	56 (35, 82)

[a]n = 32 at baseline, n = 30 at Wk 12 and n = 25 at Wk 48; [b]HIV-RNA < 50 copies/mL at Wk 48 (or at Wks 36 and 52 if a Wk 48 sample was not available), n = 19.

was 337 (98, 812) and 398 (119, 812) cells/mm^3, respectively. In virologically suppressed patients, the CD4+% increased significantly from baseline to Week 48 ($P < .03$; Figure 1). The median (range) CD8+ count at baseline for the total patient population was 912.5 (288, 3131) cells/mm^3, while the median (range) CD8+ count in virologically suppressed patients at baseline was 1037 (288, 3131) cells/mm^3. The CD8+% decreased significantly from baseline to Week 48 ($P < .01$) in virologically suppressed patients (Figure 1). The median (range) CD4+/CD8+ ratio at baseline was 0.22 (0.01, 0.70) in all patients and 0.22 (0.01, 0.70) in virologically suppressed patients. The CD4+/CD8+ ratio at Weeks 12 and 48 is displayed in Figure 1 and Table 2. The CD4+/CD8+ ratio increased significantly from baseline to Week 48 ($P < .01$) in suppressed patients. The percentage of CD4+ and CD8+ cells at Weeks 12 and 48 in suppressed patients is shown over 48 weeks in Figure 1. The percentage of CD4+ cells significantly increased ($P < .01$) and CD8+ cells significantly decreased ($P = .03$) from baseline to Week 48.

Improvements in immune activation, as measured by decreases in CD38 and HLA-DR expression on CD4+ and CD8+ cells over the course of the study, were observed in both the total patient population (Table 2) and in virologically suppressed patients (Table 2; Figure 2).

The percentage of apoptotic (CD95+) CD4+ cells in suppressed patients significantly increased from baseline to Week 48 ($P = .0142$; Table 2; Figure 2). The percentage of apoptotic CD8+ cells, on the other hand, significantly decreased from baseline to Week 48 in suppressed patients ($P = .0025$; Table 2; Figure 2).

Changes in immune replicative senescence were measured by changes in the frequency of CD4+/CD28− or CD8+/CD28− cells (Table 2). There was little change in the expression of costimulatory marker CD28+ on CD4+ cells from baseline to Week 48 in the total patient population or the virologically suppressed group (Table 2). There was a small decrease in the expression of CD28+ on CD8+ cells in the total patient population and the virologically suppressed population from baseline to Week 48 (Table 2).

3.3. Immune Function. The ability of CD4+ lymphocytes to respond to mitogens and recall antigens improved in GRACE patients over the course of the study. Proliferation in response to CD3+/CD28+ and PHA was at, or near, normal levels by Week 12 in virologically suppressed patients, and proliferation in response to pokeweed and *Candida* was at normal levels by Week 48 (Figure 3). Intracellular production of TNF-α and IL-2 also increased during the study. Tumor necrosis factor-alpha and IL-2 significantly increased in staphylococcal enterotoxin B-stimulated CD4+ cells of virologically suppressed patients by Week 48; there

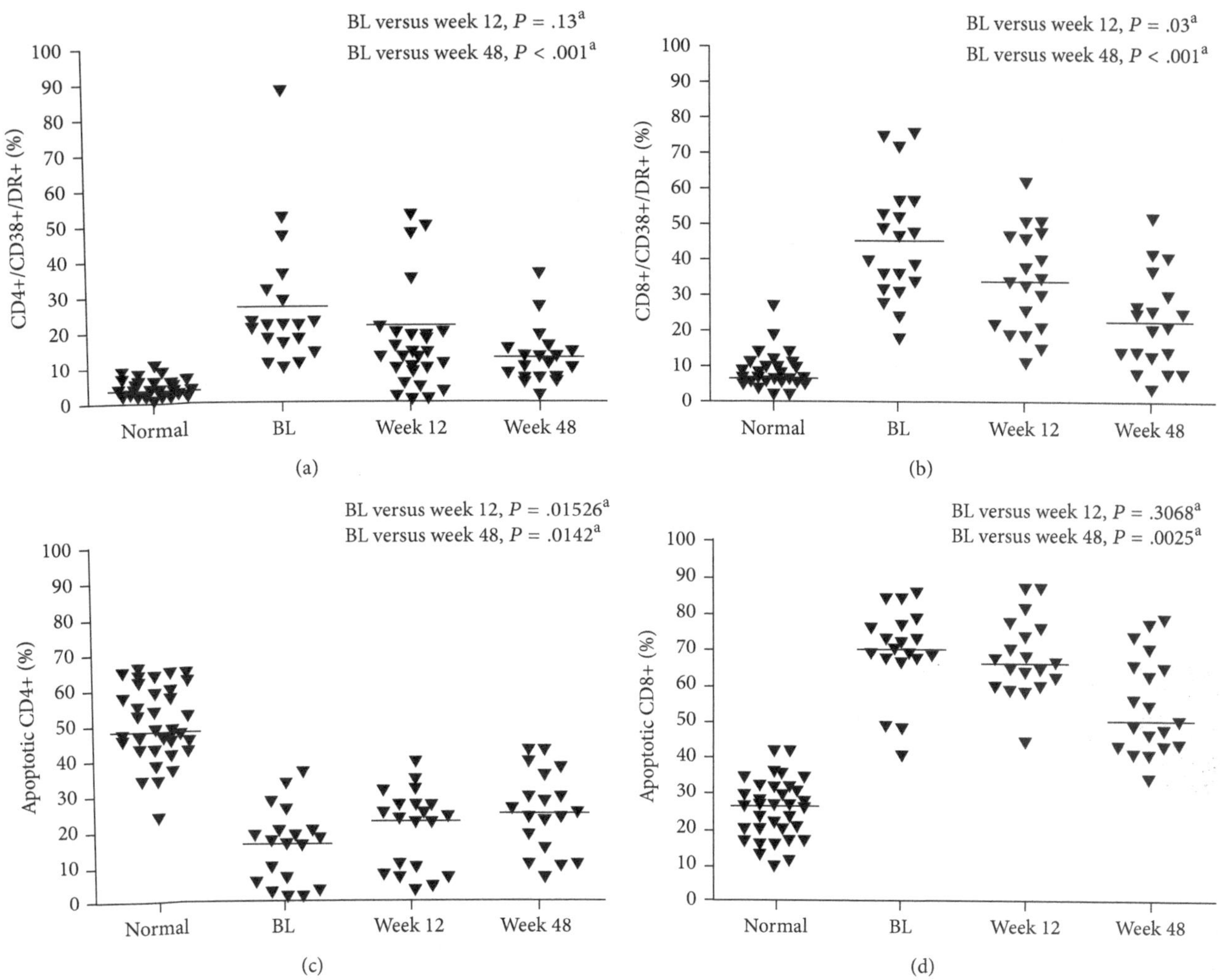

FIGURE 2: (a) CD4+/CD38+/DR+, (b) CD8+/CD38+/DR+, percentage of apoptotic T cells, (c) CD4+/CD95+, (d) CD8+/CD95+. Line represents median; [a]Wilcoxon rank-sum test; BL: baseline.

was no significant change in IFN-γ in the stimulated CD4+ cells (Figure 4).

4. Discussion

Few published studies within clinical trials have prospectively assessed in vitro changes in immune function as measured by lymphocyte proliferation [34, 35], and none of these assessed intracellular cytokine production in response to ARV therapy. This substudy from the GRACE trial evaluated T-cell function in a racially diverse, treatment-experienced population comprised of more than 30% women. As expected, based on results from previous studies [24, 27, 28], DRV/r-based therapy resulted in increases in CD4+ cell counts and decreases in CD8+ counts in virologically suppressed patients, with an improved CD4+/CD8+ ratio. In addition, we found that DRV/r-based ARV therapy was associated with progressive functional immune recovery over 48 weeks in virologically suppressed patients, as demonstrated by improved lymphocyte response to mitogens and recall antigens. This suggests that not only do the CD4+ cell counts of HIV-1-infected patients improve during DRV/r-based therapy, but their ability to respond in vitro to immune stimuli may improve as well. Results from this report are consistent with a recent study that demonstrated significant decreases in immune activation and apoptosis in CD4+ and CD8+ T cells and a decrease in immune CD8+ senescence following ARV therapy [36].

While there have been studies evaluating the influence of ARV therapy on immune parameters, data typically represent class-specific rather than regimen-specific treatment approaches. For example, therapy with integrase inhibitors has been shown to result in larger CD4+ cell count increases compared with other ARV classes [29, 37, 38]. The work shown here represents a regimen-specific study, with combination DRV/r treatment in addition to an optimized background regimen that could differ across patients. Unfortunately, we cannot assess differences between regimens, as our study was not comparative.

The reduction in T-cell activation seen here has previously been shown to correlate with the reduction in viral load, as well as an improved response to recall antigens

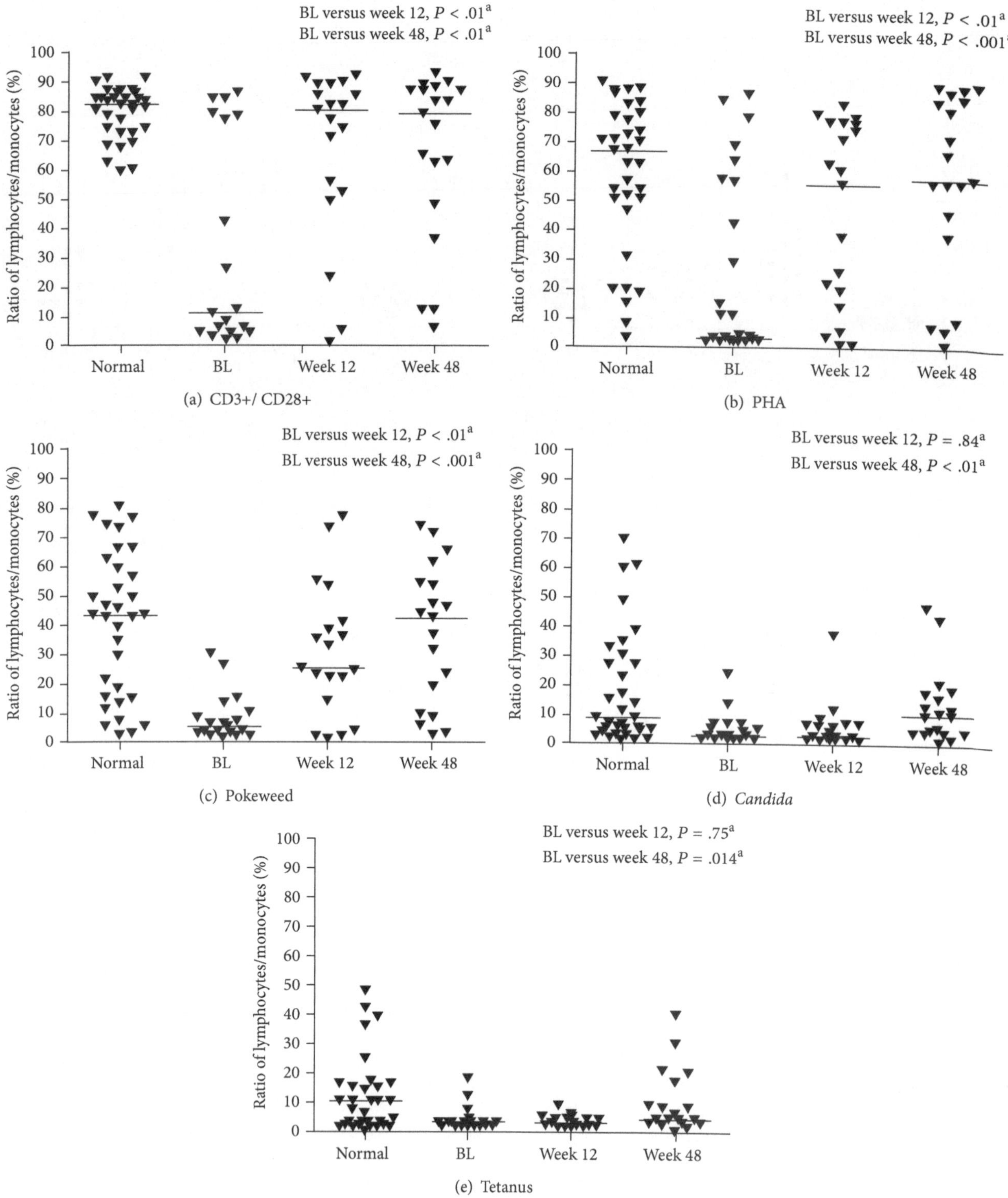

FIGURE 3: CD4+ lymphocyte proliferation in (a) CD3+/CD28+, (b) phytohemagglutinin, (c) pokeweed, (d) *Candida*, and (e) tetanus. Line represents median; [a]Wilcoxon rank-sum test; BL: baseline; PHA: phytohemagglutinin.

[24]. The observed HIV-1-induced increase in apoptotic CD95+/CD4+ cells has been suggested to be independent of ARV activity; the PI saquinavir has been shown to decrease CD95 expression in CD4+ cells from healthy donors whose cells were previously briefly incubated with HIV-1 virus [25]. Although anti-CD95-induced apoptosis declines with therapy, this change is only occasionally associated with a reduction in expression of CD95 on T lymphocytes [39]. It is thus not surprising that in our study CD95 expression on T cells did not decline. In the GRACE study, no improvement

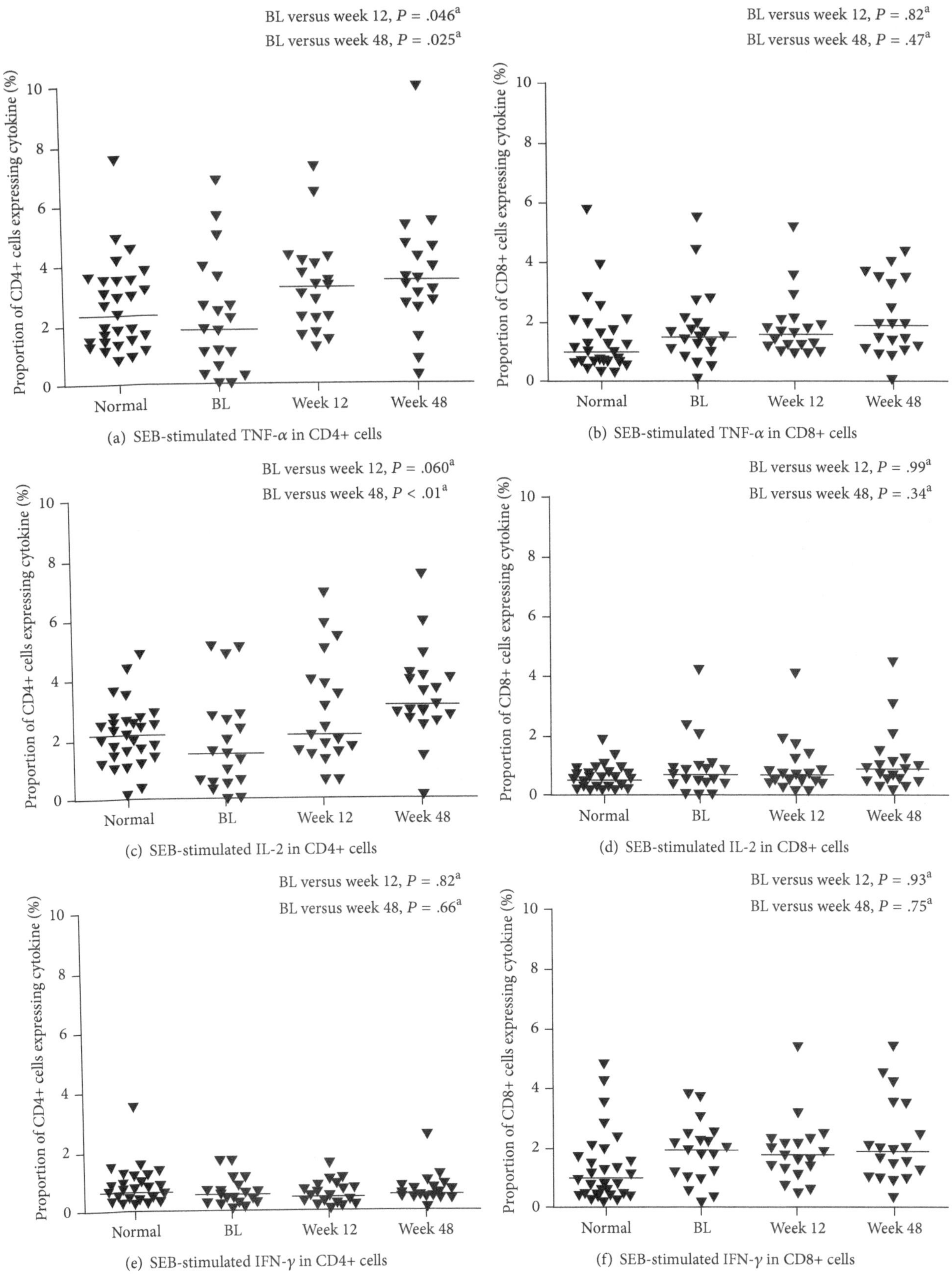

(a) SEB-stimulated TNF-α in CD4+ cells

(b) SEB-stimulated TNF-α in CD8+ cells

(c) SEB-stimulated IL-2 in CD4+ cells

(d) SEB-stimulated IL-2 in CD8+ cells

(e) SEB-stimulated IFN-γ in CD4+ cells

(f) SEB-stimulated IFN-γ in CD8+ cells

Figure 4: Staphylococcal enterotoxin B-stimulated cytokine expression in virologically suppressed patients. Line represents median; [a]Wilcoxon rank-sum test; TNF-α: tumor necrosis factor-alpha; IL-2: interleukin-2; IFN-γ: interferon-gamma; SEB: staphylococcal enterotoxin B; BL: baseline.

in the CD4+/CD28− or CD8+/CD28− phenotype was seen, consistent with other studies that have suggested that CD28 expression is not normalized in HIV-1–infected patients who have undergone up to 3 years of ARV therapy [40, 41].

One possible limitation to this study is the small sample size, which may limit data interpretation. The study aimed to enroll 50 women and 50 men, but, due to a delayed start date, after initiation of the GRACE study, the patient pool for this substudy was limited and the enrollment goal was not reached. Nonetheless, the data obtained are similar to those of other trials. Both immune phenotype and function of CD4+ and CD8+ cells were significantly improved in treatment-experienced patients receiving DRV/r-based therapy, as evidenced by positive changes in the capacity to proliferate and the expression of intracellular cytokines by CD4+ cells. The functional recovery observed in virologically suppressed patients, as assessed by proliferative response and intracellular cytokine expression, was also seen in nonsuppressed patients, although to a lesser degree.

Antiretroviral therapy has been available for 25 years; however, there has been limited research on immune recovery after long-term treatment. Furthermore, the focus of immune recovery has historically been an assessment of CD4+ cell counts. In the current study, in addition to the evaluation of CD4+ cell counts, CD4+ cell activation (CD38+/HLA-DR+, CD95+), function, and senescence (CD28−) were measured as well as CD8+ cell counts, activation, function, and senescence. It should be noted that, as observed in this trial, despite the improvements in immune phenotype and function seen with ARV therapy, complete normalization of CD4+ and CD8+ parameters is rarely achieved in HIV-1-infected individuals [24, 42]. However, we hypothesize that there may be some clinical benefit even in patients who do not experience measurable or significant increases in CD4+ cell counts. It is feasible that, in patients with higher baseline CD4 levels, measurable increases in CD4+ cell counts may not be observed [43].

Previous studies have shown that despite CD4+ cell count normalization, the pretreatment nadir CD4+ count and level of CD28 CD4+ coexpressing lymphocytes determine ongoing immune competence, including responses to immunization [40]. Despite the successful HIV therapy noted in the GRACE substudy, there seemed to be a higher frequency of the CD8+ CD28− phenotype. This possible treatment-resistant expansion and persistence of cells with a senescence phenotype may have potential for long-term cardiovascular [44], metabolic, and other aging-associated consequences.

This GRACE substudy demonstrates that DRV/r-based therapy improved CD4+ cell recovery and was associated with progressive functional immune recovery over the 48-week study period. Thus, initiation of ARV therapy may be required not only to restore immune function, but also to diminish the effects of chronic inflammation.

Disclosure

This paper was presented at the 5th International AIDS Society Conference on HIV pathogenesis, Treatment and Prevention. Cape Town, South Africa, July 19–22, 2009, Poster TUPD203.

Conflict of Interests

Dr. Tsoukas is a consultant for Merck, Abbott, Boehringer Ingelheim, GlaxoSmithKline, Bristol-Myers Squibb, Gilead, Tibotec/Johnson & Johnson, Novartis, Roche, and Talecris. Ms. Gilbert and Mr. Lewis have no financial conflict of interests. Dr. Hatzakis receives grant/research support from Masimo Biotech. Dr. Falcon is an employee and stockholder of Johnson & Johnson. Dr. Mrus is an employee and stockholder of Johnson & Johnson.

Acknowledgments

The authors would like to thank the patients and their families, the study sites, and the principal investigators for their participation in the trial. The authors would like to acknowledge Gilead for supplying emtricitabine, tenofovir, and emtricitabine/tenofovir. The authors would additionally like to acknowledge internal study support staff, as well as Samantha Taylor, Ph.D., Medicus International New York, for her editorial assistance.

References

[1] L. Kestens, G. Vanham, C. Vereecken et al., "Selective increase of activation antigens HLA-DR and CD38 on CD4+ CD45RO+ T lymphocytes during HIV-1 infection," *Clinical and Experimental Immunology*, vol. 95, no. 3, pp. 436–441, 1994.

[2] M. Levacher, F. Hulstaert, S. Tallet, S. Ullery, J. J. Pocidalo, and B. A. Bach, "The significance of activation markers on CD8 lymphocytes in human immunodeficiency syndrome: staging and prognostic value," *Clinical and Experimental Immunology*, vol. 90, no. 3, pp. 376–382, 1992.

[3] J. V. Giorgi, H.-N. Ho, K. Hirji et al., "CD8+ lymphocyte activation at human immunodeficiency virus type 1 seroconversion: development of HLA-DR+ CD38- CD8+ cells is associated with subsequent stable CD4+ cell levels," *Journal of Infectious Diseases*, vol. 170, no. 4, pp. 775–781, 1994.

[4] S. A. Klein, J. M. Dobmeyer, T. S. Dobmeyer et al., "Demonstration of the Th1 to Th2 cytokine shift during the course of HIV-1 infection using cytoplasmic cytokine detection on single cell level by flow cytometry," *AIDS*, vol. 11, no. 9, pp. 1111–1118, 1997.

[5] Z. Liu, W. G. Cumberland, L. E. Hultin, H. E. Prince, R. Detels, and J. V. Giorgi, "Elevated CD38 antigen expression on CD8+ T cells Is a stronger marker for the risk of chronic HIV disease progression to AIDS and death in the multicenter AIDS Cohort study than CD4+ cell count, soluble immune activation markers, or combinations of HLA-DR and CD38 expression," *Journal of Acquired Immune Deficiency Syndromes and Human Retrovirology*, vol. 16, no. 2, pp. 83–92, 1997.

[6] M.-L. Dion, J.-F. Poulin, R. Bordi et al., "HIV infection rapidly induces and maintains a substantial suppression of thymocyte proliferation," *Immunity*, vol. 21, no. 6, pp. 757–768, 2004.

[7] A. Landay, B. Ohlsson-Wilhelm, and J. V. Giorgi, "Application of flow cytometry to the study of HIV infection," *AIDS*, vol. 4, no. 6, pp. 479–497, 1990.

[8] J. B. Margolick, A. Munoz, A. D. Donnenberg et al., "Failure of T-cell homeostasis preceding AIDS in HIV-1 infection. The Multicenter AIDS Cohort study," *Nature Medicine*, vol. 1, no. 7, pp. 674–680, 1995.

[9] L. Kestens, G. Vanham, P. Gigase et al., "Expression of activation antigens, HLA-DR and CD38, on CD8 lymphocytes during HIV-1 infection," *AIDS*, vol. 6, no. 8, pp. 793–797, 1992.

[10] V. Appay, J. R. Almeida, D. Sauce, B. Autran, and L. Papagno, "Accelerated immune senescence and HIV-1 infection," *Experimental Gerontology*, vol. 42, no. 5, pp. 432–437, 2007.

[11] S. P. Aries, B. Schaaf, C. Muller, R. H. Dennin, and K. Dalhoff, "Fas (CD95) expression on CD4+ T cells from HIV-infected patients increases with disease progression," *Journal of Molecular Medicine*, vol. 73, no. 12, pp. 591–593, 1995.

[12] T. H. Mogensen, J. Melchjorsen, C. S. Larsen, and S. R. Paludan, "Innate immune recognition and activation during HIV infection," *Retrovirology*, vol. 7, article 54, 2010.

[13] M. E. Peter, A. Ehret, C. Berndt, and P. H. Krammer, "AIDS and the death receptors," *British Medical Bulletin*, vol. 53, no. 3, pp. 604–616, 1997.

[14] Z. Bentwich, A. Kalinkovich, Z. Weisman, and Z. Grossman, "Immune activation in the context of HIV infection," *Clinical and Experimental Immunology*, vol. 111, no. 1, pp. 1–2, 1998.

[15] Z. Grossman, M. Meier-Schellersheim, W. E. Paul, and L. J. Picker, "Pathogenesis of HIV infection: what the virus spares is as important as what it destroys," *Nature Medicine*, vol. 12, no. 3, pp. 289–295, 2006.

[16] M. D. Hazenberg, D. Hamann, H. Schuitemaker, and F. Miedema, "T cell depletion in HIV-1 infection: how CD4+ T cells go out of stock," *Nature Immunology*, vol. 1, no. 4, pp. 285–289, 2000.

[17] L. A. Trimble, P. Shankar, M. Patterson, J. P. Daily, and J. Lieberman, "Human immunodeficiency virus-specific circulating CD8 T lymphocytes have down-modulated CD3ζ and CD28, key signaling molecules for T-cell activation," *Journal of Virology*, vol. 74, no. 16, pp. 7320–7330, 2000.

[18] J. H. Vingerhoets, G. L. Vanham, L. L. Kestens et al., "Increased cytolytic T lymphocyte activity and decreased B7 responsiveness are associated with CD28 down-regulation on CD8+ T cells from HIV-infected subjects," *Clinical and Experimental Immunology*, vol. 100, no. 3, pp. 425–433, 1995.

[19] S. T. Parish, J. E. Wu, and R. B. Effros, "Sustained CD28 expression delays multiple features of replicative senescence in human CD8 T lymphocytes," *Journal of Clinical Immunology*, vol. 30, no. 6, pp. 798–805, 2010.

[20] V. I. Avelino-Silva, Y.-L. Ho, T. J. Avelino-Silva, and S. D. S. Santos, "Aging and HIV infection," *Ageing Research Reviews*, vol. 10, no. 1, pp. 163–172, 2011.

[21] K. L. Wood, H. L. Twigg III, and A. I. Doseff, "Dysregulation of CD8+ lymphocyte apoptosis, chronic disease, and immune regulation," *Frontiers in Bioscience*, vol. 14, no. 10, pp. 3771–3781, 2009.

[22] J. V. Giorgi, Z. Liu, L. E. Hultin, W. G. Cumberland, K. Hennessey, and R. Detels, "Elevated levels of CD38+CD8+ T cells in HIV infection add to the prognostic value of low CD4+ T cell levels: results of 6 years of follow-up," *Journal of Acquired Immune Deficiency Syndromes*, vol. 6, no. 8, pp. 904–912, 1993.

[23] M. Clerici and G. M. Shearer, "A $T_H1 \rightarrow T_H2$ switch is a critical step in the etiology of HIV infection," *Immunology Today*, vol. 14, no. 3, pp. 107–111, 1993.

[24] B. Autran, G. Carcelain, T. S. Li et al., "Positive effects of combined antiretroviral therapy on CD4+ T cell homeostasis and function in advanced HIV disease," *Science*, vol. 277, no. 5322, pp. 112–116, 1997.

[25] J. Estaquier, J.-D. Leliévre, F. Petit et al., "Effects of antiretroviral drugs on human immunodeficiency virus type 1-induced CD4+ T-cell death," *Journal of Virology*, vol. 76, no. 12, pp. 5966–5973, 2002.

[26] A. D. Badley, K. Parato, D. W. Cameron et al., "Dynamic correlation of apoptosis and immune activation during treatment of HIV infection," *Cell Death and Differentiation*, vol. 6, no. 5, pp. 420–432, 1999.

[27] M. Goicoechea, D. M. Smith, L. Liu et al., "Determinants of CD4+ T cell recovery during suppressive antiretroviral therapy: association of immune activation, T cell maturation markers, and cellular HIV-1 DNA," *Journal of Infectious Diseases*, vol. 194, no. 1, pp. 29–37, 2006.

[28] S. A. Riddler, R. Haubrich, A. G. DiRienzo et al., "Class-sparing regimens for initial treatment of HIV-1 infection," *The New England Journal of Medicine*, vol. 358, no. 20, pp. 2095–2106, 2008.

[29] M. Pichenot, S. Deuffic-Burban, L. Cuzin, and Y. Yazdanpanah, "Efficacy of new antiretroviral drugs in treatment-experienced HIV-infected patients: a systematic review and meta-analysis of recent randomized controlled trials," *HIV Medicine*, vol. 13, no. 3, pp. 148–155, 2012.

[30] J. M. Llibre, M. J. Buzón, M. Massanella et al., "Treatment intensification with raltegravir in subjects with sustained HIV-1 viraemia suppression: a randomized 48-week study," *Antiviral Therapy*, vol. 17, no. 2, pp. 355–364, 2012.

[31] H. Hatano, T. L. Hayes, V. Dahl et al., "A randomized, controlled trial of raltegravir intensification in antiretroviral-treated, HIV-infected patients with a suboptimal CD4+ T cell response," *Journal of Infectious Diseases*, vol. 203, no. 7, pp. 960–968, 2011.

[32] H. Byakwaga, M. Kelly, D. F. J. Purcell et al., "Intensification of antiretroviral therapy with raltegravir or addition of hyperimmune bovine colostrum in HIV-infected patients with suboptimal CD4+ T-cell response: a randomized controlled trial," *Journal of Infectious Diseases*, vol. 204, no. 10, pp. 1532–1540, 2011.

[33] J. Currier, D. A. Bridge, D. Hagins et al., "Sex-based outcomes of Darunavir-Ritonavir therapy: a single-group trial," *Annals of Internal Medicine*, vol. 153, no. 6, pp. 349–357, 2010.

[34] J. B. Angel, K. G. Parato, A. Kumar et al., "Progressive human immunodeficiency virus-specific immune recovery with prolonged viral suppression," *Journal of Infectious Diseases*, vol. 183, no. 4, pp. 546–554, 2001.

[35] H. Ullum, T. Katzenstein, H. Aladdin et al., "Immunological changes in Human Immunodeficiency Virus (HIV)-infected individuals during HIV-specific protease inhibitor treatment," *Scandinavian Journal of Immunology*, vol. 49, no. 5, pp. 539–547, 1999.

[36] R. C. Kaplan, C. M. Parrinello, H. N. Hodis et al., "Impact of HAART initiation on immune regulation (activation/senescence) in aging HIV-infected women: Women's Interagency HIV study," in *Proceedings of the 19th Conference on Retroviruses and Opportunistic Infections*, Seattle, Wash, USA, 2012.

[37] C. Garrido, N. Rallón, V. Soriano et al., "Mechanisms involved in CD4 gains in HIV-infected patients switched to raltegravir," *AIDS*, vol. 26, no. 5, pp. 551–557, 2012.

[38] R. T. Steigbigel, D. A. Cooper, P. N. Kumar et al., "Raltegravir with optimized background therapy for resistant HIV-1 infection," *The New England Journal of Medicine*, vol. 359, no. 4, pp. 339–354, 2008.

[39] M.-L. Gougeon, H. Lecoeur, and Y. Sasaki, "Apoptosis and the CD95 system in HIV disease: impact of Highly Active Anti-Retroviral Therapy (HAART)," *Immunology Letters*, vol. 66, no. 1–3, pp. 97–103, 1999.

[40] C. G. Lange, M. M. Lederman, K. Medvik et al., "Nadir CD4+ T-cell count and numbers of CD28+ CD4+ T-cells predict functional responses to immunizations in chronic HIV-1 infection," *AIDS*, vol. 17, no. 14, pp. 2015–2023, 2003.

[41] T. Niehues, G. Horneff, S. Knipp, O. Adams, and V. Wahn, "Treatment-resistant expansion of CD8+CD28-cells in pediatric HIV infection," *Pediatric Research*, vol. 47, no. 3, pp. 418–421, 2000.

[42] C. G. Lange and M. M. Lederman, "Immune reconstitution with antiretroviral therapies in chronic HIV-1 infection," *Journal of Antimicrobial Chemotherapy*, vol. 51, no. 1, pp. 1–4, 2003.

[43] A. Hill, J. Montaner, M. Lederman, A. Cutrell, S. Tortell, and D. Thorborn, "Discordant CD4/RNA responses to HAART are strongly associated with high baseline CD4 count and low HIV RNA: analysis of 406 naive patients," in *Proceedings of the 3rd International Workshop on HIV Drug Resistance and Treatment Strategies*, San Diego, Calif, USA, 1999.

[44] R. C. Kaplan, E. Sinclair, A. L. Landay et al., "T cell activation and senescence predict subclinical carotid artery disease in HIV-infected women," *Journal of Infectious Diseases*, vol. 203, no. 4, pp. 452–463, 2011.

20

Moderate-Intensity Exercise Improves Body Composition and Improves Physiological Markers of Stress in HIV-Infected Men

Wesley David Dudgeon,[1] Jason Reed Jaggers,[2] Kenneth Doyle Phillips,[3] John Larry Durstine,[2] Stephanie E. Burgess,[4] George William Lyerly,[5] John Mark Davis,[2] and Gregory Alan Hand[2]

[1] *Department of Health, Exercise, and Sport Science, The Citadel, 171 Moultrie Street, Charleston, SC 29403, USA*
[2] *Department of Exercise Science, Arnold School of Public Health, University of South Carolina, 1300 Wheat Street, Columbia, SC 29208, USA*
[3] *College of Nursing, University of Tennessee, 4520 Ivy Rose Drive, Knoxville, TN 37918, USA*
[4] *College of Nursing, University of South Carolina, 1601 Greene Street, Columbia, SC 29208, USA*
[5] *Department of Health, Kinesiology, and Sports Studies, Coastal Carolina University, P.O. Box 261954, Conway, SC 29528-6054, USA*

Correspondence should be addressed to Wesley David Dudgeon, wes.dudgeon@citadel.edu

Academic Editors: D. Aunis, R. L. D. Machado, and J. Poudrier

HIV/AIDS and its treatment often alter body composition and result in poorer physical functioning. The aim of this study was to determine the effects of a moderate-intensity exercise program on body composition and the hormones and cytokines associated with adverse health outcomes. HIV-infected males ($N = 111$) were randomized to an exercise group (EX) who completed 6 weeks of moderate-intensity exercise training, or to a nonintervention control group (CON). In pre- and postintervention, body composition was estimated via DXA, peak strength was assessed, and resting blood samples were obtained. There was a decrease in salivary cortisol at wake ($P = 0.025$) in the EX and a trend ($P = 0.07$) for a decrease 1 hour after waking. The EX had a significant increase in lean tissue mass (LTM) ($P < 0.001$) following the intervention. Those in the EX below median body fat (20%) increased LTM ($P = 0.014$) only, while those above 20% decreased fat mass ($P = 0.02$), total fat ($N = 0.009$), and trunk fat ($P = 0.001$), while also increasing LTM ($P = 0.027$). Peak strength increased between 14% and 28% on all exercises in the EX group. These data indicate that 6 weeks of moderate-intensity exercise training can decrease salivary cortisol levels, improve physical performance, and improve body composition in HIV-infected men.

1. Introduction

Over 33.3 million people are living with HIV-1 [1]. Since it was introduced in the mid to late 1990s, highly active antiretroviral therapy (HAART) has increased the time from HIV infection to acquired immunodeficiency syndrome (AIDS) diagnosis by 3 years and life expectancy of those with AIDS by up to 15 years [2]. In fact, these advances have allowed those living with HIV-1, and receiving treatment, to have life expectancies similar to uninfected persons with lifestyles that include smoking, heavy drinking, and obesity [3]. Mortality rates of HIV-infected persons dropped drastically within 18 months after the introduction of HAART, from 29.4 deaths per 100 person years to 8.8 deaths per 100 person years [4]. In fact, in younger (~30 years of age) persons with favorable disease markers (i.e., high CD4+ cell counts and low viral load) survival has been estimated at 31 years, with 45% of deaths attributable to non-HIV-related conditions, such as cardiovascular disease and cancer [5]. This brings about new challenges in treating persons with HIV-1, changing the focus from purely survival to improving quality of life by decreasing risk factors for other chronic conditions. Thus, it is important to understand how exercise training, which has been shown to be beneficial at reducing risk factors for both cardiovascular disease and cancer in uninfected populations, affects those persons living with HIV-1.

While HAART has been able to significantly increase the survival of HIV-infected patients, HAART-associated cardiometabolic risks are increasing. HAART regimens, specifically those using protease inhibitors (PI), have been shown to cause lipodystrophy as well as metabolic changes that result in an increased risk for cardiovascular disease. It has been previously observed that patients with lipodystrophy show increases in total serum and low-density lipoprotein cholesterol, triglycerides, and insulin resistance [6].

A complication of HIV disease that has remained, even with the implementation of HAART, is HIV/AIDS-related wasting, which effects nearly 20% of those living with HIV-1 [7]. HIV/AIDS-associated wasting is characterized by reductions in fat mass, lean body mass (LBM), muscular strength, and functional performance and is associated with disease progression [8].

The pathophysiology behind these somatic changes increases the risk for cardiometabolic diseases possibly due to the proinflammatory process exhibited. Further, there is a strong association between HIV/AIDS-related wasting and increased mortality [9], impaired functional status [10], accelerated disease progression [11], and a declining ability to carry out activities of daily living [12]. HIV-infected persons also demonstrate an increased susceptibility to infection [13] and show a progressive depletion of metabolically active tissue near death [14].

The mechanisms behind HIV-associated wasting appear to be abnormal levels of circulating catabolic and anabolic hormones, cytokines, and binding proteins. Cortisol, which is elevated in HIV-infected persons [15–17], is a potent catabolic hormone, which increases rates of protein degradation and slows protein synthesis rates, especially in skeletal muscle [18]. Serum cortisol levels also appear to be the best predictor for insulin resistance followed by interleukin-6 (IL-6) in persons with inflammatory conditions [19]. Insulin-like growth factor 1 (IGF-1) is the mechanism by which growth hormone (GH) influences skeletal muscle and is a potent regulator of muscle mass [20]. Those persons suffering from HIV/AIDS wasting frequently demonstrate GH resistance, which manifests itself in increased GH levels and decreased IGF-1 levels, and may be attributed to malnutrition [21]. Insulin-like growth factor binding protein 3 (IGFBP-3) is the major IGF-1 binding protein in circulation and can extend the half-life of circulating IGF-1 from minutes to several hours thereby maintaining constant IGF-1 levels. HIV-1 infection increases the proteolysis of IGFBP-3, thus decreasing IGFBP-3 levels and in turn reducing the amount of IGF-1 in circulation [22]. Another hormone of interest is testosterone, which is low in 30–50% of HIV-infected men [23] and is of significance because testosterone is a potent regulator of skeletal muscle mass that acts, via multiple pathways, to increase protein synthesis [24–26].

Inflammation is a prominent component in HIV/AIDS wasting and is also linked to cardiometabolic conditions. While inflammation is a necessary process for muscle generation [27], it may be catabolic if found in excess levels for prolonged periods. Cytokines of note in this inflammatory process include tumor necrosis factor alpha (TNF-α), interleukin one beta (IL-1-β), and IL-6. However, IL-6 may also exhibit anti-inflammatory functions, as it can inhibit TNF-α and IL-1-β [28]. TNF-α has been associated with muscle wasting in many diseased populations [29–31] including HIV-1 [32] and HIV-infected persons have been shown to have elevated TNF-α levels [33, 34].

Elevated levels of these proinflammatory markers are also known to be associated with an increased risk of chronic disease. Relationships have consistently been identified among atherosclerosis and cardiovascular disease with greater levels of C-reactive protein (CRP), TNF-α, and IL-6 [35, 36]. Further, IL-1-β has been implicated in numerous disease states including rheumatoid arthritis [37], atherosclerosis [38], and type I diabetes [39]. Studies looking at patients with metabolic disorders have also shown increased levels of IL-6 and CRP among type II diabetics, obese individuals, and patients experiencing metabolic syndrome [40–42].

An emerging treatment that has the potential to improve the circulating abnormalities (e.g., low anabolic hormone levels and high proinflammatory markers) of those with HIV-1 is exercise training. Before further discussing the potential beneficial effects of exercise in HIV-infected populations, it should first be recognized that research has shown exercise to be safe in this population. Low- to moderate-intensity exercise does not alter CD4 cell counts or viral load, nor does it increase the prevalence of opportunistic infection [43]. Additionally, no reports of adverse side effects to exercise interventions have been reported.

Resistance exercise training is known to increase skeletal muscle mass and muscular strength in numerous healthy and clinical populations regardless of gender, age, or race [44]. Aerobic exercise is also known to prevent or manage chronic diseases such as insulin resistance, cardiovascular disease, and cancer. This could possibly be a result of the protective effects aerobic exercise has shown to have against inflammation. Studies have repeatedly shown the benefits of aerobic exercise against inflammation by decreasing CRP, IL-6, TNF-α, among other proinflammatory markers [45–47]. Further, limited data in HIV-infected populations have shown similar effects. Progressive resistance exercise alone has produced significant increases in muscular strength and lean body mass in HIV-infected persons with and without wasting [48–50]. Similarly, the combination of resistance exercise and aerobic exercise has also increased strength and lean mass in HIV-infected populations [51–53] and produced transient increases in anabolic hormones [54]. Thus, it appears that resistance exercise training has the potential to be a complimentary therapy to pharmacological treatments for maintaining and increasing lean body mass and muscular strength in HIV-infected persons.

However, what remains to be seen is the effect of a lower dose (lower volume and lesser intensity) of combined resistance and aerobic exercise on body composition, strength and inflammation in HIV-infected persons. Further, this type of intervention may improve subject compliance. Therefore, the aim of this study was to determine the effect of an American College of Sports Medicine- (ACSM-) based low-volume, moderate-intensity resistance and aerobic exercise training program on the strength, body composition, and circulating hormone and inflammatory cytokine profile in a sample of HIV-infected men.

2. Methods

2.1. Sample. HIV-infected men over 18 years of age free of any known opportunistic infections, currently receiving antiretroviral therapy (ART), and physically able to complete the exercise intervention were recruited from local HIV/AIDS service organizations in the Columbia, SC metropolitan area. Flyers were placed in the waiting areas of clinics, and research team members enlisted the assistance of HIV/AIDS case workers in recruiting subjects.

Individuals who met the above criteria were excluded from the study following a physician's screening if (1) their medical history revealed current opportunistic infection(s), (2) they were found to be currently using, or had used in the past, hormone therapy, (3) they scored 5 or greater on the Drug Abuse Screening Test (DAST) and/or the Michigan Alcohol Screening Test (MAST), (4) they were found to be currently involved in a structured exercise program, or (5) any contraindications for graded exercise stress testing, as specified by the American College of Sports Medicine [55] were identified.

2.2. Procedure. All procedures, including testing and exercise training, were completed in the Clinical Research Laboratory in the Department of Exercise Science at the University of South Carolina. After signing the informed consent statement, subjects were assigned an identification number and then were assisted in completing a demographic data sheet (age, race, CDC disease stage, and current health status) and a cardiovascular risk factor survey that addressed current medications (including HIV medications), family history of cardiovascular disease, smoking habits, physical activity habits, any significant health concerns (other than HIV infection), and other pertinent health information. Medical personnel then reviewed the risk factor survey, and if no contraindications for exercise stress testing were identified, subjects were cleared to receive a graded treadmill stress test (GXT). Following successful completion of the GXT, subjects were randomized, using a random number table, to the intervention group (EX) or a nonintervention control (CON) group. Following the completion of study requirements, those randomized to the CON group (who did not receive intervention) then received the aerobic and resistance exercise intervention twice weekly for six weeks. The Office of Research Compliance at the University of South Carolina approved the study and its procedures.

2.3. Body Composition Assessment. Dual energy X-ray absorptiometry (DXA) scans (GE Medical Instruments, Madison, WI) for body composition were administered before the first exercise session and within 1-week following the last exercise session. A state certified DXA technician calibrated the equipment, performed each scan, and analyzed the results yielding lean mass and fat mass data, both for the entire body and by region.

2.4. Peak Strength Assessment. All subjects had peak strength determined on upper body resistance exercises (chest press, lat pull down) and lower body resistance exercises (leg extension, leg curl). Subjects were instructed on the proper techniques for each exercise and then were given one warm-up set of 8–12 repetitions (minimal weight was selected for this set) to become comfortable with the exercise. Subjects were then instructed to complete three repetitions on each exercise with the most weight possible while maintaining proper form. Weight selection was based on subject input and observation by the investigator. Since this population was untrained and unfamiliar with resistance training, a three-repetition maximum (3-RM) was used instead of the standard 1-RM, which has been used by others in clinical populations [7, 56, 57]. Using the standard conversion set forth by Brzycki [58], a 3-RM is approximately 94% of the 1-RM. Sixty percent of this 3-RM was then used as the initial weight for the resistance exercises.

2.5. Design. A randomized control group experimental design was used to determine the effects of moderate-intensity exercise training on circulating hormone, cytokine, and binding protein levels in HIV-infected men. All EX subjects were scheduled to attend 2 exercise sessions per week during the 6-week study. Exercise sessions were separated by at least 48 hours to allow for adequate recovery. Subjects had to complete 10 of the 12 sessions over the study duration to be included in the final analysis. Following the last exercise or control session, subjects were given three salivettes to take home. They were instructed to collect saliva samples immediately after waking (W), 1 hour after waking (W+1), and 2 hours after waking (W+2) on the day they were scheduled to return for posttesting. On the pre- and posttesting days, subjects were instructed to arrive fasted and were scheduled to arrive at the same time of the day so as to avoid hormonal variation due to normal cycles. Blood was collected and saliva samples were returned at this time.

2.6. Exercise Intervention. Those subjects randomized to the EX group completed 30 minutes of aerobic exercise training, on a treadmill or stationary cycle, in the intensity range of 60–75% of their age predicted maximum heart rate (208×0.7 (age in years)) twice weekly, for 6 weeks. Heart rate during exercise was monitored using Polar Heart Rate Monitors. Each exercise session consisted of a 3–5 minute warm up period followed by 30 minutes of training within the prescribed intensity range, and then a 3 to 5 minute cool down. Treadmill speed and grade were adjusted during each session to keep subjects within their prescribed intensity range.

Following aerobic exercise subjects completed upper body and lower body resistance training exercises. Movements targeting the chest, upper back, triceps, upper anterior and posterior legs, and lower legs were performed on resistance training machines, while movements targeting the biceps brachii and deltoids were performed using free weights. Sets were alternated in a circuit such that one particular muscle group was not exercised in consecutive sets. Subjects were given approximately one minute recovery time between sets. Resistance was adjusted so subjects could complete 12 repetitions per set of each exercise while maintaining proper form. As strength increased, resistance was changed so as to keep the subjects at the prescribed training intensity. Exercise training sessions were separated by at least 48 hours to allow for recovery and a trained exercise physiologist monitored all exercise sessions.

2.7. Sample Analysis

2.7.1. Saliva. Saliva was collected using salivettes, which contain small cotton swabs. Subjects were given the cotton swabs and instructed on appropriate placement of the swab in their mouths. The saliva was recovered by inserting a saturated cotton swab into the salivette and centrifuging the container at a relative centrifuge force of 39,000 kg for 5 minutes. The particulate free saliva sample was then obtained from the bottom of the salivette and saliva aliquots were frozen and stored at −80°C until analyzed. Salivary cortisol (CORT) was analyzed using a colorimetric sandwich ELISA (R&D Systems, Minneapolis, MN, USA).

2.7.2. Blood. Blood (3 mL) was collected at the specified times into serum separator tubes via venipuncture in an antecubital vein in the lower arm. All blood samples were taken with subjects in a seated position. The remaining whole blood was then centrifuged at a relative centrifuge force of 39,000 kg for 20 minutes, and the resulting supernatant was removed, alliquoted, and frozen at −80°C until needed for analysis. Commercially available colorimetric sandwich enzyme immunoassays (R&D Systems, Minneapolis, MN, USA) were used for the analysis of IL-6, sTNFrII, IGF-1, IGFBP-3, and GH. IL-1β was measured with a solid phase enzyme amplified sensitivity immunoassay (BioSource Europe, Nivelles, Belgium).

2.7.3. Urine. Urine was collected in urine collection containers over 24-hour periods in which no exercise was performed, both before and after the 6-week exercise training period. Subjects were given the urine collection container and instructed on the proper procedures for collection. After waking on the day in which the urine was to be collected, the first urination of the day was not collected, but each subsequent urination for the next 24-hours was to be collected in the urine collection container. Subjects were instructed to keep the urine cool until returned to the research facility, at which time it was alliquoted and frozen at −80°C until needed for analysis.

GH and CORT are released in a pulsatile fashion into the circulation throughout the day [59]. Therefore, to better estimate the total amount of hormone released, these hormones were measured in one milliliter samples of the urine, which provides the amount per milliliter. This value was then multiplied by the volume of urine produced during the day to yield the total amount produced over a 24-hour period. Urinary CORT and GH were both analyzed using a colorimetric sandwich ELISA (R&D Systems, Minneapolis, MN, USA). Normal urine production varies greatly between individuals, and is influenced by many factors. For the purposes of this study, only those subjects who collected at least 500 mL of urine (1/3 the mean production for participants) at each time point were included in the final analysis.

2.8. Quantification of Exercise Protocol. Caloric expenditure of physical work was quantified during the aerobic exercise portion of the exercise protocol using the formula published by Keytel et al. [60]. This method estimates caloric expenditure per minute of activity based on the heart rate recorded during the previous minute and includes the age, gender, body weight, and VO_2 max of the subject. The calories expended per minute were then multiplied by the duration of the exercise session yielding the total calories burned per session. There is no accepted method of estimating the caloric expenditure of resistance exercise, therefore the resistance portion of the exercise protocol was quantified based on total weight moved per session.

2.9. Measurement of Physical Activity. The Physical Activity Scale for the Elderly (PASE) was used to assess physical activity levels to determine if the aerobic and resistance exercise program had an effect on leisure and occupational physical activity levels in the exercise group. The PASE, which asks the participant to recall their activities over the previous 7 days, was administered at the pretesting session and again at the posttesting session.

2.10. Statistical Analysis. Repeated measures analysis of variance (ANOVA) was used to compare salivary cortisol within groups. Tukey post hoc analysis of treatment means was used to identify differences between groups. All other within-group variables were assessed using a paired t-test and comparison of variables between groups was done with an unpaired t-test. The significance level of all statistical tests was set at $\alpha = .05$. All values are expressed as mean $\pm$ standard error (SE). Upon completion of the initial analysis, the exercise group data was divided at the median body fat percentage, which was 20% body fat, and the data from these two groups was analyzed.

3. Results

3.1. Demographic Data. One hundred eleven (111) HIV-infected males were cleared for study participation while 17 subjects were excluded at screening based on the previously mentioned criteria. After oversampling of the control group and subject attrition, 59 subjects were randomly assigned to the control group and 52 subjects were randomized to the EX group. Forty (40) subjects completed the exercise intervention and 36 subjects in the control group finished the study. Body composition data were collected on 31 subjects in the exercise group and 27 persons in the control group. Hormone data were collected on 16 subjects in the exercise group and 27 persons in the control group. Demographic data for each group are presented in Tables 1 and 2.

3.2. Quantification of Exercise Protocol. The number of calories burned per week of aerobic exercise was not different

Table 1: Demographic data for subjects who completed the training study.

Exercise (MOD) group ($N = 16$)	Variable	Control (CON) group ($N = 10$)
43.1 ± 1.3	Age	46.6 ± 1.5
12	African American	6
4	Caucasian	4
373 ± 60 (7)	T-cell count	406 ± 76 (8)
8	HIV + symptomatic	6
3	HIV − symptomatic	1
3	AIDS	2
2	Did not answer	1
2	Excellent health	0
9	Good health	7
2	Fair health	2
1	Poor health	0
2	Did not answer	1

HIV status is based on 1993 CDC criteria.

Table 2: Demographic data for subjects who completed body composition assessment.

Exercise group ($N = 31$)	Variable	control Group ($N = 27$)
43.6 ± 1.3	Age	45.1 ± 1.5
20	African American	17
10	Caucasian	10
1	Other	0
28	ART Yes	25
3	ART No	2
17	HIV + symptomatic	19
4	HIV − symptomatic	1
7	AIDS	4
3	Did not answer	3
6	Excellent health	2
18	Good health	18
4	Fair hearth	6
1	Poor health	0
2	Did not answer	1

HIV status is based on 1993 CDC criteria. "ART Yes" refers to those subjects who reported taking at least 1 antiretroviral therapy during the study period.

between weeks; it ranged from a high of 523.3 ± 41.1 calories during week 4 to a low of 467.3 ± 54.5 calories during week 6. There was a difference in the total weight moved during each week of the resistance exercise portion of the protocol, with total pounds increasing over time. As expected, the total pounds lifted during week 6 was greater than week 1 ($P < .001$), week 2 ($P < .001$), week 3 ($P < .001$), and week 4 ($P = .02$). Similarly, the pounds lifted during week 5 were greater than week 1 ($P < .001$), week 2 ($P < .001$), and week 3 ($P = .005$).

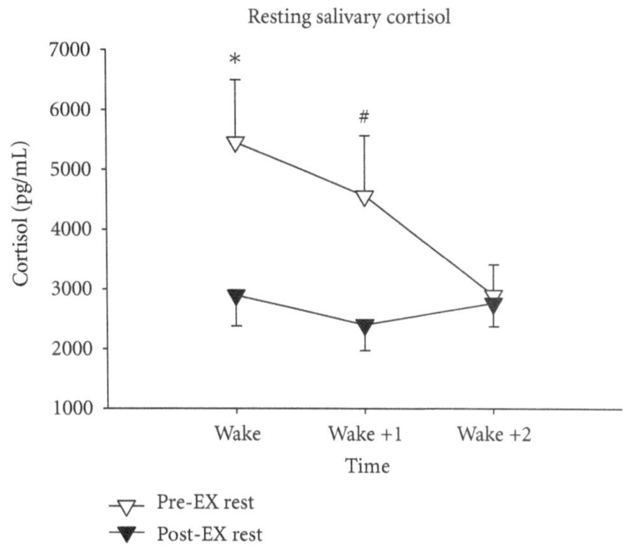

Figure 1: Salivary cortisol in exercise group. Salivary cortisol in MOD group ($N = 13$) subjects measured immediately after waking, 1 hour after waking, and 2 hours after waking. *Indicates difference from Pre-EX test with $P < .05$. #Indicates difference from Pre-EX test with $P = .07$.

3.3. Physical Activity Measurement. Following the 6-week moderate-intensity exercise intervention, there was no change in leisure and occupational physical activity levels (as measured by the PASE) in either the exercise group ($P = .38$) or the control group ($P = .42$). Additionally, there were no differences in baseline leisure and occupational physical activity levels between the exercise and control groups ($P = .29$).

3.4. Hormone and Cytokine Variables. There was a decrease in salivary cortisol at wake in the exercise group following the intervention, and there was a trend for a decrease one hour after waking in the exercise group (see Figure 1). There were no other changes from pre- to postintervention in either the exercise group or the control group in any of the hormone and cytokine variables measured (see Table 3).

3.5. Body Composition. At study initiation, there were no differences between groups regarding any of the body composition variables, including body mass index (see Table 4). Following the training period, the exercise group had an increase in lean tissue mass, while no change was seen in the control group (see Figure 2). Neither group exhibited changes in fat mass, total percentage of body fat, trunk percentage of fat, or any other body composition variable measured.

The exercise group was then divided at the median body fat percentage: those with a preintervention body fat above 20% (+20), and those below 20% (−20) (see Table 5). Following the intervention, subjects in the +20 group exhibited a significant increase in lean tissue mass ($P = .027$), as did the −20 group ($P = .014$). Further, the +20 group decreased total fat mass ($P = .02$), percentage of total

TABLE 3: Resting hormone values and normal ranges.

Variable	MOD group (N = 16)			CON group (N = 10)			Normal range
	Pre	Post	P value	Pre	Post	P value	
IL-6 (pg/mL)	3.6 ± 1.0	3.1 ± 0.6	.6	3.6 ± 1.0	6.7 ± 2.0	.08	1–10
IL-1-β (pg/mL)	5.9 ± 0.5	7.5 ± 1.7	.9	6.2 ± 0.6	6.1 ± 0.5	.3	0–2.5
sTNFrII (ng/mL)	2.2 ± 0.3	2.4 ± 0.4	.6	2.6 ± 0.5	2.5 ± 0.5	.4	0.28–7
IGF-1 (ng/mL)	128 ±10.5	132 ±10.8	.4	118 ± 10.7	137 ±17.5	.2	100–500
IGFBP-3 (ng/mL)	1897 ± 224	1934 ± 871	.7	1824 ± 247	1769 ± 218	.6	835–3778
Growth hormone (ng/day)	8.9 ± 1.7	7.1 ± 1.2	.3	15.1 ± 7.1	18.9 ± 11.8	.5	1–81
Cortisol (μg/mL)	55.6 ± 5.9	61.2±9	.3	45.5 ± 7.2	57.7 ± 8.8	.1	10–100
Testosterone (saliva) (pg/mL)	101.1 ± 16.4	65.1 ± 4.7	.06	95.1 ± 29.3	61.6 ± 8.9	.3	30–100

TABLE 4: Body composition of exercise and control group subjects.

	Exercise group (N = 31)			Control group (N = 27)		
	Pre	Post	P value	Pre	Post	P value
Height (m)	1.76 ± 0.01	1.76 ± 0.01	—	1.74 ± 0.02	1.74 ± 0.02	—
Mass (kg)	71.4 ± 2.1	71.8 ± 2.1	.08	72.5 ± 2.5	72.9 ± 2.5	.847
BMI (m/kg)	23.1	23.2		24.0	24.1	
LTM (kg)	56.3 ± 1.1	57.1 ± 1.1	<.001*	55.9 ± 1.15	55.9 ± 1.6	.915
FM (kg)	14.3 ± 1.9	14.1 ± 1.9	.295	14.1 ± 1.7	13.9 ± 1.7	.178
% Total body fat	18.5 ± 1.9	18.2 ± 1.8	.182	18.1 ± 1.8	18.0 ± 1.8	.317
% Fat trunk	21.7 ± 2.2	21.1 ± 2.1	.058	21.7 ± 2.1	21.7 ± 2.1	.239
% Fat ARM	13.7 ± 1.8	13.7 ± 1.8	1.0	14.1 ± 1.5	14.1 ± 1.7	.683
% FatLEG	16.3 ± 1.9	15.9 ± 1.9	.347	16.6 ± 1.7	16.0 ± 1.7	.847
LTM ARM (kg)	6.8 ± 0.2	6.9 ± 0.2	.244	6.8 ± 0.2	6.9 ± 0.2	1.0
LTM LEG (kg)	18.4 ± 0.5	18.8 ± 0.5	.107	18.3 ± 0.4	18.4 ± 0.4	.811
LTM TRK (kg)	27.2 ± 0.7	27.4 ± 0.6	.430	27.3 ± 0.9	27.1 ± 0.7	.695

*Indicates a significant change within groups from pre- to postintervention.

body fat (P = .009), and percentage of trunk fat (P = .001). No changes in these variables were seen in the −20 group. However, the −20 group did show an increase in total body mass (P = .007). The −20 group also had a significant increase in BMI (P = .007) following the intervention, while no change was observed in the +20 group (see Figures 3 and 4).

3.6. Peak Strength. Following the intervention, both the exercise and the control groups showed an increase in lower body strength. The exercise group had an increase in peak leg extension strength (P < .001) and an increase in peak leg curl strength (P = .001), while the control group also had increase in leg extension (P = .03) and leg curl strength (P = .006). The control group, however, did not show a change in lat pull down strength or chest press strength, while the exercise group did improve both lat pull down (P < .001) and chest press strength (P < .001) following the intervention (see Table 6).

3.7. Girth. There were no detectable changes in the exercise group for arm girth, leg girth, or chest girth following the training session. Additionally, there were no changes in arm girth, leg girth, or chest girth in the control group. Further, there were no differences between the two groups in any of the three girth measurements.

4. Discussion

Recent work has suggested that aerobic and resistance exercise interventions can cause beneficial physiologic responses and adaptations in HIV-infected populations [48, 61–63]. Specifically, we have shown that ACSM-based moderate-intensity aerobic and resistance exercise can cause transient increases in anabolic factors (GH) and decreases in catabolic factors (sTNFrII). Thus, the goal of this study was to determine if 6-weeks of a similar ACSM-based exercise program caused body composition, hormonal, and performance benefits. The rationale for testing this intervention is that (1) it is of shorter duration than other published works, (2) it is of lower intensity than other published works, (3) it combines both aerobic and resistance exercise, (4) it is an industry-recognized exercise prescription that benefits cardiovascular health in the apparently uninfected population, and (5) it has already been shown to stimulate positive humoral changes in an HIV-infected population [61].

There have been few original randomized controlled studies that have examined the effects of progressive resistance exercise interventions in HIV+ populations [48, 49, 64, 65]. Fewer yet are studies combining progressive resistance training and aerobic training [51–53]. However, results have been encouraging, with increases in total body mass [48, 51, 52, 65], lean mass [48, 49, 51], and peak strength [48, 49, 51–53, 65] being reported.

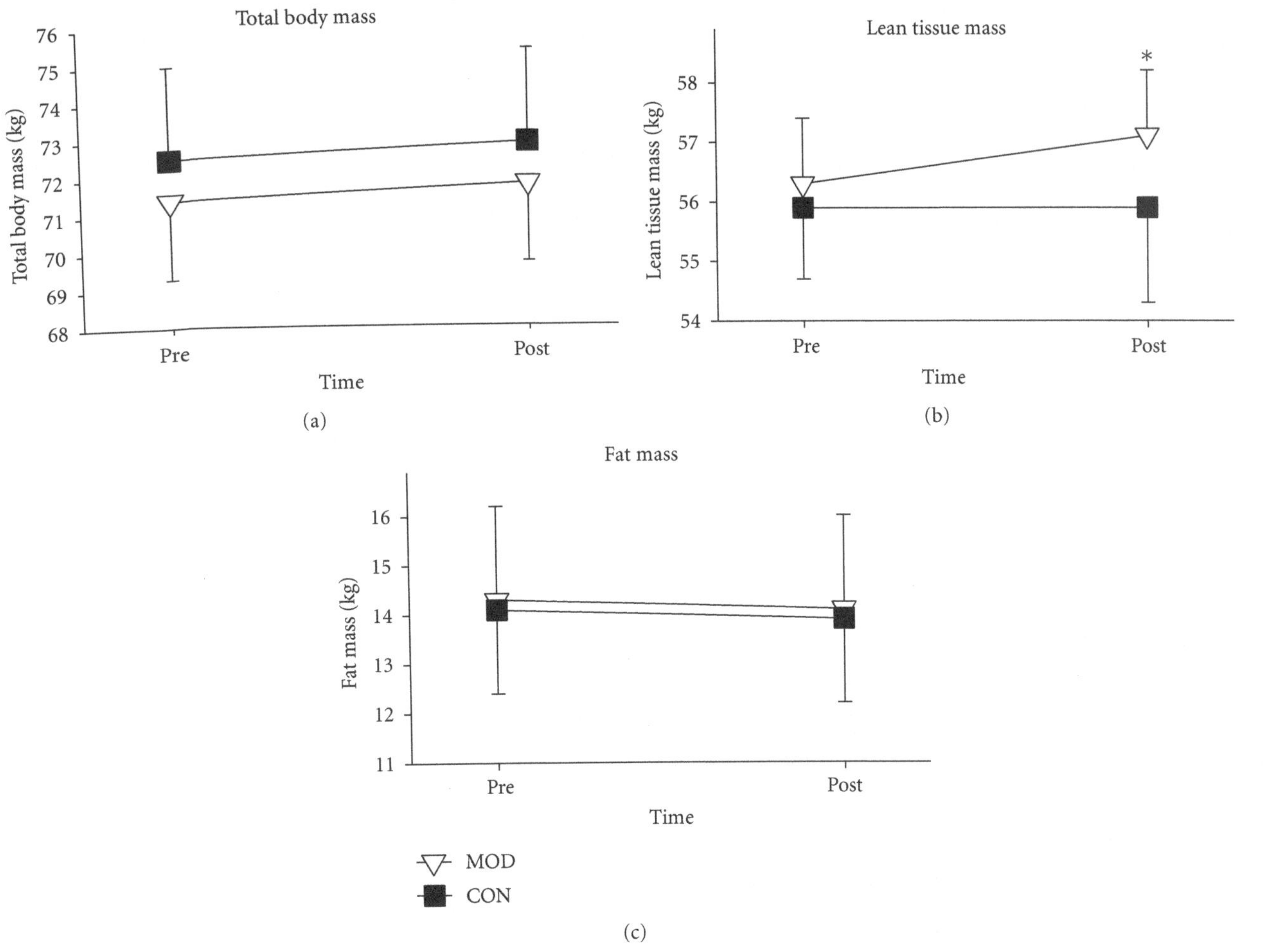

Figure 2: Lean tissue, fat, and total body mass of exercise and control group subjects. Body composition measurements taken via DXA in the exercise ($N = 31$) and control ($N = 27$) group before (pre) and after (post) the 6-week exercise intervention. *Indicates a significant change in the exercise group from Pre- to post-test.

Table 5: Body composition of exercise subjects above and below 20% body fat. Body composition variables, and within group changes, of exercise subjects as they are stratified into groups of above 20% total body fat (+20) and below 20% total body fat (−20), based on preintervention DXA testing.

	+20% Fat group ($N = 14$)			−20% Fat group ($N = 17$)		
	Pre	Post	P value	Pre	Post	P value
Height (m)	1.76 ± 0.01	1.76 ± 0.01	—	1.74 ± 0.02	1.74 ± 0.02	—
Mass (kg)	78.1 ± 2.7	78.0 ± 3.0	.665	65.8 ± 2.4	66.7 ± 2.4	.007*
BMI (m/kg)	25.4 ± 0.9	25.3 ± 1.0	.664	21.3 ± 0.8	21.6 ± 0.9	.007*
LTM (kg)	56.4 ± 1.7	57.1 ± 1.7	.027*	56.3 ± 1.5	57.1 ± 1.5	.014*
FM (kg)	23.4 ± 2.4	22.71 ± 2.4	.02*	6.7 ± 0.9	7.0 ± 1.0	.143
% Total Body Fat	28.6 ± 1.5	27.7 ± 1.6	.009*	10.1 ± 1.1	10.4 ± 1.1	.269
% Fat Trunk	33.7 ± 1.3	32.2 ± 1.4	.001*	11.8 ± 1.5	12.1 ± 1.5	.299
% Fat ARM	22.3 ± 2.4	22.0 ± 2.4	.619	6.6 ± 0.8	6.8 ± 1.1	.757
% FatLEG	24.3 ± 2.7	24.0 ± 2.8	.269	9.7 ± 1.2	9.3 ± 0.9	.578
LTM ARM (kg)	6.9 ± 0.3	6.9 ± 0.3	.746	6.8 ± 0.3	6.9 ± 0.3	.189
LTM LEG (kg)	18.4±.0.6	18.6 ± 0.6	.660	18.5 ± 0.7	19.1 ± 0.8	.014*
LTM TRK (kg)	27.3 ± 1.1	27.8 ± 0.9	.268	27.0 ± 0.8	27.0 ± 0.7	.898

* Indicates a significant change from pre- to postintervention within groups.

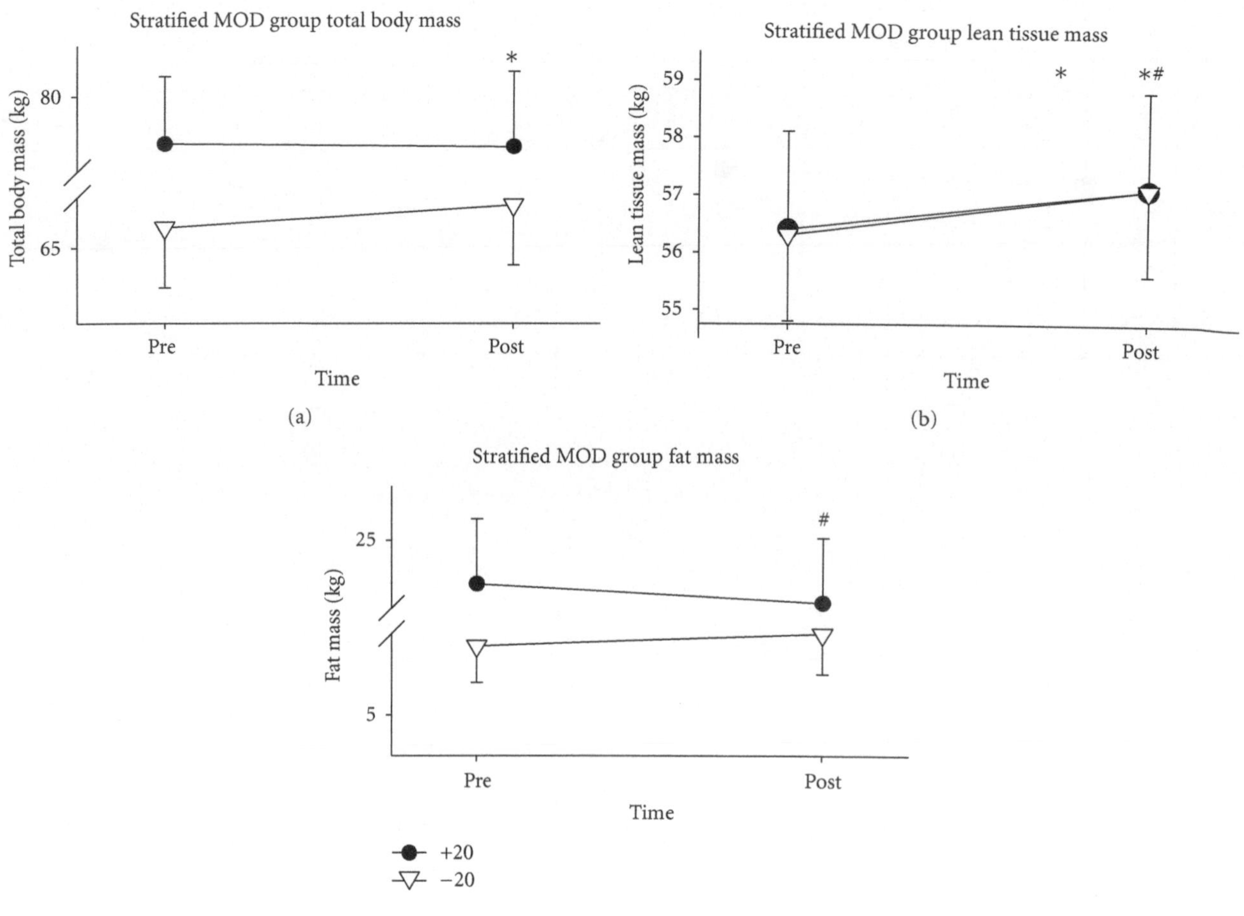

(c)

FIGURE 3: Lean tissue, fat, and total body mass of exercise subjects above and below 20% body fat. Body composition measurements taken via DXA in the +20 ($N = 14$) and −20 ($N = 17$) exercise groups before (pre) and after (post) the 6-week exercise intervention. *Indicates a significant change in the −20 group; #indicates a significant change in the +20 group.

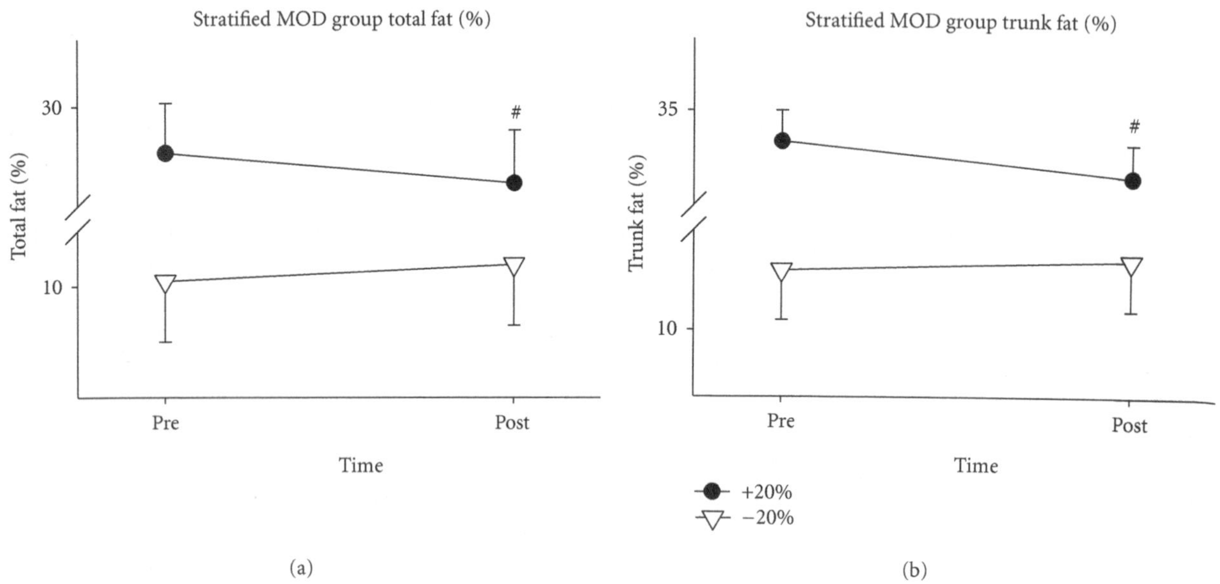

FIGURE 4: Total percentage of body fat and trunk percentage of body fat in exercise subjects above and below 20% Body Fat. Body fat percentage of measurements taken via DXA in the +20 ($N = 14$) and −20 ($N = 14$) exercise groups before (pre) and after (post) the 6-week exercise intervention. #Indicates a change in the +20 group.

Table 6: Strength changes in exercise and control group subjects. Peak strength results, and within group changes, for the exercise and control groups.

Exercise	Exercise Group (n = 17)			Control Group (n = 11)		
	Pre	Post	P Value	Pre	Post	P Value
Leg Extension	153.8 ± 13.3	185.3 ± 13.5	<.001*	140 ± 11.3	161.4 ± 13.9	.03*
Leg Curl	120.4 ± 9	143.2 ± 7.9	.001*	105.5 ± 6.1	128.2 ± 7.1	.006*
Lat Pull	132.4 ± 7.4	148.8 ± 7.2	<.001*	120.9 ± 7.6	124.1 ± 7.4	.532
Chest Press	118.5 ± 6.2	135.3 ± 7	<.001*	111.6 ± 8.7	109.6 ± 6.1	.782

* Indicates a significant change from pre to post test.

The majority of these interventions have required subjects to participate in three exercise sessions per week, and with the exception of one study [65], all have been 8–16 weeks in duration, with 12 weeks being the most common [48, 51–53]. The interventions have generally required the subjects to start resistance exercise at 60% of their 1-RM, then increased resistance to anywhere from 80% to 90% 1-RM near the end of the study.

4.1. Body Composition. The effect of exercise training on total body mass in HIV-infected persons has been ambiguous, with some showing an increase [48, 52, 65], while others [49, 51] have failed to detect a change. We did not show a difference in total body mass following training. Results similar to our findings were reported by Grinspoon and colleagues [51] and Roubenoff and colleagues who did not show an exercise effect on total body mass following 8 weeks of exercise training at intensities of 80% 1-RM and higher. Conversely, Spence et al. [65] reported a 1.7 kg increase in body weight following 6 weeks of three weekly progressive resistance exercise sessions. However, these subjects had recently recovered from *Pneumocystis carinii* pneumonia and were examined before HAART was available. Similarly, Lox and colleagues [52] reported a 2.2 kg increase in total body mass following 12 weeks of three weekly progressive resistance exercise sessions in men receiving ART. A 2.2 kg increase in total body mass was also seen by Bhasin et al. [48] in men (all receiving ART) following 16 weeks (3 sessions/wk.) of progressive resistance exercise with resistance progressing from 60% 1-RM to 90%. The discrepancy in total body mass changes following exercise is difficult to interpret for the following reasons: subjects in all the above studies had similar total body mass at study initiation, study duration did not appear to have an effect as both shorter [65] and longer [48, 52] durations showed increases, lower progressive resistance exercise intensities [65] and higher intensities [48] produced changes, and changes were seen in those who were on ART [48] and who were not [52, 65].

Our detection of a 0.8 kg increase in lean tissue mass is consistent with the findings of others. Grinspoon and colleagues [51] (2.3 kg), Bhasin and colleagues [48] (2.0 kg), and Roubenoff and colleagues [49] (1.8 kg) all showed significant increases in lean tissue mass using DXA, while Lox [52] showed a 2.3 kg increase in nonfat tissue using the skin-fold technique. While our change is significant, it appears to be less than the other studies mentioned. However, it should be noted that the subjects in our study trained at a lower intensity, less frequently, and for a shorter time period than the other studies showing increases in lean tissue mass. Of the other three studies mentioned, only Roubenoff et al. [49] (8 weeks) trained subjects for less than 12 weeks, and the reported change in lean tissue mass (1.8 kg) was less than the other studies (2.3 kg, 2.3 kg, and 2.0 kg) of longer duration. Additionally, of the other studies mentioned, only Lox et al. trained subjects at a lower intensity (60% 1-RM), but still observed similar lean tissue mass gains. It appears that ART does not influence lean tissue mass gains, as those subjects not using ART [52] and those subjects using ART [48, 49, 51] both showed an increase in lean tissue mass. However, it appears that the length of the intervention may affect lean tissue mass gains, in that interventions of longer duration may result in larger lean tissue mass gains.

To our knowledge, we are the first to stratify subjects based on preintervention body fat percentage. The rationale for this action was based on our finding of a significant increase in lean tissue mass in the exercise group, with no changes in total body mass or fat mass. When looking at the exercise group in this fashion it can be seen that the +20 did not change total body mass and the −20 gained total body mass, thus explaining the no change in total body mass the entire exercise group. Similarly, the +20 group lost total fat mass while the −20 group did not change in these variables, so again no overall change was seen. This suggests a differential effect of exercise training based on preintervention body composition.

The only group to show a regional change in LTM was the −20 group, who exhibited an increase in leg lean tissue mass. Using CT, Grinspoon et al. [51] showed an increase in thigh muscle area, and using MRI, Bhasin et al. [48] found and increase in thigh muscle volume. Though no direct mass measurements were taken, Spence et al. [65] showed an increase in thigh girth. Thus, it seems consistent across the literature that resistance training is capable of increasing lean tissue mass in the legs. However, what remains uncertain is why we only found an increase in leg lean tissue mass in the −20 group, and not the +20 group.

Only Roubenoff et al. [49] reported a decrease in total fat mass following their exercise intervention. This change in fat, however, could stem from the extended exercise time prescribed in the study (20 minutes of aerobic training in addition to 1 hour of resistance training). Our study, along with the remainder of the studies included in this discussion, only prescribed exercise regimens lasting approximately 60 minutes. The 0.92 ± 2.22 kg decrease in total fat mass reported by Roubenoff et al. [49] is similar to the 0.73 ± 0.3 kg decrease seen in our study. However, the decrease in our study was only observed in men with body fat above 20%. A possible explanation for this could be that the subjects in the Roubenoff et al. [49] study had 20.3 ± 2.3 kg of body fat at study initiation, while our exercise group as a whole had only 14.3 ± 1.9 kg, and our +20 group had 23.4 ± 2.4 kg. Therefore, when similar populations are compared, it appears that the exercise effect on total body fat is consistent. Further, our finding of a decrease in trunk fat in the +20 group suggests additional health benefits, as trunk fat is associated with numerous cardiometabolic diseases which are common in HIV disease [5].

4.2. Physical Functioning. Following our exercise training program, those in the exercise group showed significant increases in all four strength exercises tested: leg extension (25 ± 6.2%), leg curl (27.6 ± 9.5%), lat pull (13.8 ± 3.3%), and chest press (14.3 ± 1.8%). Bhasin et al. [48] (29–36%), Roubenoff et al. [49] (31–50%), and Lox et al. [52] also showed increased strength using conventional isotonic testing equipment. Rigsby et al. [53] showed upper and lower body strength increases using a hydraulic dynamometer. Only Grinspoon et al. [51] failed to show a change in strength following the exercise intervention; however, this study used isometric testing which, as the authors suggest, may not have detected a strength change if it existed [66]. These findings indicate that, even at moderate intensities, resistance exercise training can cause an increase in strength in HIV-infected men, independent of ART usage.

4.3. Resting Hormones and Cytokines. The only change detected within groups at the conclusion of the intervention was a decrease in salivary cortisol from pre- to posttest in the exercise group at the waking time point, and there was a trend for a decrease one hour after waking. There were no other changes detected in CORT, TEST, IGF-1, IGFBP-3, GH, IL-6, STNFrII, or IL-1-β in the CON or exercise groups.

In light of the changing landscape of HIV disease, namely, the shift towards a chronic disease, it is important to determine how HIV-infected persons who have yet to develop AIDS respond to exercise training. This population is now dealing with the same chronic diseases as their noninfected counterparts, specifically cancer and cardiometabolic diseases which are the leading non-HIV related causes of death [5]. While certain causes of these diseases (physical inactivity, stress, poor diet, etc.) undoubtedly are involved in their development in HIV-infected persons, the chronic immune activation and inflammatory state found in these persons may also be contributing factors [67]. Thus, it is prudent to examine exercise training in this population given the effect of exercise on body composition, hormone, and cytokine profiles, as well as the established benefits of exercise in reducing the risk for developing cardiometabolic diseases and cancer.

There is no research outlining the effects of exercise training on resting hormone and cytokine levels in HIV-infected persons. However, data does exist in other populations suggesting that exercise can influence many of the anabolic and catabolic factors implicated in the altered metabolic environment of those with HIV [68, 69]. The measurement of resting cytokines in the circulation is difficult, thus little research in this area is available. One of the major factors influencing cytokine levels is immune function, thus, whether the individual is currently ill or recovering from illness, cytokine levels are not "normal" [70]. Further, it appears that the primary impact of exercise on cytokine levels occurs during, and immediately following exercise sessions.

IL-6 levels have been shown to increase immediately following exercise that is not of sufficient intensity to induce muscle damage [71, 72] and this increase may provide anti-inflammatory effects [28]. This is the proposed rationale for the association that has been discovered between increased physical activity levels and decreased systemic inflammation in healthy persons [73–76]. Though we did see elevated resting levels of one inflammatory marker (IL-1-β) in our population, we did not see a change in IL-6 following exercise. It should be noted that IL-6 levels (3.6 ± 0.7 pg/mL) were found to be within a normal range in our sample and we have previously shown that IL-6 levels rise acutely following exercise [54], thus fitting with the hypothesis that the anti-inflammatory effects of exercise in this population are the result of acute changes.

We anticipated a change in sTNFrII and IL-1-β following the exercise intervention given that basal levels in HIV-infected populations have been shown to be elevated and acute exercise appears to decrease these levels [77]. We found sTNFrII to be within normal range in our population, thereby potentially explaining our lack of a detectable change because these levels were not elevated. By contrast, we found resting IL-1-β to be well above normal, which would fit with other literature. However, the theoretical anti-inflammatory effects of exercise are dependent upon another cytokine, IL-6, which we also found not to change following our training. Thus, if IL-6 did not increase, it would not directly block TNF-α and IL-1-β production, nor would it inhibit these inflammatory cytokines by inducing production of the anti-inflammatory agents IL-10 and IL-1ra production.

Normal daily urine production is highly variable and can range 700–2000 mL/day, with males typically producing approximately 1500 mL/day. The subjects in our study averaged 772 ± 118 mL/day, with a range from 300 mL to 2800 mL. We had access to our subjects only during the testing days, and the exercise sessions, thus in order to get a representation of total GH production we measured GH levels in 24-hour urine samples. We found an average of 8.6 ± 1.2 ng/day in our subjects, which fits within the 1–81 ng/day reported in healthy populations [78]. The consensus in the literature is that basal GH levels do not change following exercise training in healthy populations [69, 79, 80]. Therefore, our lack of change fits with the current literature.

Our resting IGF-1 levels were in the lower range of normal values for uninfected populations. Our results show no change in resting levels of IGF-1 following the exercise intervention. This finding, in combination with the reported presence of a change in elderly men [81] that often suffer the same decrease in lean tissue mass as HIV-infected persons, makes the absence of a change in resting IGF-1 levels in our population somewhat surprising. However, other clinical populations have failed to show a change in IGF-1 levels following exercise training, and some have even reported a decrease [82].

In addition to the lack of a change in IGF-1, the major binding protein, IGFBP-3, was also unchanged following our 6-week moderate-intensity exercise training intervention. The effects of individual exercise sessions on circulating IGFBP-3 levels are just now being realized, and the effect of exercise training on resting IGFBP-3 is largely unknown. Individual exercise sessions of moderate-intensity exercise appear to increase IGFBP-3 levels [83]. Combined with the increased IGFBP-3 proteolysis reported in HIV-infected persons, we anticipated an increase in resting IGFBP-3 levels. However, we did not see a change in IGFBP-3 following our intervention, and we found IGFBP-3 levels to be normal.

It appears that training status is a factor in the response of resting cortisol levels to exercise training. Prolonged exercise training does not appear to influence cortisol levels in trained persons [84, 85]; however, cortisol was lower following training in many populations, including sedentary adult males. Thus, it was unexpected that we did not see decreases in 24-hour cortisol levels following exercise training in our exercise naïve population. Additionally, it should be noted that resting cortisol levels in our population were within a normal range. However, our untrained population did exhibit a decrease in salivary cortisol following training at the wake time point and showed a trend for a decrease 1 hour after waking.

The literature clearly demonstrates that persons infected with HIV are prone to multiple hormone and cytokine abnormalities. However, the use of ART, which slows disease progression, can also normalize some of the hormone and cytokine levels in this population [86]. Thus, in our population receiving ART, and in whom a majority classified themselves as HIV-positive and asymptomatic, it is logical to see mostly normal hormone and cytokine profiles. Therefore, it is possible that these normal circulating levels explain the lack of changes following the exercise intervention.

A limitation that affects many training studies, not just those involving HIV-infected persons, is subject retention and adherence to exercise. The high incidence of opportunistic infections in this population adds difficulty to subject retention, as does the poverty and lack of reliable transportation that so often is present in this population. Further, the stigma of HIV that is pervasive in this country dissuades many HIV-infected persons from responding to research opportunities. Given these circumstances, plus the 3–5 weekly exercise sessions required in other studies, poor retention rates and small sample sizes can be explained. However, our 77% retention rate suggests that (1) our sampled population was not burdened with the problems of other studied HIV-infected populations, (2) our twice weekly sessions were manageable, and (3) our moderate-intensity exercise regimen lessened the fatigue and muscle soreness that accompanies higher intensity regimens.

5. Conclusion

This research further strengthens the evidence for the safety and efficacy of prescribing resistance and aerobic exercise to HIV-infected men. No adverse events were reported, and there was a very low attrition rate. The only circulating hormone or cytokine we found in abnormal levels was IL-1-β, which was more than twice as high as the upper limit of the normal range. Aside from IL-1-β, our findings of "normal" circulating levels of hormones and cytokines in our population may explain our inability to detect changes in all these variables, except cortisol. It may be that those HIV-infected persons experiencing chronic low-grade inflammation may respond differently to the prescribed exercise intervention. Even in healthy populations, it is common to not detect changes in these variables, thus our HIV-infected population may be responding to exercise training the same as uninfected persons. Also, these data suggest that the benefits of exercise training in HIV-infected men using ART may be attributable to the transient decrease in resting CORT, the accumulation of hormone and cytokine changes following individual exercise sessions, or to factors yet to be investigated. Additionally, these results indicate that low-volume moderate-intensity exercise training, consistent with ACSM guidelines, is sufficient to produce beneficial physiological adaptations and the resulting performance improvements (increase in upper and lower body strength) in HIV-infected men receiving ART. Further, this study is the first to report differential effects of exercise training based on preintervention body composition. Both the +20 and −20 groups realized the health benefits of increasing lean tissue mass, without gaining fat mass, while the +20 group also experienced the health benefit of losing trunk fat. Taken together, these results provide evidence for the effectiveness of combined moderate-intensity aerobic and resistance exercise training at decreasing the risk for cardiometabolic diseases and increasing lean tissue mass; thus, strongly suggesting its inclusion in the standardized treatment plan of those infected with HIV-1.

Acknowledgments

Support for this work was provided by the American College of Sports Medicine Carl V. Gisolfi Memorial Research Fund and NIH/NCMHD (1 P20 MD001770-030003). The views expressed are those of the authors and should not be assumed to be an endorsement of the ACSM.

References

[1] UNIADS, "UNAIDS global report on the AIDS epidemic," Tech. Rep., 2010.

[2] R. P. Walensky, A. D. Paltiel, E. Losina et al., "The survival benefits of AIDS treatment in the United States," *Journal of Infectious Diseases*, vol. 194, no. 1, pp. 11–19, 2006.

[3] M. Zwahlen, R. Harris, M. May, R. Hogg, D. Costagliola, F. de Wolf et al., "Mortality of HIV-infected patients starting potent antiretroviral therapy: comparison with the general population in nine industrialized countries," *International Journal of*

Epidemiology, vol. 38, no. 6, Article ID dyp306, pp. 1624–1633, 2009.

[4] F. J. Palella Jr., K. M. Delaney, A. C. Moorman et al., "Declining morbidity and mortality among patients with advanced human immunodeficiency virus infection," *New England Journal of Medicine*, vol. 338, no. 13, pp. 853–860, 1998.

[5] R. S. Braithwaite, A. C. Justice, C. C. H. Chang et al., "Estimating the proportion of patients infected with HIV who will die of comorbid diseases," *American Journal of Medicine*, vol. 118, no. 8, pp. 890–898, 2005.

[6] S. Grinspoon and A. Carr, "Cardiovascular risk and body-fat abnormalities in HIV-infected adults," *New England Journal of Medicine*, vol. 352, no. 1, pp. 48–62, 2005.

[7] C. A. Wanke, M. Silva, T. A. Knox, J. Forrester, D. Speigelman, and S. L. Gorbach, "Weight loss and wasting remain common complications in individuals infected with human immunodeficiency virus in the era of highly active antiretroviral therapy," *Clinical Infectious Diseases*, vol. 31, no. 3, pp. 803–805, 2000.

[8] A. J. S. Coats, "Origin of symptoms in patients with cachexia with special reference to weakness and shortness of breath," *International Journal of Cardiology*, vol. 85, no. 1, pp. 133–139, 2002.

[9] A. Schwenk, A. Beisenherz, K. Romer, G. Kremer, B. Salzberger, and M. Elia, "Phase angle from bioelectrical impedance analysis remains an independent predictive marker in HIV-infected patients in the era of highly active antiretroviral treatment," *American Journal of Clinical Nutrition*, vol. 72, no. 2, pp. 496–501, 2000.

[10] S. Grinspoon, C. Corcoran, D. Rosenthal et al., "Quantitative assessment of cross-sectional muscle area, functional status, and muscle strength in men with the acquired immunodeficiency syndrome wasting syndrome," *Journal of Clinical Endocrinology and Metabolism*, vol. 84, no. 1, pp. 201–206, 1999.

[11] P. Guenter, N. Muurahainen, G. Simons et al., "Relationships among nutritional status, disease progression, and survival in HIV infection," *Journal of Acquired Immune Deficiency Syndromes*, vol. 6, no. 10, pp. 1130–1138, 1993.

[12] M. C. Gelato and R. A. Frost, "IGFBP-3: functional and structural implications in aging and wasting syndromes," *Endocrine*, vol. 7, no. 1, pp. 81–85, 1997.

[13] M. S. Dworkin and J. M. Williamson, "AIDS wasting syndrome: trends, influence on opportunistic infections, and survival," *Journal of Acquired Immune Deficiency Syndromes*, vol. 33, no. 2, pp. 267–273, 2003.

[14] D. P. Kotler, A. R. Tierney, J. Wang, and R. N. Pierson, "Magnitude of body-cell-mass depletion and the timing of death from wasting in AIDS," *American Journal of Clinical Nutrition*, vol. 50, no. 3, pp. 444–447, 1989.

[15] A. Biglino, P. Limone, B. Forno et al., "Altered adrenocorticotropin and cortisol response to corticotropin-releasing hormone in HIV-1 infection," *European Journal of Endocrinology*, vol. 133, no. 2, pp. 173–179, 1995.

[16] N. Christeff, S. Gharakhanian, N. Thobie, W. Rozenbaum, and E. A. Nunez, "Evidence for changes in adrenal and testicular steroids during HIV infection," *Journal of Acquired Immune Deficiency Syndromes*, vol. 5, no. 8, pp. 841–846, 1992.

[17] J. M. Villette, P. Bourin, C. Doinel et al., "Circadian variations in plasma levels of hypophyseal, adrenocortical and testicular hormones in men infected with human immunodeficiency virus," *Journal of Clinical Endocrinology and Metabolism*, vol. 70, no. 3, pp. 572–577, 1990.

[18] R. Breitkreutz, J. Wagner, M. Tokus et al., "Flux of amino acids and energy substrates across the leg in weight-stable HIV-infected patients with acute opportunistic infections: indication of a slow protein wasting process," *Journal of Molecular Medicine*, vol. 79, no. 11, pp. 671–678, 2001.

[19] M. Lehrke, U. C. Broedl, I. M. Biller-Friedmann et al., "Serum concentrations of cortisol, interleukin 6, leptin and adiponectin predict stress induced insulin resistance in acute inflammatory reactions," *Critical Care*, vol. 12, no. 6, article no. R157, 2008.

[20] M. Hameed, R. W. Orrell, M. Cubbold, G. Goldspink, and S. D. R. Harridge, "Expression of IGF-I splice variants in young and old human skeletal muscle after high resistance exercise," *Journal of Physiology*, vol. 547, no. 1, pp. 247–254, 2003.

[21] S. Grinspoon, C. Corcoran, K. Lee et al., "Loss of lean body and muscle mass correlates with androgen levels in hypogonadal men with acquired immunodeficiency syndrome and wasting," *Journal of Clinical Endocrinology and Metabolism*, vol. 81, no. 11, pp. 4051–4058, 1996.

[22] M. C. Gelato and R. A. Frost, "IGFBP-3: functional and structural implications in aging and wasting Syndromes," *Endocrine*, vol. 7, no. 1, pp. 81–85, 1997.

[23] A. S. Dobs, "Androgen therapy in AIDS wasting," *Bailliere's Clinical Endocrinology and Metabolism*, vol. 12, no. 3, pp. 379–390, 1998.

[24] R. C. Griggs, D. Halliday, W. Kingston, and R. T. Moxley, "Effect of testosterone on muscle protein synthesis in myotonic dystrophy," *Annals of Neurology*, vol. 20, no. 5, pp. 590–596, 1986.

[25] R. J. Urban, Y. H. Bodenburg, C. Gilkison et al., "Testosterone administration to elderly men increases skeletal muscle strength and protein synthesis," *American Journal of Physiology*, vol. 269, no. 5, part 1, pp. E820–E826, 1995.

[26] F. C. W. Wu, "Endocrine aspects of anabolic steroids," *Clinical Chemistry*, vol. 43, no. 7, pp. 1289–1292, 1997.

[27] T. A. Robertson, M. A. L. Maley, M. D. Grounds, and J. M. Papadimitriou, "The role of macrophages in skeletal muscle regeneration with particular reference to chemotaxis," *Experimental Cell Research*, vol. 207, no. 2, pp. 321–331, 1993.

[28] R. Schindler, J. Mancilla, S. Endres, R. Ghorbani, S. C. Clark, and C. A. Dinarello, "Correlations and interactions in the production of interleukin-6 (IL-6), IL-1, and tumor necrosis factor (TNF) in human blood mononuclear cells: IL-6 suppresses IL-1 and TNF," *Blood*, vol. 75, no. 1, pp. 40–47, 1990.

[29] S. D. Anker and M. Rauchhaus, "Insights into the pathogenesis of chronic heart failure: immune activation and cachexia," *Current Opinion in Cardiology*, vol. 14, no. 3, pp. 211–216, 1999.

[30] M. O. Farber and E. T. Mannix, "Tissue wasting in patients with chronic obstructive pulmonary disease, the acquired immune deficiency syndrome, and congestive heart failure," *Neurologic Clinics*, vol. 18, no. 1, pp. 245–262, 2000.

[31] M. J. Tisdale, "Wasting in cancer," *Journal of Nutrition*, vol. 129, no. 1, supplement, pp. 243S–246S, 1999.

[32] L. L. Moldawer and F. R. Sattler, "Human immunodeficiency virus-associated wasting and mechanisms of cachexia associated with inflammation," *Seminars in Oncology*, vol. 25, no. 1, supplement 1, pp. 73–81, 1998.

[33] D. R. Luke, B. J. McCreedy, T. P. Sarnoski et al., "Phase I/II study of pentoxifylline with zidovudine on HIV-1 growth in AIDS patients," *International Journal of Clinical Pharmacology Therapy and Toxicology*, vol. 31, no. 7, pp. 343–350, 1993.

[34] N. Wig, P. Anupama, S. Singh et al., "Tumor necrosis factor-α levels in patients with HIV with wasting in South Asia," *AIDS Patient Care and STDs*, vol. 19, no. 4, pp. 212–215, 2005.

[35] P. T. Larsson, S. Hallerstam, S. Rosfors, and N. H. Wallén, "Circulating markers of inflammation are related to carotid artery atherosclerosis," *International Angiology*, vol. 24, no. 1, pp. 43–51, 2005.

[36] P. M. Ridker, J. E. Buring, N. R. Cook, and N. Rifai, "C-reactive protein, the metabolic syndrome, and risk of incident cardiovascular events: an 8-year follow-up of 14 719 initially healthy American women," *Circulation*, vol. 107, no. 3, pp. 391–397, 2003.

[37] J. H. Schwab, S. K. Anderle, R. R. Brown, F. G. Dalldorf, and R. C. Thompson, "Pro- and anti-inflammatory roles of interleukin-1 in recurrence of bacterial cell wall-induced arthritis in rats," *Infection and Immunity*, vol. 59, no. 12, pp. 4436–4442, 1991.

[38] G. Ku, C. E. Thomas, A. L. Akeson, and R. L. Jackson, "Induction of interleukin 1β expression from human peripheral blood monocyte-derived macrophages by 9-hydroxyoctadecadienoic acid," *Journal of Biological Chemistry*, vol. 267, no. 20, pp. 14183–14188, 1992.

[39] T. Mandrup-Poulsen, S. Helqvist, J. Molvig, L. D. Wogensen, and J. Nerup, "Cytokines as immune effector molecules in autoimmune endocrine diseases with special reference to insulin-dependent diabetes mellitus," *Autoimmunity*, vol. 4, no. 3, pp. 191–218, 1989.

[40] U. N. Das, "Is obesity an inflammatory condition?" *Nutrition*, vol. 17, no. 11-12, pp. 953–966, 2001.

[41] J. M. Fernández-Real and W. Ricart, "Insulin resistance and chronic cardiovascular inflammatory syndrome," *Endocrine Reviews*, vol. 24, no. 3, pp. 278–301, 2003.

[42] A. D. Pradhan, J. E. Manson, N. Rifai, J. E. Buring, and P. M. Ridker, "C-reactive protein, interleukin 6, and risk of developing type 2 diabetes mellitus," *Journal of the American Medical Association*, vol. 286, no. 3, pp. 327–334, 2001.

[43] W. D. Dudgeon, K. D. Phillips, C. M. Bopp, and G. A. Hand, "Physiological and psychological effects of exercise interventions in HIV disease," *AIDS Patient Care and STDs*, vol. 18, no. 2, pp. 81–98, 2004.

[44] B. F. Hurley, R. A. Redmond, R. E. Pratley, M. S. Treuth, M. A. Rogers, and A. P. Goldberg, "Effects of strength training on muscle hypertrophy and muscle cell disruption in elder men," *International Journal of Sports Medicine*, vol. 16, no. 6, pp. 378–384, 1995.

[45] M. L. Kohut, D. A. McCann, D. W. Russell et al., "Aerobic exercise, but not flexibility/resistance exercise, reduces serum IL-18, CRP, and IL-6 independent of β-blockers, BMI, and psychosocial factors in older adults," *Brain, Behavior, and Immunity*, vol. 20, no. 3, pp. 201–209, 2006.

[46] M. L. M. P. Jorge, V. N. de Oliveira, N. M. Resende et al., "The effects of aerobic, resistance, and combined exercise on metabolic control, inflammatory markers, adipocytokines, and muscle insulin signaling in patients with type 2 diabetes mellitus," *Metabolism: Clinical and Experimental*, vol. 60, no. 9, pp. 1244–1252, 2011.

[47] E. S. Ford, "Does exercise reduce inflammation? Physical activity and C-reactive protein among U.S. adults," *Epidemiology*, vol. 13, no. 5, pp. 561–568, 2002.

[48] S. Bhasin, T. W. Storer, M. Javanbakht et al., "Testosterone replacement and resistance exercise in HIV-infected men with weight loss and low testosterone levels," *Journal of the American Medical Association*, vol. 283, no. 6, pp. 763–770, 2000.

[49] R. Roubenoff, A. McDermott, L. Weiss et al., "Short-term progressive resistance training increases strength and lean body mass in adults infected with human immunodeficiency virus," *AIDS*, vol. 13, no. 2, pp. 231–239, 1999.

[50] R. Roubenoff and I. B. Wilson, "Effect of resistance training on self-reported physical functioning in HIV infection," *Medicine and Science in Sports and Exercise*, vol. 33, no. 11, pp. 1811–1817, 2001.

[51] S. Grinspoon, C. Corcoran, K. Parlman et al., "Effects of testosterone and progressive resistance training in eugonadal men with AIDS wasting: a randomized, controlled trial," *Annals of Internal Medicine*, vol. 133, no. 5, pp. 348–355, 2000.

[52] C. L. Lox, E. McAuley, and R. S. Tucker, "Aerobic and resistance exercise training effects on body composition, muscular strength, and cardiovascular fitness in an HIV-1 population," *International Journal of Behavioral Medicine*, vol. 3, no. 1, pp. 55–69, 1996.

[53] L. W. Rigsby, R. K. Dishman, A. W. Jackson, G. S. Maclean, and P. B. Raven, "Effects of exercise training on men seropositive for the human immunodeficiency virus-1," *Medicine and Science in Sports and Exercise*, vol. 24, no. 1, pp. 6–12, 1992.

[54] W. D. Dudgeon, K. D. Phillips, J. L. Durstine et al., "Individual exercise sessions alter circulating hormones and cytokines in HIV-infected men," *Applied Physiology, Nutrition and Metabolism*, vol. 35, no. 4, pp. 560–568, 2010.

[55] *ACSM'S Guidelines for Exercise Testing and Prescription*, Lippincott, Williams & Wilkins, Philadelphia, Pa, USA, 2005.

[56] A. Menkes, S. Mazel, R. A. Redmond et al., "Strength training increases regional bone mineral density and bone remodeling in middle-aged and older men," *Journal of Applied Physiology*, vol. 74, no. 5, pp. 2478–2484, 1993.

[57] S. Welle, C. Thornton, and M. Statt, "Myofibrillar protein synthesis in young and old human subjects after three months of resistance training," *American Journal of Physiology*, vol. 268, no. 3, part 1, pp. E422–E427, 1995.

[58] M. Brzycki, "Strength Testing—predicting a one-rep max from reps to fatigue," *Journal of Physical Education, Recreation, and Dance*, vol. 64, no. 1, pp. 88–90, 1993.

[59] E. N. Marieb, "Endocrine system," in *Human Anatomy & Physiology*, pp. 603–643, Pearson Education, 2006.

[60] L. R. Keytel, J. H. Goedecke, T. D. Noakes et al., "Prediction of energy expenditure from heart rate monitoring during submaximal exercise," *Journal of Sports Sciences*, vol. 23, no. 3, pp. 289–297, 2005.

[61] W. D. Dudgeon, K. D. Phillips, J. L. Durstine et al., "Individual exercise sessions alter circulating hormones and cytokines in HIV-infected men," *Applied Physiology, Nutrition and Metabolism*, vol. 35, no. 4, pp. 560–568, 2010.

[62] W. D. Dudgeon, K. D. Phillips, J. A. Carson, R. B. Brewer, J. L. Durstine, and G. A. Hand, "Counteracting muscle wasting in HIV-infected individuals," *HIV Medicine*, vol. 7, no. 5, pp. 299–310, 2006.

[63] G. A. Hand, K. D. Phillips, W. D. Dudgeon, G. W. Lyerly, J. L. Durstine, and S. E. Burgess, "Moderate intensity exercise training reverses functional aerobic impairment in HIV-infected individuals," *AIDS Care*, vol. 20, no. 9, pp. 1066–1074, 2008.

[64] D. Agin, D. Gallagher, J. Wang, S. B. Heymsfield, R. N. Pierson, and D. P. Kotler, "Effects of whey protein and resistance exercise on body cell mass, muscle strength, and quality of life in women with HIV," *AIDS*, vol. 15, no. 18, pp. 2431–2440, 2001.

[65] D. W. Spence, M. L. A. Galantino, K. A. Mossberg, and S. O. Zimmerman, "Progressive resistance exercise: effect on muscle function and anthropometry of a select AIDS population,"

Archives of Physical Medicine and Rehabilitation, vol. 71, no. 9, pp. 644–648, 1990.
[66] T. Hortobágyi, N. J. Lambert, and J. P. Hill, "Greater cross education following training with muscle lengthening than shortening," *Medicine and Science in Sports and Exercise*, vol. 29, no. 1, pp. 107–112, 1997.
[67] D. A. Cooper, "Life and death in the cART era," *The Lancet*, vol. 372, no. 9635, pp. 266–267, 2008.
[68] R. R. Kraemer, J. L. Kilgore, G. R. Kraemer, and V. D. Castracane, "Growth hormone, IGF-I, and testosterone responses to resistive exercise," *Medicine and Science in Sports and Exercise*, vol. 24, no. 12, pp. 1346–1352, 1992.
[69] W. J. Kraemer, K. Häkkinen, R. U. Newton et al., "Effects of heavy-resistance training on hormonal response patterns in younger versus older men," *Journal of Applied Physiology*, vol. 87, no. 3, pp. 982–992, 1999.
[70] L. R. Watkins, S. F. Maier, and L. E. Goehler, "Immune activation: the role of pro-inflammatory cytokines in inflammation, illness responses and pathological pain states," *Pain*, vol. 63, no. 3, pp. 289–302, 1995.
[71] M. A. Febbraio and B. K. Pedersen, "Muscle-derived interleukin-6: mechanisms for activation and possible biological roles," *FASEB Journal*, vol. 16, no. 11, pp. 1335–1347, 2002.
[72] A. M. W. Petersen and B. K. Pedersen, "The anti-inflammatory effect of exercise," *Journal of Applied Physiology*, vol. 98, no. 4, pp. 1154–1162, 2005.
[73] J. L. Abramson and V. Vaccarino, "Relationship between physical activity and inflammation among apparently healthy middle-aged and older US adults," *Archives of Internal Medicine*, vol. 162, no. 11, pp. 1286–1292, 2002.
[74] K. E. Fallon, S. K. Fallon, and T. Boston, "The acute phase response and exercise: court and field sports," *British Journal of Sports Medicine*, vol. 35, no. 3, pp. 170–173, 2001.
[75] D. F. Geffken, M. Cushman, G. L. Burke, J. F. Polak, P. A. Sakkinen, and R. P. Tracy, "Association between physical activity and markers of inflammation in a healthy elderly population," *American Journal of Epidemiology*, vol. 153, no. 3, pp. 242–250, 2001.
[76] D. E. King, P. Carek, A. G. Mainous, and W. S. Pearson, "Inflammatory markers and exercise: differences related to exercise type," *Medicine and Science in Sports and Exercise*, vol. 35, no. 4, pp. 575–581, 2003.
[77] A. M. W. Petersen and B. K. Pedersen, "The anti-inflammatory effect of exercise," *Journal of Applied Physiology*, vol. 98, no. 4, pp. 1154–1162, 2005.
[78] L. M. Winer, M. A. Shaw, and G. Baumann, "Urinary growth hormone excretion rates in normal and acromegalic man: a critical appraisal of its potential clinical utility," *Journal of Endocrinological Investigation*, vol. 12, no. 7, pp. 461–467, 1989.
[79] K. Häkkinen, A. Pakarinen, W. J. Kraemer, R. U. Newton, and M. Alen, "Basal concentrations and acute responses of serum hormones and strength development during heavy resistance training in middle-aged and elderly men and women," *Journals of Gerontology. Series A*, vol. 55, no. 2, pp. B95–B105, 2000.
[80] J. O. Marx, N. A. Ratamess, B. C. Nindl et al., "Low-volume circuit versus high-volume periodized resistance training in women," *Medicine and Science in Sports and Exercise*, vol. 33, no. 4, pp. 635–643, 2001.
[81] E. T. Poehlman, C. J. Rosen, and K. C. Copeland, "The influence of endurance training on insulin-like growth factor-1 in older individuals," *Metabolism: Clinical and Experimental*, vol. 43, no. 11, pp. 1401–1405, 1994.
[82] B. C. Nindl, S. A. Headley, A. P. Tuckow et al., "IGF-I system responses during 12 weeks of resistance training in end-stage renal disease patients," *Growth Hormone and IGF Research*, vol. 14, no. 3, pp. 245–250, 2004.
[83] L. Di Luigi, L. Guidetti, M. Nordio, C. Baldari, and F. Romanelli, "Acute effect of physical exercise on serum insulin-like growth factor-binding protein 2 and 3 in healthy men: role of exercise-linked growth hormone secretion," *International Journal of Sports Medicine*, vol. 22, no. 2, pp. 103–110, 2001.
[84] J. P. Ahtiainen, A. Pakarinen, M. Alen, W. J. Kraemer, and K. Häkkinen, "Short vs. long rest period between the sets in hypertrophic resistance training: influence on muscle strength, size, and hormonal adaptations in trained men," *Journal of Strength and Conditioning Research*, vol. 19, no. 3, pp. 572–582, 2005.
[85] I. Smilios, T. Pilianidis, M. Karamouzis, and S. P. Tokmakidis, "Hormonal responses after various resistance exercise protocols," *Medicine and Science in Sports and Exercise*, vol. 35, no. 4, pp. 644–654, 2003.
[86] N. Amirayan-Chevillard, H. Tissot-Dupont, Y. Obadia, H. Gallais, J. L. Mege, and C. Capo, "Highly active antiretroviral therapy (HAART) and circulating markers of immune activation: specific effect of HAART on Neopterin," *Clinical and Diagnostic Laboratory Immunology*, vol. 7, no. 5, pp. 832–834, 2000.

Motivating Factors and Psychosocial Barriers to Condom Use among out-of-School Youths in Dar es Salaam, Tanzania: A Cross Sectional Survey Using the Health Belief Model

E. Katikiro[1] and B. Njau[2]

[1] *National AIDS Control Programme Division, Ministry of Health and Social Welfare, P.O. Box 11857, Dar es Salaam, Tanzania*
[2] *Community Health Department, Kilimanjaro Christian Medical University College, P.O. Box 2240, Moshi, Tanzania*

Correspondence should be addressed to B. Njau, biesein2007@gmail.com

Academic Editors: D. Aunis, M. Gherardi, S. Kravcik, H. C. Mwandumba, and J. Poudrier

Condoms remain a cost-effective and relatively simple intervention to prevent HIV infection. However, condom use is still very low, particularly among youths aged 15 to 24. 348 individuals (186 males and 162 females) completed a pre-tested questionnaire. Logistic regression analysis was used to identify factors associated with condom use. Out of 348 respondents, 296 (85.0%) were sexually experienced, and 260 (87.8%) reported noncondom use in the past 3 months prior to the study. Among men, noncondom use was independently associated with feeling shy to buy condoms (AOR = 1.16; 95% CI 1.12–1.34), condoms reducing sexual pleasure (AOR = 8.19; 95% CI 3.98–17.01), and HIV is a serious and deadly disease (AOR = 0.36; 95% CI 0.28–0.46). Among women, experiencing forced sex (AOR = 1.16; 95% CI 1.10–2.78), condoms reduce sexual pleasure (AOR = 8.29; 95% CI 3.36–20.73), and inability to convince a partner to use condoms (AOR = 1.14; 95% CI 1.04–1.28) were predictors of noncondom use. In conclusion, sexually active youths in this population practice risky sexual behaviours, with low condom use practices. Strategies to improve condom use should address these psychosocial barriers associated with noncondom use.

1. Background

One of the current challenges on the prevention and control of HIV/AIDS faced worldwide is among youths aged 15–24 years. In fact, the global population of adolescents has reached over one billion, the largest in human history [1]. In Tanzania, almost two-thirds (65%) of the population is under the age of 24 and almost 20% are aged 15 to 24 [2, 3]. In fact, these young women and men are the future of Tanzania, and thus, an important age group for the growth and prosperity of the country.

Globally, it is estimated that 5.4 million young people aged 15 to 24 are living with HIV, 3.2 million of whom live in Sub-Saharan Africa [4]. In sub-Saharan Africa (SSA), youth lack access to HIV prevention education programes. For example, only 8 percent of out-of-school youth, have access to prevention education programes [5]. Overall HIV prevalence of 7.9% among youth aged 15 to 24 in Tanzania indicates that the HIV infection is two to three times higher among females than males (7% versus 3%), particularly in urban populations [2, 3]. Indicators of sexual activity among young people in Tanzania have revealed that a substantial proportion (46%) of unmarried youths aged 15–24 years is sexually experienced [2, 3]. A host of environmental, economic, and legal factors, together with social norms, are likely to influence early sexual debut and tendency for adolescents to be engaged in high-risk sexual behavior. In Tanzania, HIV prevention programes have been developed to target school youths and exclude out-of-school youths, increasing the risk of HIV infection among this risk age group [2, 6].

Several studies have documented the cost-effectiveness of condoms as a relatively simple intervention to prevent HIV infection [5]. However, studies on adolescent sexuality have shown a significant increase in sexual experiences at a younger age associated with inconsistent condom use

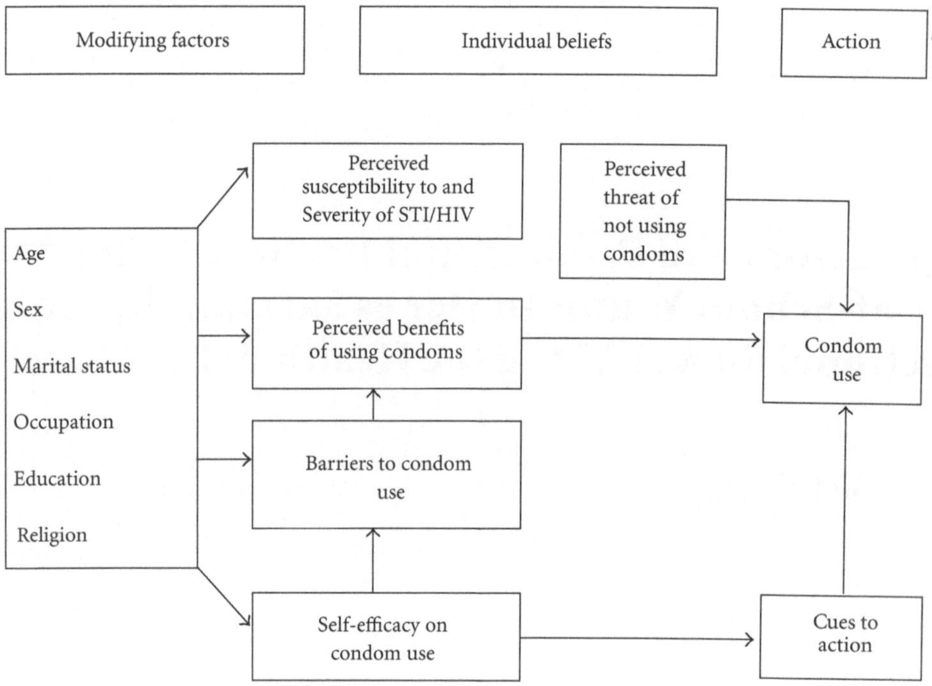

FIGURE 1: Operational description of the Health Belief Model.

[5, 7–9]. Several psychosocial and cultural barriers have been associated with noncondom use among youths aged 15 to 24 [6, 10, 11]. Moreover, more than 200 myths, misconceptions, and fears that may hinder access to or use of condoms have been noted [5]. A major challenge facing HIV prevention efforts among out-of-school youths aged 15 to 24 in Tanzania is inadequate research on factors that influence youth's intention to use condom. Studies conducted on factors associated with condom use among youths and adolescents in Tanzania were mainly on knowledge, attitudes, and practices (KAP), which did not use behavioral change models such as the Health Belief Model (HBM). This study therefore aims to identify factors that motivate or hinder condom use among out-of-school youths in an urban setting. Considering that the HBM is a behavioral change framework, which addresses several constructs influencing health behaviors (e.g., condom use), it is expected that the findings from this analysis will provide a basis for designing an effective HIV prevention programme for out-of-school youths aged 15–24 years in urban communities of Tanzania.

2. Conceptual Framework

This study, which was conducted in Kinondoni Municipality, Dar es Salaam, Tanzania used the Health Belief Model (HBM) as a conceptual framework to address the study objectives. The Health Belief Model postulates that an individual's actions are based on beliefs. According to the HBM, several factors, such as perceived susceptibility or vulnerability, perceived severity of an outcome or condition, perceived efficacy or benefits of a preventive measure, and the perceived barriers are important factors in decision making [12, 13] (see Figure 1).

3. Methods

3.1. Study Setting. The study was conducted in Dar es Salaam, one of the 30 regions of Tanzania mainland, with a population of more than three million. Kinondoni Municipality is one of three municipal councils with a population of 1.4 million and youths aged 15 to 24 are estimated to be 234,003 (17.2%) [14, 15]. The HIV prevalence in Dar es Salaam in 2009 was estimated to be 9.3%, which is comparatively higher than the national prevalence of 5.9% [2, 3]. This study was done in Kinondoni municipality of Dar es Salaam's three municipal councils. Data was collected in 12 randomly selected wards (administrative areas) out of 27 wards. This study was conducted from April to May, 2010.

3.2. Sample and Sample Size Determination. The sample size was calculated using Epi Info version 6.0 statistical software. The result of a previous study conducted in Nigeria, which showed condom use among out-of-school youths to be 29% was used to calculate the sample size for the present study [16]. To detect a 10% difference in the rate of condom use with 95% confidence interval (CI) and 80% power, a sample of 316 was needed. With the addition of a 10% nonresponse rate, the final sample size became 348.

A multistage sampling method was applied in this study. A list of all wards in all four divisions within Kinondoni Municipality was used to randomly select 12 wards out of a total of 27 wards. Out of the 12 wards, an average of 29 households per ward was randomly selected to participate into the study. Using the local government register a list of all out-of-school 15–24-year-olds was made and stratified by age groups and gender. Proportional sampling was used to select equal numbers of eligible males and females for participation in the study. Consent was obtained after the potential participants and their parents (for those below 18 years) were informed of the study's objectives.

3.3. Ethical Clearance. Approval for this study was obtained from the Kilimanjaro Christian Medical University College Research Ethics Committee. Permission to conduct the study was sought from the Kinondoni Municipal authority.

3.4. Measurements. The survey questionnaire was designed as an adaptation from the instrument used in Benin for assessing key constructs of Health Belief Model related to condom use among youths aged 15–24 years [17]. Social demographic characteristics, proportions of condom use, and individual risk factors were also noted. A pretest of the tool was carried out on a convenience sample of 30 out-of-school youths of both genders for clarity and to ascertain internal consistency. Respondents were given a self-administered questionnaire in Kiswahili, a language well known to the participants. Confidentiality was assured by providing a private room or other place. Four trained research assistants (2 males; 2 females) who were about the same age (range 15–24 years old) and the same gender assisted those unable to read or write. The completed questionnaires were checked by the research assistants for errors and missing data before participants were allowed to go.

The dependent variable for this study was measured by asking respondents if they have had sex without condom in the past 3 months (1 = yes, 2 = no). A response of "yes" indicated sexual risk behavior.

Social-demographic characteristics included: age categorized into two groups (15–19 and 20–24), sex, marital status divided into two categories (married and unmarried), ability to read divided into 2 categories (able to read or read with difficulties), occupation was categorized into two groups (employed or unemployed), and religion. Behavioral risk factors included number of lifetime sexual partners, use of condoms in the first sexual contact, whether a partner has demanded unprotected sex, whether respondent had experienced forced sex, whether the respondent had had sex under the influence of alcohol, and whether the respondent had ever had sex under the influence of substances. Each of the questions required a response of 1 = yes, 2 = no.

Psychosocial barriers to condom use were assessed with the following questions: My religion prohibits condom use, I do not like condoms, condoms reduce sexual pleasure, condoms offer no protection, and I feel shy to buy condoms. Each of the questions required a response of 1 = yes, 2 = no.

Motivational factors to condom use were assessed by the following questions: whether respondents perceived HIV as a severe and deadly disease, perceived benefits of condom to prevent STIs/HIV, whether respondent feels confident to discuss condom use prior to sexual intercourse, and whether respondent is able or not to convince a partner to use condoms. Each of the questions required a response of 1 = yes, 2 = no.

3.5. Statistical Analysis. Data were edited, cleaned, coded, entered, and analysed using Statistical Package for Social Sciences version-12.0.1 (SPSS for Windows; SPSS, Chicago, IL, USA). The assessment included descriptive and multivariate analyses. Probability values (P values) were calculated at the 0.05 level of significance, odds ratios (OR) and 95% confidence intervals (CI) were provided in bivariate analysis. Two-sided chi-square tests for association were computed to detect differences in categorical variables and logistic regressions were calculated when testing the relationships between categorical variables. To identify independently associated factors, two logistic regression models (women and men) were performed, with noncondom use in the past 3 months as the outcome variable. All explanatory variables that were associated with the outcome variable in bivariate analysis, variables with a P-value of ≤ 0.05 were included in the logistic models.

4. Results

4.1. Characteristics of Respondents. The study was based on a sample of 348 randomly selected respondents. A total of 186 men and 162 women respondents were interviewed, yielding a response rate of 100%. The mean age for men was 20.37 ± 2.58 (mean ± SD) years while it was 19.56 ± 2.60 (mean ± SD) for women. The sociodemographic characteristics are summarized in Table 1.

4.2. Behavioral Risk Factors. Two hundred and ninety six participants reported had had sex in the past 3 months prior to the study. Out of 296 sexually active participants, 260 (87.8%), reported noncondom use in the past 3 months prior to the study. Males were marginally more likely to use a condom compared to their female counterparts (41.3% versus 36.7%). In addition, females were more likely to have unprotected sexual intercourse due to a demand from a sexual partner compared to males (53.7% versus 38.7%; $P < 0.01$). Furthermore, the study revealed that more females than males experienced forced sex (44.9% versus 18.7%; $P < 0.001$). There were no significant differences between males and females in the other behavioral risk factors (data not shown).

4.3. Psychosocial Barriers to Condom Use. As depicted in Table 2, there was significant difference in perceived psychosocial barriers to condom use among condom users (n = 36) and noncondom users (n = 260) in the past 3 months prior to the study. Participants who agreed that their religion prohibits condom use were more likely to report having sex without a condom (odds ratio (OR) = 5.08; 95% CI 2.22–11.86; $P < 0.001$). In addition, sex without a condom was associated with a belief that condoms reduced sexual pleasure (OR) = 15.00; 95% CI 5.58–41.87; $P < 0.001$), condoms offer no protection (OR) = 7.83; 95% CI 3.32–18.95; $P < 0.001$),

TABLE 1: Sociodemographic characteristics of respondents ($n = 348$).

Characteristics of the respondents	Total $N = 348$ (%)	Males $n = 186$ (53.4)	Females $n = 162$ (46.6)
Age group (years)			
15–19	146 (42.0)	68 (36.6)	78 (48.1)
20–24	202 (58.0)	118 (63.4)	84 (51.9)
Marital status			
Unmarried	260 (74.7)	142 (76.3)	118 (72.8)
Married	88 (25.3)	44 (23.7)	44 (27.2)
Ability to read			
Able to read	291 (83.6)	156 (83.9)	135 (83.3)
Read with difficulty/not at all	57 (16.4)	30 (16.1)	27 (16.7)
Occupation			
Employed	84 (24.1)	48 (25.8)	36 (22.2)
Unemployed	264 (75.9)	138 (74.2)	126 (77.8)
Religion			
Christian	201 (57.8)	106 (57.0)	95 (58.6)
Muslim	128 (36.8)	69 (37.1)	59 (36.4)
Other	19 (5.4)	11 (5.9)	8 (5.0)

TABLE 2: Psychosocial barriers to condom use among condom users and noncondom users in the past 3 months ($n = 296$).

	Sex without condom past 3 months		OR [95% CI]; P value
	Yes ($n = 260$)	No ($n = 36$)	
My religion prohibits condom use			
Yes	172 (66.2)	10 (27.8)	1
No	88 (33.8)	26 (72.2)	5.08 (2.22–11.86), $P < 0.001$
I do not like condoms			
Yes	164 (63.1)	28 (77.8)	1
No	96 (36.9)	8 (22.2)	0.49 (0.20–1.18), $P = 0.08$
Condoms reduce sexual pleasure			
Yes	231 (88.8)	6 (16.7)	1
No	21 (11.2)	30 (83.3)	15.00 (5.58–41.87), $P < 0.001$
Condoms offer no protection			
Yes	188 (73.8)	9 (25.0)	1
No	72 (26.2)	27 (75.0)	7.83 (3.32–18.95), $P < 0.001$
I feel shy to buy condoms			
Yes	229 (88.1)	6 (16.7)	1
No	31 (11.9)	30 (83.3)	25.78 (13.27–36.94), $P < 0.001$

and feeling shy to buy a condom (OR) = 25.78; 95% CI 13.27–36.94; $P < 0.001$).

4.4. Determinants of Condom Use. Table 3 presents a summary of selected determinants of behavioral change associated with noncondom use among male and female participants in the past 3 months prior to the study. In the bivariate analyses for men, five variables (experiencing forced sex, demanded unprotected sex by a partner, feeling shy to buy condoms, condoms reducing sexual pleasure, and perceiving HIV as a serious and deadly disease) were found to be associated with noncondom use. Males who had experienced forced sex were more likely to report sex without a condom compared to those who had never experienced forced sex (odds ratio (OR) = 1.66; 95% CI 1.12–2.35; $P = 0.02$). Additionally, males who were asked not to use condoms by a partner were more likely to report sex without a condom (OR = 1.58; 95% CI 1.10–2.27; $P = 0.01$). Males who agreed that they felt shy to buy condoms were more likely to report sex without a condom compared to those who did not feel shy (OR = 1.12; 95% CI 1.10–1.24; $P = 0.001$). Furthermore, males who perceived that condoms reduce sexual pleasure were more likely to report sex without a condom compared

TABLE 3: Unadjusted odds ratios (OR) and adjusted odds ratios (AOR) from logistic regression analyses that examined the association between selected determinants of behavioural change and noncondom use in past 3 months by gender (n = 296).

Variables	[a]Males (n = 160)			[b]Females (n = 136)		
Bivariate analysis	P value	OR	95% CI	P-value	OR	95% CI
Had sex while drunk	0.480	0.87	0.58–1.30	<0.001†	0.39	0.20–0.75
Experienced forced sex	<0.01*	1.66	1.12–2.35	<0.01*	1.43	1.14–2.77
Demanded unprotected sex from partner	<0.01*	1.58	1.10–2.27	0.765	0.94	0.60–1.45
I feel shy to buy condoms	<0.001†	1.12	1.10–1.24	<0.001†	1.30	1.05–1.17
Condoms reduce sexual pleasure	<0.001†	1.20	1.13–1.27	<0.001†	1.27	1.05–1.54
Cannot convince partner to use condoms	0.063	0.94	0.84–1.06	<0.01*	1.10	1.02–1.18
Discussed condom use prior to sex	0.521	0.91	0.82–1.95	<0.001†	0.57	0.49–0.67
HIV is a serious and deadly disease	<0.001†	0.40	0.18–0.63	<0.001†	0.51	0.33–0.78
Multivariate analysis§	P-value	AOR	95% CI	P-value	AOR	95% CI
Had sex while drunk	0.520	0.91	0.62–1.34	<0.001†	0.16	0.13–0.21
Experienced forced sex	0.574	1.14	0.73–1.76	<0.01*	1.16	1.10–2.78
I feel shy to buy condoms	<0.001†	1.16	1.12–1.34	0.58	0.78	0.29–2.10
Condoms reduce sexual pleasure	<0.001†	8.19	3.98–17.01	<0.001†	8.29	3.39–20.73
Cannot convince partner to use condoms	0.071	0.92	0.76–1.16	<0.01*	1.14	1.04–1.28
Discussed condoms use prior to sex	0.561	0.45	0.11–1.05	<0.001†	0.41	0.18–0.63
HIV is a serious and deadly disease	<0.001†	0.36	0.28–0.46	<0.001†	0.39	0.21–0.66

† $P < 0.001$; * $P < 0.01$.
[a]2 Log likelihood test: 176.5; R^2 .224; [b]2 Log likelihood test: 138.5; R^2 .257.
§ Adjusted for sociodemographic, risky behaviours, psychosocial and motivating variables.

to those who did not perceive so (OR = 1.20; 95% CI 1.13–1.27; P = 0.001). On the other hand, males who perceived HIV as a serious and deadly disease were less likely to report sex without a condom compared to those who did not perceive so (OR = 0.40; 95% CI 0.18–0.63; $P < 0.001$).

For females, seven variables (experiencing forced sex, feeling shy to buy condoms, condoms reducing sexual pleasure, cannot convince partner to use a condom, prior discussion about condom use, perceiving HIV as a serious and deadly disease and having sex while drunk,) were found to be significantly associated with condom use. Females who had experienced forced sex were more likely to report sex without a condom compared to those who had not (OR = 1.43; 95% CI 1.14–2.77; P = 0.02). In addition, females who agreed that they felt shy to buy condoms were more likely to report sex without a condom compared to those who did not feel shy (OR = 1.30; 95% CI 1.05–1.17; P = 0.001). Furthermore, females who perceived that condoms reduce sexual pleasure (OR = 1.27; 95% CI 1.05–1.54; P = 0.001), or that they cannot convince a partner to use condoms (OR = 1.10; 95% CI 1.02–1.18; P = 0.02) were more likely to report sex without a condom. Females who discussed condom use prior to having sex were less likely to report sex without a condom compared to those who never had prior discussion (OR = 0.57; 95% CI 0.49–0.67; $P < 0.001$). Lastly, perceiving that HIV is a serious and deadly disease (OR = 0.51; 95% CI 0.33–0.78; $P < 0.001$) and having sex while drunk (OR = 0.39; 95% CI 0.20–0.75; P = 0.001) were negatively associated with condom use among females participants.

In the multivariate logistic regression analyses for men, three variables (feeling shy to buy condoms, condoms reducing sexual pleasure, and perceiving HIV as a serious and deadly disease), were found to be associated with noncondom use (Table 3). Males who were shy to buy condoms had an increased odd to report sex without a condom, in comparison to those who were not shy (adjusted odds ratio (AOR) = 1.16; 95% CI 1.12–1.34). Among male respondents, the strongest predictor of having sex without a condom was the perception that condoms reduce sexual pleasure (AOR = 8.19; 95% CI 3.98–17.01). On the other hand, males' respondents who perceived that HIV is a serious and deadly disease were less likely to report having sex without a condom compared to those who did not perceive so (AOR = 0.36; 95% CI 0.28–0.46).

For females, six variables (having sex while drunk, experiencing forced sex, condoms reduce sexual pleasure, cannot convince partner to use a condom, prior discussion about condom use and perceiving HIV as a serious and deadly disease) were found to be significantly associated with having sex without a condom. As depicted in Table 3, females who reported not having sex while drunk were less likely to report having sex without a condom compared to those who had sex while drunk (AOR = 0.16; 95% CI 0.13–0.21). Females who had experienced forced sex were more likely to report having sex without a condom (AOR = 1.16; 95% CI 1.10–2.78). Among female respondents, the strongest predictor of having sex without a condom was the perception that condoms reduce sexual pleasure (AOR = 8.29; 95% CI 3.39–20.73). Females who agreed that they cannot convince a partner to use condoms were more likely to report having sex without a condom than those who did not (AOR = 1.14; 95% CI 1.04–1.28).

Females who did not report prior discussion about condoms with their partners were 59% less likely to use a condom, in comparison with those who reported having prior discussion (AOR = 0.41; 95% CI 0.18–0.63). Lastly, females who perceived that HIV is a serious and deadly disease were less likely to report having sex without a condom than those who did not perceive HIV as a serious and deadly disease (AOR = 0.39; 95% CI 0.21–0.66).

5. Discussion

The aim of the study was to determine factors that motivate or hinder condom use among out-of-school youths aged 15 to 24 in an urban setting in Tanzania. The majority (85%) of out-of-school youths in this study reported engaging in premarital sex. In addition, 87.8% of the sexually experienced respondents reported having unprotected intercourse in the past 3 months, with male respondents marginally more likely to report condom use than their female counterparts. This finding substantiates national data gathered by the 2006-2007 Demographic Health Survey (DHS) for Tanzania, whereby 24% of unmarried youths aged 15–24 years reported unprotected intercourse [2] and may reflect a more fundamental problem that condom use decreases among adolescents as sexual experiences increases, despite of the high risk of HIV infection [2, 10]. This observation supports the need for an innovative community outreach HIV prevention services for out-of-school youths in Tanzania [5, 6]. This study used the Health Belief Model (HBM) to assess factors associated with condom use among the sample population. According to the HBM framework, perceived barriers to prevention are regarded as the single most powerful predictor for decision making [12, 13, 17]. Consistent with studies conducted elsewhere, the study findings confirmed that the psychosocial barriers are associated with noncondom use among sexually experienced respondents [5, 17, 18]. The psychosocial factors associated with noncondom use in this study were as follows: my religion prohibits condoms, condoms reduce sexual pleasure, condoms offer no protection, and feeling shy to buy a condom. The strongest psychosocial barrier to condom use, for both men and women was their concern regarding condoms' reduction of sexual pleasure. Respondents who perceived that a condom reduces sexual pleasure were more likely to report having sex without a condom when compared to those who did not perceive that a condom reduces sexual pleasure. Generally, adolescents tend to believe that a condom reduces sexual pleasure and this belief discourages condom use. According to existing literature on sexuality, there are four basic reasons why an individual may want to have sex. The first is sex for pleasure; the second is sex for procreation; the third is sex for money/or gifts; and the fourth is sex for cultural rituals [5]. The finding suggests that the interventions designed to increase condom use, should address the belief that condoms reduce pleasure among out-of-school youths. An intervention designed to increase motivation for condom use while addressing this salient barrier may be an effective approach [5, 11, 19–21].

Using the HBM to assess motivating factors associated with condom use among out-of-school youths, we found that perceiving HIV as a serious and deadly disease was strongly associated with condom use in both male and female models. Respondents who perceived HIV as a serious and deadly disease were less likely to report having sex without a condom when compared to those who did not perceive HIV as a serious and deadly disease. This finding supports one of the important constructs of the HBM, which postulates that perceived susceptibility and severity of a condition (e.g., HIV infection) or disease is an important component, which may induce action or inaction and emphasize that behavioral change will be successful, if people feel threatened by their current behavioral patterns [13]. There is thus a need to strengthen current strategies based on increasing perceived severity of HIV as a deadly disease to encourage condom use among out-of-school youths in this population.

Champion and Skinner observed that self-efficacy and cues for action are the key components of HBM framework and are important determinants for an individual in taking an action and the degree of persistence they would demonstrate in the face of failure and/or adversity [13, 22]. However, in this study self-efficacy was not predictive of condom use and thus was eliminated from the analysis. This observation is contrary to other studies in other settings, which observed an association between high self-efficacy and condom use. Self-efficacy, which is defined as a confidence in individual's capacity to perform a desired behavior was observed to be a driving force in consistent condom use [6, 17, 21]. Thus further research, perhaps with combined theoretical frameworks, such as social learning theories [23], may help to assess the association between self-efficacy and condom use among this population [19, 20, 22, 24].

In this study, discussion on condom use prior to having sex was associated with condom use among female participants. Females who reported to discuss condom use prior to having sex were less likely to report having sex without a condom when compared to those who did not discuss condom use. These findings are consistent with the HBM, which postulates that discussion on health behavior (e.g., condom use) can act as a trigger for action. From the HBM perspectives, human behavior depends on cues that elicit certain response and that maintenance of the desired behavior, such as condom use may occur by automation after sufficient repetition [13]. The finding suggests that perhaps a goal-oriented method of communication designed to potentiate readiness to condom use may be an effective approach [19].

Experiencing forced sex was independently associated with noncondom use among female respondents. Females who had experienced forced sex were more likely to report having sex without a condom when compared to those who had not experienced forced sex. In addition, female respondents who had sex while drunk were more likely not to use condoms. As expected, females who agreed to have sex while drunk were more likely to report having sex without a condom when compared to those who did not had sex while drunk. Although this observation does not support any construct of the HBM, it underscores the role of risky behaviors in understanding the progression towards health behavior change [19, 21, 25] and underscores the importance of addressing the risk behavior of mixing unprotected sexual intercourse and alcohol and skill development for safer sex among out-of-school youths.

This study has certain limitations. First, the study asked respondents to recall events that may have happened in the distant past. Recall bias is more likely among older youths who may be unable to remember the exact timing of their first sexual intercourse and condom use. Second, the study was limited in that it relied on self-report. It is known that the self-reported behavior is subject to reporting bias. Third, the study did not assess the grades that out-of-school participants had completed. Future research among out-of-school participants needs to include this variable in order to identify the influence of educational attainment on behavioral change in this population. Fourth, HIV knowledge was not assessed in this study, which may have affected the study findings particularly in a setting where many myths related to HIV do exist. Item level analyses were limited due to the low internal reliability of items. Future studies needs to assess important constructs related to condom use attitudes and intention. Lastly, cross-sectional studies are not adequate for measuring the directionality of associations found and therefore this cannot account for potential confounders. Nevertheless, the study findings provide very important insight into perspectives of out-of-school youths on condom use in Kinondoni Municipality in Dar es Salaam, Tanzania. The findings emphasize the extent to which noncondom use remains an important issue and the need to focus additional attention on this issue, particularly among out-of-school youths.

6. Conclusions

In this study the majority of out-of-school youths were sexually experienced, while condom use was low. Furthermore, most sexually experienced participants had unprotected intercourse in the past 3 months prior to the study. This observation may reflect a fundamental problem of noncondom use as sexual experiences increases, irrespective of perceived risk of HIV infection among out-of-school youths in Tanzania. Our finding supported some of the HBM constructs, such as perceived barriers, perceived severity of HIV infection, and cues for action, but also highlighted constructs of other theoretical frameworks. Our findings confirmed that psychosocial barriers are associated with noncondom use in both men and women. This finding pinpoints the importance of addressing psychosocial barriers associated with noncondom use and suggests strategies which will increase motivation for condom use in this population. Perceiving HIV as serious and deadly disease was strongly associated with condom use and suggests that the fear of a disease outcome may influence a successful behavioral change. In addition, discussion on condom use prior to having sex was associated with condom use, particularly among women. These findings emphasize the importance of cues for action as triggers to potentiate readiness to action, such as condom use. On the other hand, self-efficacy on intention to use a condom was not predictive of condom use in this sample. This suggests that further research is required to determine the association between self-efficacy on intention to use a condom and condom use among out-of-school youths. Additionally, having sex while drunk was associated with noncondom use, particularly among females respondents. This observation underscores the importance of addressing the risk behavior of mixing unprotected sexual intercourse and alcohol among this population. In conclusion, therefore, it is important that HIV programme planners and policy makers understands the importance of focusing on identified HBM constructs that have the greatest probability of influencing condom use by providing accurate information about benefits of condoms and address gender norms and skills to overcome HIV risk behaviors in efforts to dispel psychosocial barriers to condom use among out-of-school youths in Tanzania.

Competing Interests

The author(s) declare that they have no competing interest.

Authors' Contribution

E. Katikiro participated in the design, data collection, and interpretation of results and drafting of the paper. B. Njau participated in the design, interpretation of results and drafting of the paper. The authors have read and approved the final paper.

Acknowledgments

The authors thank all the individuals who accepted to participate in this study. The authors also thank leaders of NGAO and Tandale youth group for their participation during the sampling of participants. Their gratitude goes to Kinondoni Municipal authorities and KCMU College for granting permission to conduct the study. The authors acknowledge the Tanzania Ministry of Health and Social Welfare financial support for MK. Lastly, the authors also thank Drs. Melissa Watt and Ayaba Worjoloh of Duke University, USA for critical review and editing of the paper.

References

[1] UNFPA, "Youth and HIV/AIDS Fact Sheet: State of the World population," http://www.unfpa.org/swp/.../factsheets/facts_youth.htm, 2009.

[2] Tanzania Commission for AIDS (TACAIDS), Zanzibar AIDS Commission (ZAC), National Bureau of Statistics (NBS), and Office of the Chief Government Statistician (OCGS) & Inc, *Tanzania HIV/AIDS and Malaria Indicator Survey 2007-08*, TACAIDS, ZAC, NBS, OCGS, and Macro International Inc, Dar es Salaam, Tanzania, 2008.

[3] UNGASS/TACAIDS, "UNGASS reporting for 2010: Tanzania Mainland & Zanzibar," http://www.unaids.org/.../country-progressreports/2010, 2010.

[4] International Youth Foundation website, http://www.iyfnet.org/document.cfm/748.

[5] UNAIDS/WHO, "Epidemiological Fact sheet on HIV and AIDS (pdf)," http://apps.who.int/globalatlas/predefinedReports/EFS2008/full/EFS2008_IN.pdf, 2010.

[6] B. Njau, S. Mtweve, L. Barongo et al., "The influence of peers and other significant persons on sexuality and condom-use among young adults in nothern Tanzania," *African Journal of AIDS Research*, vol. 5, no. 3, pp. 33–40, 2006.

[7] G. Calazanz, R. Dias, G. Venturi, and V. Paiva, "Age and condom use at first secual intercourse of Brazilian adolescents," *Revista de Saude Publica*, vol. 42, no. 1, pp. 45–53, 2008.

[8] H. Alemu, D. H. Mariam, K. A. Belay, and G. Davey, "Factors predisposing out-of-school youths to HIV/AIDS-related risky sexual behaviour in northwest Ethiopia," *Journal of Health, Population and Nutrition*, vol. 25, no. 3, pp. 344–350, 2007.

[9] L. A. Lema, R. S. Katapa, and A. S. Musa, "Knowledge on HIV/AIDS and sexual behaviour among youths in Kibaha District, Tanzania," *Tanzania journal of health research*, vol. 10, no. 2, pp. 79–83, 2008.

[10] N. Prata, L. Morris, E. Mazive, F. Vahidnia, and M. Stehr, "Relationship between HIV risk perception and condom use: Evidence from a population-based survey in Mozambique," *International family planning perspectives*, vol. 32, no. 4, pp. 192–200, 2006.

[11] S. M. Noar, "Behavioral interventions to reduce HIV-related sexual risk behavior: Review and synthesis of meta-analytic evidence," *AIDS and Behavior*, vol. 12, no. 3, pp. 335–353, 2008.

[12] S. H. Muela, J. M. Ribera, and I. Nyamongo, "Health seeking behaviour and health system response," DCPP Working Paper 14, 2003.

[13] V. L. Champion and C. S. Skinner, "The Heath Belief Model," in *Health Behavior & Health Education: Theory, Research and Practice*, Glanz et al., Ed., pp. 45–65, Jossey-Bass, San Francisco, Calif, USA, 4th edition, 20082008.

[14] National Bureau of Statistics (NBS), "Population and Housing Census 2002," General Report, National Bureau of Statistics, Dar es Salaam, Tanzania, 2002.

[15] Kinondoni Municipal Profile, http://www.kmc.go.tz/, 2008.

[16] A. O. Adebiyi and M. C. Asuzu, "Condom use amongst out of school youths in a local government area in Nigeria," *African Health Sciences*, vol. 9, no. 2, pp. 92–97, 2009.

[17] S. H. Hounton, H. Carabin, and N. J. Henderson, "Towards an understanding of barriers to condom use in rural Benin using the health belief model: a cross sectional survey," *BMC Public Health*, vol. 5, no. 8, pp. 1471–2458, 2005.

[18] O. O. Lawoyin and R. M. Kanthula, "Factors that influence attitudes and sexual behavior among constituency youth workers in Oshana Region, Namibia," *African Journal of Reproductive Health*, vol. 14, no. 1, pp. 55–69, 2010.

[19] J. L. Lauby, L. Bond, D. Eroğlu, and H. Batson, "Decisional balance, perceived risk and HIV testing practices," *AIDS and Behavior*, vol. 10, no. 1, pp. 83–92, 2006.

[20] J. O. Prochaska, "Moving beyond the transtheoretical model," *Addiction*, vol. 101, no. 6, pp. 768–774, 2006.

[21] A. Outlaw, S. Naar-King, H. Janisse, and J. T. Parsons, "Predictors of condom use in a multisite study of high-risk youth living with HIV," *AIDS Education and Prevention*, vol. 22, no. 1, pp. 1–14, 2010.

[22] A. Bandura, *Social Learning Theories*, Printice-Hall, Englewood Cliffs, NJ, USA, 1997.

[23] J. D. Fisher and W. A. Fiseher, "Theoretical approaches to individual-level change in HIV risk behaviours," in *Handbook of HIV Prevention, (AIDS Prevention and Mental Health)*, J. L. Peterson and R. J. DiClemente, Eds., pp. 3–48, Kluwer Academic/Plenum, New York, NY, USA, 2000.

[24] K. L. Hall and J. S. Rossi, "Meta-analytic examination of the strong and weak principles across 48 health behaviors," *Preventive Medicine*, vol. 46, no. 3, pp. 266–274, 2008.

[25] L. M. Romero, J. S. Galbraith, L. Wilson-Williams, and K. M. Gloppen, "HIV prevention among African American Youth: how well have evidence-based interventions addressed key theoretical constructs?" *AIDS and Behavior*, pp. 1–16, 2010.

Permissions

The contributors of this book come from diverse backgrounds, making this book a truly international effort. This book will bring forth new frontiers with its revolutionizing research information and detailed analysis of the nascent developments around the world.

We would like to thank all the contributing authors for lending their expertise to make the book truly unique. They have played a crucial role in the development of this book. Without their invaluable contributions this book wouldn't have been possible. They have made vital efforts to compile up to date information on the varied aspects of this subject to make this book a valuable addition to the collection of many professionals and students.

This book was conceptualized with the vision of imparting up-to-date information and advanced data in this field. To ensure the same, a matchless editorial board was set up. Every individual on the board went through rigorous rounds of assessment to prove their worth. After which they invested a large part of their time researching and compiling the most relevant data for our readers. Conferences and sessions were held from time to time between the editorial board and the contributing authors to present the data in the most comprehensible form. The editorial team has worked tirelessly to provide valuable and valid information to help people across the globe.

Every chapter published in this book has been scrutinized by our experts. Their significance has been extensively debated. The topics covered herein carry significant findings which will fuel the growth of the discipline. They may even be implemented as practical applications or may be referred to as a beginning point for another development. Chapters in this book were first published by Hindawi Publishing Corporation; hereby published with permission under the Creative Commons Attribution License or equivalent.

The editorial board has been involved in producing this book since its inception. They have spent rigorous hours researching and exploring the diverse topics which have resulted in the successful publishing of this book. They have passed on their knowledge of decades through this book. To expedite this challenging task, the publisher supported the team at every step. A small team of assistant editors was also appointed to further simplify the editing procedure and attain best results for the readers.

Our editorial team has been hand-picked from every corner of the world. Their multi-ethnicity adds dynamic inputs to the discussions which result in innovative outcomes. These outcomes are then further discussed with the researchers and contributors who give their valuable feedback and opinion regarding the same. The feedback is then collaborated with the researches and they are edited in a comprehensive manner to aid the understanding of the subject.

Apart from the editorial board, the designing team has also invested a significant amount of their time in understanding the subject and creating the most relevant covers. They scrutinized every image to scout for the most suitable representation of the subject and create an appropriate cover for the book.

The publishing team has been involved in this book since its early stages. They were actively engaged in every process, be it collecting the data, connecting with the contributors or procuring relevant information. The team has been an ardent support to the editorial, designing and production team. Their endless efforts to recruit the best for this project, has resulted in the accomplishment of this book. They are a veteran in the field of academics and their pool of knowledge is as vast as their experience in printing. Their expertise and guidance has proved useful at every step. Their uncompromising quality standards have made this book an exceptional effort. Their encouragement from time to time has been an inspiration for everyone.

The publisher and the editorial board hope that this book will prove to be a valuable piece of knowledge for researchers, students, practitioners and scholars across the globe.

List of Contributors

Musie Ghebremichael
Harvard Medical School and Ragon Institute of MGH, MIT and Harvard, 400 Technology Square, Room 857, Cambridge, MA 02129, USA

Rubeshan Perumal, Nesri Padayatchi and Kogieleum Naidoo
Centre for the AIDS Programme of Research in South Africa (CAPRISA), University of KwaZulu-Natal, Durban 4000, South Africa

Stephen Knight
Department of Public Health Medicine, University of KwaZulu-Natal, Durban 4000, South Africa

Rajesh T. Patil
Department of Microbiology, Azeezia Institute of Medical Sciences & Research, Kollam, Kerala, India

Rajiv M. Gupta
DDGMS (IT) Office of Directorate General ofMedical Services (Army) Integrated HQ ofMoDAG's Branch, L Block, New Delhi, India

Sourav Sen
Department of Microbiology, Army Hospital (Research& Referral), Delhi, India

Srikanth P. Tripathy
National JALMA Institute of Leprosy and other Mycobacterial Diseases (Indian Council of Medical Research), Agra, India

Devidas N. Chaturbhuj, Nitin K. Hingankar and Ramesh S. Paranjape
National AIDS Research Institute (Indian Council of Medical Research), Pune, India

W. Massavon
Department of Paediatrics, University of Padua, Via Giustiniani 3, 35128 Padua, Italy
St. Raphael of St. Francis Hospital (Nsambya Hospital), Kampala, Uganda

L. Barlow-Mosha, D. Wabwire and M. Mubiru
Makerere University, Johns Hopkins University Research Collaboration, Kampala, Uganda

L. Mugenyi
Infectious Diseases Research Collaboration, Mulago Hospital Complex, Kampala, Uganda

W. McFarland
Department of Global Health Sciences, University of California San Francisco, 50 Beale Street, 12th

G. Gray
University ofWitwatersrand, 1 Jan Smuts Avenue, Braamfontein 2000, Johannesburg, South Africa

R. Lundin, P. Costenaro, M. Penazzato, D. Bilardi and C. Giaquinto
Department of Paediatrics, University of Padua, Via Giustiniani 3, 35128 Padua, Italy

M. M. Nannyonga, C. P. Namisi and S. Kironde
St. Raphael of St. Francis Hospital (Nsambya Hospital), Kampala, Uganda

D. Bagenda
Makerere University, Johns Hopkins University Research Collaboration, Kampala, Uganda
Department of Global Heath and Population, Harvard University School of Public Health, Boston, MA, USA

A. Mazza
Santa Chiara Hospital, Via Largo GoldMedals 9, 38122 Trento, Italy

M. G. Fowler
Makerere University, Johns Hopkins University Research Collaboration, Kampala, Uganda
Department of Pathology, Johns Hopkins School of Medicine 600 N.Wolfe Street/Carnegie 43 Baltimore, MD 21287, USA

P. Musoke
Makerere University, Johns Hopkins University Research Collaboration, Kampala, Uganda
Department of Paediatrics and Child Health, Makerere University, Kampala, Uganda

C. Shumba, L. Atuhaire, R. Imakit, R. Atukunda, and P. Memiah
Uganda Program, Institute of Human Virology, University of Maryland, 124 Luthuli Avenue, Bugolobi, Kampala, Uganda

Mitiku Teshome Hambisa and Yadeta Dessie
Department of Public Health, College of Health and Medical Sciences, Haramaya University, P.O. Box 235, Harar, Ethiopia

Ahmed Ali
Department of Epidemiology and Biostatistics, School of Public Health, Addis Ababa University, P.O. Box 25819/1000, Addis Ababa, Ethiopia

Spinello Antinori
Department of Biomedical and Clinical Sciences Lvigi Sacco, Universit`a degli Studi di Milano, Via GB Grassi 74, 20157 Milano, Italy

D. R. Arora
Department of Microbiology, SGT Medical College, Budhera, Gurgaon, Haryana 123505, India

Megha Maheshwari
Department of Microbiology, SGT Medical College, Budhera, Gurgaon, Haryana 123505, India
Shri Guru Gobind Singh Tricentenary Medical College, Village Budhera, Gurgaon, Haryana 123505, India

B. Arora
Department of Pathology, SGT Medical College, Budhera, Gurgaon, Haryana 123505, India

Zelalem Teklemariam, Degu Abate and Habtamu Mitiku
Department of Medical Laboratory Sciences, College of Health and Medical Sciences, Haramaya University, P.O. Box 235, Harar, Ethiopia

Yadeta Dessie
Department of Public Health, College of Health and Medical Sciences, Haramaya University, P.O. Box 235, Harar, Ethiopia

Debjani Guha and Velpandi Ayyavoo
Department of Infectious Diseases and Microbiology, Graduate School of Public Health, University of Pittsburgh, 130 Desoto Street, Pittsburgh, PA 15261, USA

Habtamu Mitiku and Zelalem Teklemariam
Department of Medical Laboratory Sciences, College of Health and Medical Sciences, Haramaya University, P.O. Box 235, Harar, Ethiopia

Tekabe Abdosh
College of Health and Medical Sciences, Haramaya University, School of Medicine, P.O. Box 235, Harar, Ethiopia

Denise Mudzinge and Danai Tavonga Zhou
Department of Medical Laboratory Sciences, College of Health Sciences, University of Zimbabwe, P.O. Box A 178, Harare, Zimbabwe

Tinashe Kenny Nyazika
Department of Chemical Pathology, College of Health Sciences, University of Zimbabwe, P.O. Box A 178, Harare, Zimbabwe

Tawanda Jonathan Chisango
Biotechnology Department, Chinhoyi University of Technology, P.O. Box 2274, Chinhoyi, Zimbabwe

Yemane Berhane
Axum College of Nursing, Tigray, Ethiopia

Haftu Berhe, Gerezgiher Buruh Abera and Hailemariam Berhe
Department of Nursing, College of Health Sciences, Mekelle University, Ethiopia

Ijeoma Okoronkwo, Anthonia Chinweuba and Peace Iheanacho
Department of Nursing Sciences, University of Nigeria, Enugu Campus, Enugu, Nigeria

Uchenna Okeke
Department of Nursing Sciences, University of Nigeria, Enugu Campus, Enugu, Nigeria
Nursing Services Department, Nnamdi Azikiwe University Teaching Hospital, Nnewi, Nigeria

Alessandra D'Abramo, Claudia D'Agostino, Alessandra Oliva, Marco Iannetta, Gabriella D'Ettorre, Francesco Vullo, Massimo Mancone, Maria Rosa Ciardi, Claudio Maria Mastroianni and Vincenzo Vullo
Department of Public Health and Infectious Diseases, "Sapienza" University of Rome, Viale del Policlinico 155, 00161 Rome, Italy

Patrick Baldwin, Roman Shrestha, Jessica Potrepka, and Michael Copenhaver
University of Connecticut, Department of Allied Health Sciences, 358 Mansfield Road, Unit 2101, Storrs, CT 06269-2101, USA

Christian Obirikorang
Department of Molecular Medicine, School of Medical Sciences, College of Health Sciences,
Kwame Nkrumah University of Science and Technology (KNUST), Kumasi, Ghana

Peter Kuugemah Selleh
Department of Medical Laboratory Technology, Faculty of Allied Health, College of Health Sciences,
Kwame Nkrumah University of Science and Technology (KNUST), Kumasi, Ghana

Jubilant Kwame Abledu
School of Veterinary Medicine, University of Ghana, Legon, Ghana

Chris Opoku Fofie
Ghana Health Service, UpperWest Regional Hospital,Wa, UpperWest Region, Ghana

Christos Tsoukas and Trevor Lewis
Department of Microbiology and Immunology, McGill University Health Centre, Room A5-140, 1650 Cedar Avenue, Montreal, QC, Canada H3G 1A4

Louise Gilbert
Montreal General Hospital, Flowcytometry Laboratory, 1650 Cedar Avenue, Room C10-166, Montreal, QC, Canada H3G 1A4

George Hatzakis
LAC+USC Medical Center, 1200 N State Street, Room IPT-C4E100, Los Angeles, CA 90033, USA

Ron Falcon and Joseph Mrus
Janssen Services, LLC, Clinical Affairs, 1125 Trenton-Harbourton Road, Titusville, NJ 08560, USA

Wesley David Dudgeon
Department of Health, Exercise, and Sport Science, The Citadel, 171 Moultrie Street, Charleston, SC 29403, USA

Jason Reed Jaggers, John Larry Durstine , John Mark Davis and Gregory Alan Hand
Department of Exercise Science, Arnold School of Public Health, University of South Carolina, 1300 Wheat Street, Columbia, SC 29208, USA

KennethDoyle Phillips
College of Nursing, University of Tennessee, 4520 Ivy Rose Drive, Knoxville, TN 37918, USA

Stephanie E. Burgess
College of Nursing, University of South Carolina, 1601 Greene Street, Columbia, SC 29208, USA

George William Lyerly
Department of Health, Kinesiology, and Sports Studies, Coastal Carolina University, P.O. Box 261954, Conway, SC 29528-6054, USA

E. Katikiro
National AIDS Control Programme Division, Ministry of Health and Social Welfare, P.O. Box 11857, Dar es Salaam, Tanzania

B. Njau
Community Health Department, Kilimanjaro Christian Medical University College, P.O. Box 2240, Moshi, Tanzania

Bhanu Mehra, Sonali Bhattar, Preena Bhalla, and Deepti Rawat
Department of Microbiology, Maulana Azad Medical College, New Delhi 110002, India